CO-AWV-378

Bioavailability of Drugs to the Brain and the Blood-Brain Barrier

Editors:

Jerry Frankenheim, Ph.D.
Roger M. Brown, Ph.D.

Research Monograph 120
1992

U.S. DEPARTMENT OF HEALTH AND HUMAN SERVICES
Public Health Service
Alcohol, Drug Abuse, and Mental Health Administration

National Institute on Drug Abuse
5600 Fishers Lane
Rockville, MD 20857

ACKNOWLEDGMENT

This monograph is based on the papers and discussions from a technical review on "Drug Bioavailability and the Blood-Brain Barriers" held on September 13-14, 1990, in Rockville, MD. The review meeting was sponsored by the National Institute on Drug Abuse (NIDA).

COPYRIGHT STATUS

For sale by the U.S. Government Printing Office
Superintendent of Documents, Mail Stop: SSOP, Washington, DC 20402-9328
ISBN 0-16-037914-8

Contents

Introduction

Jerry Frankenheim

In the past decade, understanding of the multifaceted importance of the blood-brain barrier (BBB) has mushroomed. One reflection of this is the recent proliferation of popular and scientific publications regarding the BBB:

- "The Sciences" (Pardridge 1987)
- 1989 Grass Instrument calendar (Cserr 1989)
- Two "Scientific American" articles (Spector and Johanson 1989; Goldstein and Betz 1986)
- "Discover" (Angier 1990)
- "Trends in Neurosciences" (Risau and Wolburg 1990)

There also have been detailed reviews in "Annual Review of Pharmacology and Toxicology" (Pardridge 1988), "Acta Neuropathologica" (Broadwell 1989), "Handbook of Neurochemistry" (Betz and Goldstein 1984), and "Basic Neurochemistry" (Betz et al. 1989) as well as several excellent books. The BBB is even part of an attraction called "Body Wars," at Epcot Center in Florida.

Without the BBB scientists who participated in this technical review and authored this monograph, these books and articles would not have been written. Each of these scientists has his or her name on at least one brick in the wall, one piece of the puzzle. It was a great privilege to welcome them to the National Institute on Drug Abuse. Their discoveries are improving the therapy of movement disorders (e.g., Parkinson's disease), epilepsy, strokes, and central nervous system (CNS) infection and tumors. Perhaps advances in the treatment of drug abuse will be next. This will be a very difficult task, since abused drugs, like almost all things that can make people feel good, are (unfortunately) remarkably soluble in fat, and they penetrate the BBB with extreme ease. Areas of possible interest include (but are certainly not limited to):

- Changes (including deficits) in BBB function caused by acute and chronic abuse of such drugs as cocaine, amphetamine, phencyclidine (PCP), and heroin

1

- Improved understanding of the reinforcing properties of abused drugs in terms of their entry into the brain and their fate at the BBB and in brain interstitium

- Other roles of the BBB (e.g., the role of its enzymes with regard to the toxicity of abused substances)

- Rational strategies for targeting potential treatment drugs (including peptides, neurotransmitter precursors, and nutrients) to the brain

The main reason for planning the technical review was to determine the importance of BBB research findings to *drug abuse* research. In planning the review, it was confirmed that drug abuse researchers must be constantly aware of findings about the BBB. The chapters herein demonstrate the importance of the BBB in understanding drug abuse and affirm that the various roles of the BBB have to be understood to fully comprehend the mechanisms of CNS effects of drugs, including drugs of abuse, and the treatment of drug abuse. The central effects of drugs are not isolated from their effects on the BBB nor from the effects of the BBB on the drugs.

REFERENCES

Angier, N. Storming the wall. *Discover* 11(5):67-72, 1990.

Betz, A.L., and Goldstein, G.W. Brain capillaries: Structure and function. In: Lajtha, A., ed. *Handbook of Neurochemistry*. Vol. 7. New York: Plenum Press, 1984. pp. 465-484.

Betz, A.L.; Goldstein, G.W.; and Katzman, R. Blood-brain-cerebrospinal fluid barriers. In: Siegel, G.J.; Agranoff, B.; Albers, R.W.; and Molinoff, P., eds. *Basic Neurochemistry*. New York: Raven Press, 1989. pp. 591-606.

Broadwell, R.D. Transcytosis of macromolecules through the blood-brain barrier: A cell biological perspective and critical appraisal. *Acta Neuropathol* 79:117-128, 1989.

Cserr, H. *Biology of the Blood-Brain Barrier*. Quincy, MA: Grass Instrument Company Calendar, 1989.

Goldstein, G.W., and Betz, A.L. The blood-brain barrier. *Sci Am* 255:74-83, 1986.

Pardridge, W.M. The gatekeeper. *The Sciences* 27:50-55, 1987.

Pardridge, W.M. Recent advances in blood-brain barrier transport. *Annu Rev Pharmacol Toxicol* 28:25-39, 1988.

Risau, W., and Wolburg, H. Development of the blood-brain barrier. *Trends Neurosci* 13:174-178, 1990.

Spector, R., and Johanson, C.E. The mammalian choroid plexus. *Sci Am* 261:68-74, 1989.

AUTHOR

Jerry Frankenheim, Ph.D.
Pharmacologist
Neuroscience Research Branch
Division of Preclinical Research
National Institute on Drug Abuse
Parklawn Building, Room 10A-31
5600 Fishers Lane
Rockville, MD 20857

The Basic Neurobiology of Addiction

Roger M. Brown

INTRODUCTION

A thorough understanding of the relationship between the brain mechanisms that underlie compulsive drug seeking and how these processes are changed by exposure to drugs is essential to understand phenomena such as drug abuse, addiction, and physical dependence and also to develop a rational biomedical treatment for the changes in central nervous system (CNS) homeostasis that are the direct result of chemical insult.

SUBSTRATE FOR ADDICTION

The discovery of endogenous opioid peptides in the brain has explained how a material from a poppy plant can induce narcosis in a human. Differences in the distribution of the endogenous opioids within the brain and spinal cord imply that they subserve specific functions. These substances have been shown to be involved with the modulation of pain by drugs, in physiological events such as trauma and acupuncture, as well as in the physical dependence induced by opiates. The opiate narcotics, as well as barbiturates and alcohol, are well known to have the ability to induce tolerance and physical dependence, the hallmark of addiction. Drug dependence has long been associated with an adaptation of the CNS to the presence of the drug so that normal functioning is only possible in the presence of the addictive substance. When this occurs, drug seeking becomes oriented toward an avoidance of the painful consequences of drug abstinence. Neuroscientists are examining the changes in presynaptic and postsynaptic receptor function that occur during drug dependence and withdrawal to intercede and "reset" the neuron to a normative state.

Brain Reward Circuitry—Basis for Drug Abuse

Although there has never been complete agreement on what constitutes drug addiction, cocaine certainly does not fit the older definition of an addictive drug. Tolerance to its effects does not occur to any appreciable extent, and it does

4

not induce a profound physical withdrawal syndrome. Yet, the abuse of this "nonaddictive" drug has reached epidemic proportions, and treatment centers are filled to capacity in attempts to help users rid themselves of it.

Over the past decade, neuropsychopharmacologists have been examining the biological basis of drug-seeking behavior and have developed a model to explain why taking certain drugs is so attractive. According to the hypothesis, drugs are sought because they directly activate the brain's reward system, a neural network responsible for the subjective experience of pleasure. The foundation for the hypothesis began in 1954, when Olds and Milner (1954) reported that animals would work for electrical stimulation of certain neuroanatomical pathways in the brain. This finding gave rise to the concept that the brain contains a system that is responsible for the experience of pleasure. Presumably, this pathway is activated physiologically by any event, activity, or stimulus that is highly reinforcing. Stated another way, these events are rewarding because this "reward" pathway is activated.

As a result of the discovery of reward centers, neuroscientists began to map regions of the brain that were positive for brain self-stimulation. Two findings resulted from this line of investigation. First, the dopaminergic projections of the ventral tegmental area (VTA), the mesolimbic and mesocortical dopamine (DA) projections, were found to be a critical link in the reward system. Second, it was found that animals would self-administer drugs directly into the reward circuit. Many types of abused drugs, including morphine, heroin, cocaine, amphetamine, and possibly nicotine, activate this system, albeit at different loci. The involvement of DA synapses is consistent with the findings that (1) neuroleptics block intracranial self-stimulation; (2) neuroleptics block the systemic self-administration of a variety of drug classes: opiates, amphetamine, cocaine, and barbiturates; and (3) systemic administration of DA blockers prevents the self-administration of drugs directly into certain regions of brain tissue (Wise 1983; Nakajima and McKenzie 1986; Goeders and Smith 1983; Koob et al. 1987).

The DA synapse is not the only link in the chain. Neuroleptics block the electrical self-stimulation of reward sites in certain regions of the cerebellum, yet there are no DA neurons there. Therefore, the DA synapse, which is critical to brain reward, may be several synapses removed from the activating source. Many drugs of abuse, including amphetamine, opiates, MDMA (3,4-methylenedioxymethamphetamine or "ecstasy"), phencyclidine (PCP or "angel dust"), pentazocine and tripelennamine (a combination known as "T's and Blues"), and nicotine, are among the drugs found to lower the threshold for electrical self-stimulation from the VTA and other rewarding sites such as the medial forebrain bundle (Bain and Kornetsky 1987; Hubner et al. 1988;

Kornetsky 1985; Unterwald and Kornetsky 1984). The facilitation of intracranial self-stimulation by these drugs is blocked by opiate antagonists such as naloxone.

Thus, the reward circuitry involves at least a dopaminergic synapse and an opioidergic synapse. Probably several others are involved as well. The cell bodies of the VTA contain opiate and nicotine receptors, and the postsynaptic receptors of the terminals are dopaminergic. Whether there is a single brain reward circuit or several is a matter of investigation in contemporary research laboratories (Koob and Bloom 1988; Wise 1983).

COCAINE: A POTENT REINFORCER

Researchers working to elucidate the chemical neuroanatomy of this reward system began to realize that drugs are sought out initially because they induce pleasure and not because of anything directly related to the development of physical dependence. Indeed, physical dependence and brain reward can be dissociated. As with cocaine, animals will self-administer opiates into their VTA. They will not, however, self-administer drugs into the periaqueductal gray (PAG) region, an anatomical relay station that is important in narcotic-induced modulation of pain transmission and that, like the VTA, is populated with opiate receptors. This demonstrates that the VTA is responsible for mediating opiate-seeking behavior. On the other hand, when opiates are continuously infused into the PAG over a 24- to 48-hour period, an abstinence syndrome is observed when naloxone is administered. In contrast, infusions of opiate into the VTA do not result in a precipitated abstinence syndrome following administration of narcotic antagonist. Thus, the PAG is responsible for physical dependence, and the VTA mediates drug self-administration (Bozarth and Wise 1984).

Abuse of a drug must be related to some positive aspect of drug action; therefore, it is believed that different classes of drugs are abused because they activate the brain's reward mechanism. For example, cocaine is potentially dangerous to health because it is rewarding (and continually used) despite its lack of physical dependence liability, whereas heroin and other opiates are dangerous because they are rewarding in addition to their ability to induce physical dependence. The positive subjective effect of several drug classes reinforces drug-seeking behavior in spite of simultaneously occurring harmful physiological effects that may not be apparent to the user.

The strength of the rewarding impact of cocaine is illustrated by the findings of many animal drug self-administration studies (see Johanson 1984). Cocaine is inherently reinforcing; that is, no priming is necessary to induce animals to self-administer the drug. Morphine, on the other hand, usually requires the

6

production of physical dependence before self-administration occurs. Also, animals do not initially self-administer barbiturates; they have to be trained on another drug first and then switched to barbiturates. In fact, cocaine is often used as the training drug when shaping animals to self-administer. Cocaine is not unique in this respect, however. Heroin, too, is inherently reinforcing and requires no manipulations to set the condition for drug self-administration.

Another way to measure the rewarding value of a drug is to conduct a "breaking point" study that asks how many lever presses an animal is willing to emit for a single infusion of a test drug. This kind of abuse liability testing has made possible the characterization (and comparison) of drugs in terms of relative potency (i.e., the amount of drug required to maintain equivalent break points relative to another drug) and/or reinforcing efficacy (i.e., the maximum break point for any dose of the test drug). Studies to date indicate that the reinforcing efficacy of cocaine far exceeds that of most other drugs. For example, among drugs tested, cocaine's breaking point exceeds that of methylphenidate, fenfluramine, amphetamine, methamphetamine, nicotine, and local anesthetics. Animals have been reported to press a lever more than 12,000 times for a single cocaine dose of 0.5 mg/kg (Yanagita 1973).

Further evidence for cocaine's potential danger to health comes from the finding that, when given unlimited access, animals will self-administer the drug to the point of toxicity and death. This is in contrast to opiate self-administration, which is self-limiting. Opiates and barbiturates are examples of drugs that are not self-administered to the point of toxicity. Again, however, cocaine is not unique in this respect. Alcohol and amphetamine also are self-administered to the point of toxicity. Thus, cocaine's abuse potential and danger to health surpasses that of morphine in two ways. First, cocaine is inherently reinforcing, whereas other drugs such as morphine are less so; second, cocaine is self-administered to the point of toxicity, whereas this is less so for opiates (Bozarth and Wise 1985).

DEFINITION OF ADDICTION BASED ON DRUG SEEKING

Concern over today's epidemic of cocaine abuse is probably the single most important factor in focusing on the neural basis for drug seeking. As pointed out above, cocaine does not appear to conform to the older concept of an addictive drug, yet its abuse liability ranks along with that of the "hard drugs" such as heroin. Because of inadequacies in the definition of addiction, Cohen (1985) pointed out the need to define addiction in behavioral terms and suggested that addiction be defined as "the loss of control over the intake of a drug that leads to its compulsive use despite harmful effects in some area of the person's functioning." Cocaine certainly falls into this category, along with other abused substances, such as nicotine, that do not induce any appreciable tolerance and physical dependence.

IMPLICATIONS OF THE BRAIN REWARD MODEL OF ADDICTION

The brain reward model explains the "why" of drug abuse and brings the concept of psychological dependence into the realm of neurobiological events. The model also may provide the rationale for developing effective pharmacotherapeutic treatment strategies. According to the model, drugs are sought because they pharmacologically activate the brain reward system to a degree that surpasses that from natural rewards. The ventral tegmental DA projection is critical in the circuitry, and a variety of drug classes activate components of the neural system. The animal models used to test and elaborate the model all have shown brain dopaminergic neurons to be critical in mediating drug self-administration. In the human cocaine abuser, however, greater success has been obtained with the use of DA agonists. The discrepancy between animal and human treatments probably exists because in the animal model the physiological reward process is the principal determinant of the drug-seeking behavior, whereas in the clinic the therapist may be dealing with drug reward, drug craving, or both.

Because bromocriptine, a DA agonist, has been reported effective in treating cocaine addiction, speculations have been made concerning cocaine-induced DA depletions (Dakis and Gold 1985). Although there is little, if any, evidence for DA depletion following cocaine use, there may be a "functional" shortage of neurotransmitter that is responsible for purported success with treatment aimed at DA agonism. The "functional" DA depletion could result from adaptive regulatory mechanisms responding to cocaine-induced excess of neurotransmitter in the synaptic cleft, the end result being an inadequate impulse-induced release of DA. It is not yet clear whether the most effective way to terminate cocaine abuse should be aimed at cocaine-induced reward (DA antagonists to block reward and possibly craving) or drug-induced transmitter deficiencies (DA agonists to correct dopaminergic receptor down-regulation). Both possibilities are being examined.

A recent pharmacotherapy investigation examined the role of DA receptor subtypes in cocaine action. The two types of DA receptors on neurons in the CNS, D_1 and D_2 DA receptors, are distinguished from each other by their localization in brain areas, their ligand affinities, and their behavioral characteristics. Recently, the development of drugs that are specific agonists or antagonists for D_1 and D_2 receptors has made it possible to separate DA neurotransmission by receptor type. One of the roles of the D_1 receptor is to enable D_2 functioning (i.e., the behavioral events following D_2 stimulation require D_1 receptor stimulation for their expression). D_1 antagonists have been shown by several investigators (Clark and White 1987; Koob and Hubner 1989; Koob et al 1987; Nakajima and McKenzie 1986) to block behavioral effects of amphetamine and cocaine. The advantage of testing D_1 receptor antagonists to counteract cocaine self-administration is that these drugs show a wide dose-response curve. This is in contrast to D_2 antagonists, which show very narrow, practically all-or-none, dose-effect curves. Although these studies are still in experimental stages, the advantage of using D_1 receptor antagonists is that it may be possible to titrate the patient so that the action against cocaine craving is maximized while the distressing neuroleptic action is minimized.

While the involvement of DA receptor subtypes in drug reward is being analyzed, other investigators are beginning to examine the processes underlying craving and/or relapse. The model, as presented, may explain why clinical treatment with dopaminergic antagonists is not as useful as initially speculated. First, the circuitry of the brain reward system is responsible for the pleasurable effects of drugs, and this is what initially drives drug seeking. Once the drug is experienced, its presence causes adaptive changes in the neuron (e.g., up- or down-regulatory alterations in postsynaptic receptors, changes in autoreceptor sensitivity, alterations in impulse flow). The perturbations in homeostasis need to be corrected before the abuser can be drug-free. What role DA neurons play in drug craving or relapse has yet to be evaluated, although some evidence suggests that neuroleptics can prevent relapse in some psychomotor stimulants (Ettenberg 1990).

Finally, much interest has been directed recently toward a methadone-like drug for cocaine. In treating opiate addiction, methadone, a weak opiate agonist, is given orally, and its presence in the body serves to prevent the development of aversive withdrawal symptoms. As long as methadone is taken, physiological processes are functional. The oral methadone is primarily a negative reinforcer, in that it prevents the occurrence of abstinence symptoms. On the other hand, quite a different situation exists in treating cocaine addiction because cocaine does not induce physical dependence but acts directly on the reward substrate. As aptly pointed out by Wise (1988), cocaine is a positive reinforcer, and any drug that partially substitutes for cocaine not only would satisfy cocaine cravings but also would simultaneously activate the brain reward mechanism and perhaps even "prime" cocaine-seeking behavior. Clearly, a cocaine substitute would not appear suitable as a treatment drug. On the other hand, if long-term cocaine use leads to down-regulation of DA receptors, how does one go about up-regulating the system without producing a "high"?

SUMMARY

This overview on cocaine's addiction liability is presented in this monograph on the blood-brain barrier (BBB) because the National Institute on Drug Abuse has been given the task of finding pharmacotherapies to treat addiction. Knowledge about the BBB might help researchers design better drugs or approaches to keep the "good" drugs inside and/or the "bad" drugs outside. It is to be hoped that the BBB community can be convinced that drug abuse is an exciting area and that work on biological barriers has something to offer.

REFERENCES

Bain, G.T., and Kornetsky, C. Naloxone attenuation of the effect of cocaine on rewarding brain stimulation. *Life Sci* 40:1119-1125, 1987.

Bozarth, M.A., and Wise, R.A. Anatomically distinct receptor fields mediate reward and physical dependence. *Science* 224:516-517, 1984.

Bozarth, M.A., and Wise, R.A. Toxicity associated with long-term intravenous heroin and cocaine self-administration in the rat. *JAMA* 254(1):16-18, 1985.

Clark, D., and White, F.J. D_1 dopamine receptor—the search for a function: A critical evaluation of the D_1/D_2 dopamine receptor classification and its functional implications. *Synapse* 1:347-388, 1987.

Cohen, S. *Cocaine: The Bottom Line*. Rockville, MD: American Council for Drug Education, 1985.

Dakis, C.A., and Gold, M.S. Bromocriptine as a treatment of cocaine abuse. *Lancet* 8438(May 18):1151, 1985.

Ettenberg, A. Haloperidol prevents the reinstatement of amphetamine-rewarded runway responding in rats. *Pharmacol Biochem Behav* 36:635-638, 1990.

Goeders, N., and Smith, J. Cortical dopaminergic involvement in cocaine reinforcement. *Science* 221:773-775, 1983.

Hubner, C.B.; Bird, M.; Rassnick, S.; and Kornetsky, C. The threshold lowering effects of MDMA (ecstasy) on brain-stimulation reward. *Psychopharmacology* 95:49-51, 1988.

Johanson, C.E. Assessment of the dependence potential of cocaine in animals. In: Grabowski, J., ed. *Cocaine: Pharmacology, Effects, and Treatment of Abuse*. National Institute on Drug Abuse Research Monograph 50. DHHS Pub. No. (ADM)87-1326. Washington, DC: Supt. of Docs., U.S. Govt. Print. Off., 1984. pp. 54-71.

Koob, G.F., and Bloom, F.E. Cellular and molecular mechanisms of drug dependence. *Science* 242:715-723, 1988.

Koob, G.F., and Hubner, C.B. Reinforcement pathways for cocaine. In: Clouet, D.; Asghar, K.; and Brown, R., eds. *Mechanisms of Cocaine Abuse and Toxicity*. National Institute on Drug Abuse Research Monograph 88.

DHHS Pub. No. (ADM)89-1585. Washington, DC: Supt. of Docs., U.S. Govt. Print. Off., 1988. pp. 137-159.

Koob, G.F.; Le, H.T.; and Creese, I. D$_1$ receptor antagonist SCH 23390 increases cocaine self-administration in the rat. *Neurosci Lett* 79:315-321, 1987.

Kornetsky, C. Brain-stimulation reward: A model for the neuronal basis for drug-induced euphoria. In: Brown, R.M.; Friedman, D.P.; and Nimit, Y., eds. *Neuroscience Methods in Drug Abuse Research.* National Institute on Drug Abuse Research Monograph 62. DHHS Pub. No. (ADM)85-1415. Washington, DC: Supt. of Docs., U.S. Govt. Print. Off., 1985. pp. 30-50.

Nakajima, S., and McKenzie, G.M. Reduction of the rewarding effect of brain stimulation by blockade of D-1 receptors with SCH-23390. *Pharmacol Biochem Behav* 24:919-923, 1986.

Olds, J., and Milner, P. Positive reinforcement produced by electrical stimulation of the septal area and other regions of the rat brain. *J Comp Physiol Psychol* 47:419, 1954.

Unterwald, E.M., and Kornetsky, C. Effects of concomitant pentazocine and tripelennamine on brain-stimulation reward. *Pharmacol Biochem Behav* 21:961-964, 1984.

Wise, R.A. Brain neuronal systems mediating reward processes. In: Smith, J.E., and Lane, J.D., eds. *The Neurobiology of Opiate Reward Process.* New York: Elsevier, 1983. pp. 405-437.

Wise, R.A. The neurobiology of craving: Implications for the understanding and treatment of addiction. *J Abnorm Psychol* 97(2):118-132, 1988.

Yanagita, T. An experimental framework for evaluation of dependence liability of various types of drugs in monkeys. *Bull Narc* 25(4):57-64, 1973.

SUGGESTED READING

Brown, R.M. Pharmacology of cocaine abuse. In: Redda, K.K.; Walker, C.A.; and Barnett, G., eds. *Cocaine, Marijuana, Designer Drugs: Chemistry, Pharmacology, and Behavior.* Boca Raton, FL: CRC Press, 1989. pp. 39-51.

Clouet, D.; Asghar, K.; and Brown, R., eds. *Mechanisms of Cocaine Abuse and Toxicity.* National Institute on Drug Abuse Research Monograph 88. DHHS Pub. No. (ADM)89-1585. Washington, DC: Supt. of Docs., U.S. Govt. Print. Off., 1988.

Kleber, H.D., and Gawin, F.H. Cocaine abuse: A review of current and experimental treatments. In: Grabowski, J., ed. *Cocaine: Pharmacology, Effects, and Treatment of Abuse.* National Institute on Drug Abuse Research Monograph Number 50. DHHS Pub. No. (ADM)87-1326. Washington, DC: Supt. of Docs., U.S. Govt. Print. Off., 1984. pp. 111-129.

Kuhar, M.J.; Ritz, M.C.; and Boja, J.W. The dopamine hypothesis of the reinforcing properties of cocaine. *Trends Neurosci* 14(7):299-301, 1991.

Stewart, J. Conditioned and unconditioned drug effects in relapse to opiate and stimulant drug self-administration. *Prog Neuropsychopharmacol Biol Psychiatry* 7:591-597, 1983.

AUTHOR

Roger M. Brown, Ph.D.
Chief
Neuroscience Branch
Division of Preclinical Research
National Institute on Drug Abuse
Parklawn Building, Room 10A-31
5600 Fishers Lane
Rockville, MD 20857

Some Relationships Between Addiction and Drug Delivery to the Brain

William H. Oldendorf

INTRODUCTION

The rapidity and abruptness of drug delivery to the brain using various routes of administration are factors in drug addiction. The shorter the interval between intake and perceived effect of a drug, the greater the propensity toward a more severe addiction. For example, severity of cigarette nicotine addiction is probably related to the approximately 3 seconds elapsing between the act of gasping smoke accumulated in the mouth and the perceived mental response.

This chapter offers some documentation in support of the following hypothesis: Some of the steps involved in taking an addicting substance are (1) the act of taking the substance into the body, (2) the period of time elapsing during which there is no subjective effect, and (3) the time at which a drug effect is perceived. The more immediate the effect after intake, the more addicting the substance is likely to be. The latter has been widely discussed in the literature and is not presented here as novel; rather, some hemodynamic data obtained from human studies related to this hypothesis are presented. Most of these studies were radioisotopic tracer studies of human brain blood flow following carotid or intravenous (IV) injection (Oldendorf 1962; Oldendorf and Kitano 1965a, 1965b).

It is assumed that substances reported in these hemodynamic studies, ^{131}I-iodohippurate (hydrophilic) and ^{131}I-iodoantipyrine (lipophilic), have no psychotropic effects in the small tracer doses used. Their blood-brain barrier (BBB) permeabilities closely resemble common drugs of abuse; it also is assumed that their early distributions in the body are representative of some drugs of addiction (i.e., nicotine, cocaine, heroin, ethanol, and morphine).

The human brain content of chromium-labeled red blood cells (^{51}Cr-RBC) and separately labeled plasma, radioiodinated serum albumin (^{131}RISA),

13

after a carotid injection is shown in figure 1. Both these labeled substances remain confined to blood and rapidly leave the brain by about 10 seconds after their abrupt carotid injection (Oldendorf et al. 1965a). These curves show that the labeled red blood cells pass through the brain more rapidly than does labeled plasma. This is a well-recognized phenomenon and is included here because it provides an indication of how rapidly blood cells and plasma pass out of the human brain after carotid injection. Cranial counts were done by external gamma counting. Only the cranial portion of the head is measured in these studies.

In animal studies, a ^{14}C test substance (such as a radiolabeled drug of abuse mixed with ^{3}HOH) has been extensively applied by rapidly injecting the mixture into the common carotid artery of a barbiturate-anesthetized rat (Oldendorf 1971). At 5 seconds, the rat is decapitated and the side of the brain injected is digested and subjected to liquid scintillation spectrometry. By 5 seconds after carotid injection, any of the test substance that did not penetrate the BBB and remained in brain was carried out of the head by continuing blood circulation. The ^{3}HOH was an internal standard that was almost completely cleared by brain. Between 0 and 100 percent of the test substance is cleared by brain during these 5 seconds. Comparison of the tritium-to-carbon ratio in the brain with the same ratio in an aliquot of the injectate permits determination of the fractional single pass clearance of the test substance, relative to the internal standard (Oldendorf 1971). For some substances, the internal standard used was ^{14}C-butanol. Many classes of substances have been studied this way: amino acids, amines, hexoses, inert polar substances, organic acids, drugs, nucleic acid precursors, and peptides (Oldendorf 1971, 1974, 1981; Oldendorf et al. 1972).

Most of the common street drugs shown in table 1 are almost completely cleared by rat brain during a single capillary passage. As a result of these animal studies, it was clear that the equilibration of many drugs with brain was essentially instantaneous through the BBB; the rapid increase in brain drug concentration was determined largely by the rate at which drug concentration rose in arterial blood following drug intake into the body.

DYNAMICS OF DRUG DELIVERY

It is of interest to consider several routes of administration and drug delivery to brain: (1) A hypothetical injection into the ascending aorta, (2) inhalation, (3) IV, (4) intranasal, and (5) ingestion. These are listed in, approximately, a progressive lengthening of time of arrival in brain and, consequently, a corresponding decrease in abruptness of delivery to brain. Other factors in drug addiction (Goldstein and Kalant 1990) as well as other routes of drug administration (Langer 1990) have been reviewed recently.

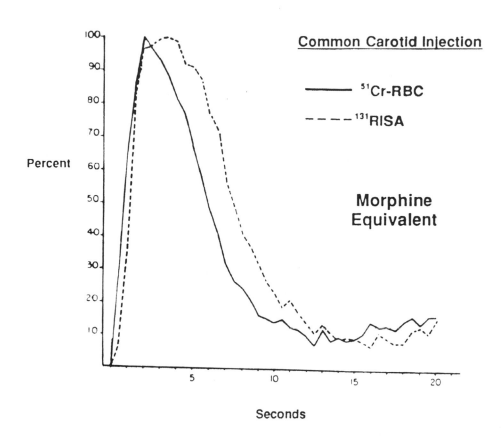

FIGURE 1. *Human brain content of ^{51}Cr-RBC (solid line) and ^{131}RISA
(dashed line) after common carotid injection (80 μc and 10 μc,
respectively). These remain intravascular and hemodynamically
would resemble morphine. In this presentation, "drug equivalent"
means that each hemodynamic curve would be similar to what
would be expected if the extensive data were transferred from
animal studies of single pass clearance by rat brain after abrupt
carotid arterial injection.*

SOURCE: Oldendorf et al. 1965a, copyright 1965, American Heart Association,
Inc.

TABLE 1.   *Single pass clearance of drug (percent of ^3HOH)*

Drug	Percent of ^3HOH
Nicotine[*]	131 ± 7
Ethanol[*]	104 ± 4
Cocaine (percent butanol)[*]	99.5 ± 3.4
Heroin[*]	90 ± 3
L-methadone[†]	68 ± 6
Codeine[*]	26 ± 2
Morphine[*]	2.6 ± 0.2

[*]Oldendorf 1981
[†]Oldendorf 1974

Injection Into the Ascending Aorta

A hypothetical injection into the ascending aorta should result in the most abrupt delivery to an entire brain.

Inhalation

It is likely that the gasp of cigarette smoke drawn into the lungs of the severely addicted smoker closely approaches the abruptness of the hypothetical aortic injection. The lung-to-brain arterial-capillary circulation time should be about 3 seconds, based on the arrival in human brain of radiographic contrast agents injected into the aorta.

The serious smoker draws smoke into the mouth with the soft palate and epiglottis closed, creating a high concentration of smoke in the mouth. The mouth is then opened and a gasp of perhaps one-half to one liter of air rapidly flushes this high concentration of smoke into the lungs. The fraction of nicotine that is taken up by lung blood has a correspondingly sharp front in its concentration curve. Three seconds after the intake gasp, about 20 percent of the nicotine front circulates to brain and all of it is lost to brain in the first microcirculatory passage.

This inhalation method probably achieves the most abrupt front of drug delivery to brain with the shortest transit time between act of intake and perceived effects. The effect is essentially immediate following the act of intake, and this is likely related to the severity and intractability of nicotine smoking. The immediate effect reinforces both the intake act and the central

16

response. Accordingly, smoking cigarettes is more addicting than is taking a similar amount of nicotine by chewing gum. An extensive report of smoking and addiction has been published recently (Surgeon General 1988).

Based on animal studies (Oldendorf 1974; Bradbury et al. 1975; Oldendorf et al. 1979), all nicotine delivered to brain after carotid injection remains there, and no measurable nicotine leaves the brain during the first minute.

Such an immediate effect in brain also may enter into the inhalation of freebase cocaine, where the inhalation is followed in 2 to 3 seconds by the central stimulation sensation. This intake interval is much shorter than would be obtained by nasal "snorting" or by IV injection; it may play a part in the rapid and severe addiction experienced by freebase cocaine users.

IV Injection

Figure 2 shows a common carotid arterial concentration of a commonly used dye, cardio-green, after its abrupt IV injection (Oldendorf 1962; Oldendorf et al. 1965b). Concentration was continually measured colorimetrically. This shows the sharpness of the arrival in the human brain after the initially abrupt bolus has been spread by cardiopulmonary passage. In figure 3, an IV injection of radiolabeled ^{131}I-iodohippurate (hydrophilic tracer) is seen (Oldendorf 1962; Oldendorf and Kitano 1963), measured by external gamma counting. Iodohippurate brain clearance resembles that of morphine, which has a single-pass clearance of about 1 percent, based on animal studies.

While working extensively with external gamma counting of human brain, a method was developed that was more accurate if the bolus was delivered into the right heart in as compact a bolus as possible. The bolus inevitably is spread longitudinally by heart and lung passage. Following a routine IV injection, the count rate from the human head normally began to rise in 8 to 10 seconds, reached a peak in about 14 seconds, and was completely gone from the head in 20 seconds.

To improve the precision of measurement, a procedure was developed for inflating the arm veins with a blood pressure cuff placed around the upper arm and inflated to diastolic pressure for about 1 minute (Oldendorf et al. 1965b). The distal venous pressure in the arm rose to this diastolic pressure, creating considerable peripheral venous distention. A small needle was placed in an antecubital vein and the blood pressure cuff raised above systolic pressure. This created a static inflated distal venous pool in the arm. The isotope was injected into the vein and then the cuff was abruptly released, allowing collapse

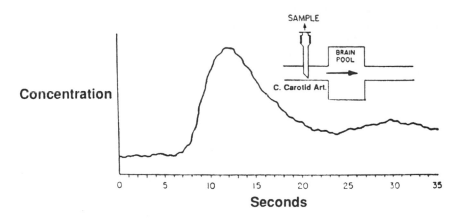

Concentration

Seconds

FIGURE 2. *Concentration of cardio-green sampled from the human common carotid artery (c. carotid art.) after IV injection. This would be expected to be hemodynamically equivalent to morphine.*

SOURCE: Oldendorf 1962, copyright 1962, The Society of Nuclear Medicine

of the distal venous pool and driving the bolus into the right heart. This created a measurably earlier and more dependable abrupt delivery of isotope into the brain (Oldendorf et al. 1965b). This procedure is now in common use in nuclear medicine laboratories to deliver an IV bolus to the right heart as abruptly as possible.

Several drugs are almost completely cleared during a single capillary passage; the amount delivered to any particular region depends on the fraction of cardiac output distributing to that region. Because skeletal muscle and skin blood flow can be altered considerably as a function of recent muscular exertion and air temperature, it should be possible to substantially alter the fraction of highly cleared drugs delivered to brain (e.g., cocaine or heroin). Thoroughly relaxed muscle may differ in blood flow by a factor of about 20 from fully active muscle blood flow.

In a wasteful scenario, the addict would, immediately after obtaining his or her drug, hurry home, run upstairs to the highest and warmest part of the house, apply a tourniquet while standing, insert the needle in a vein, and inject the drug. In a less wasteful scenario, the addict would walk home, climb as few stairs as possible, and lie down in a cool room for 5 to 10 minutes. The tourniquet then would be applied, venipuncture accomplished, and the injection made while sitting or lying prone.

18

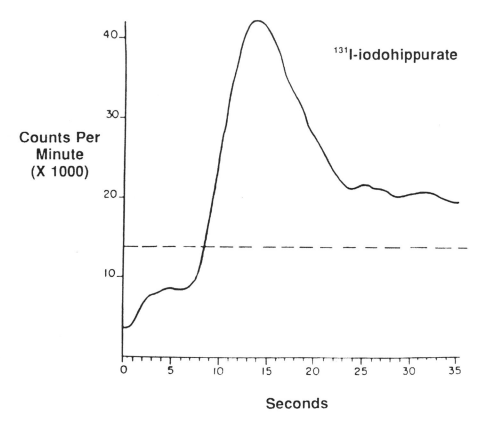

FIGURE 3. *This curve shows human brain content after IV injection of labeled*
¹³¹I-iodohippurate (400 μc), which is assumed to be
hemodynamically similar to morphine.

SOURCE: Oldendorf 1962, copyright 1962, The Society of Nuclear Medicine

In the first scenario described, muscle blood flow would be near its maximum
and might be 12 to 15 liters per minute. Blood flow to brain is constant with
exercise; thus, the greater muscle and skin blood flow would "steal" cardiac
output from brain. Cocaine or heroin, for example, in such "stolen" blood would
be lost to muscle and skin as well as all other organs. The second scenario
might deliver 2 to 3 times as much intravenously injected blood to brain,
resulting in a corresponding increase in drug deposition in brain.

One could estimate that, of a $100-per-day cocaine habit, perhaps only 2 or
3 cents worth of cocaine would find its way to human brain receptors in the

first scenario. However, in the less wasteful second scenario, perhaps 10 to 15 cents worth of cocaine would find its specific brain receptor, the remainder being dispersed elsewhere in the body, where it is nonspecifically bound, producing no central effect.

Lipophilicity of Drug

Figures 4 and 5 show the isotope content of the human brain after IV injection of a lipophilic tracer, ^{131}I-iodoantipyrine (Oldendorf and Kitano 1965b). The start of the time base is the time the tourniquet-cuff was released and the bolus began its movement centrally (figure 4). There is then a period of about 8 to 10 seconds before the head curve begins to rise. It rises to a maximum and then remains constant.

Figure 5 shows the externally gamma counted ^{131}I-iodoantipyrine averaged from 17 human subjects after IV injections (Oldendorf and Kitano 1965b). Seven of these had angiographically confirmed arteriovenous malformations; the remaining 10 were normal controls. The averaged curve with the initial peak represents a substantial amount of blood shunted around the local

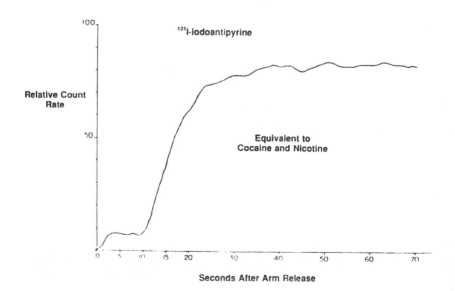

FIGURE 4. *This curve shows normal human subject brain content after IV ^{131}I-iodoantipyrine (8 µc), which is assumed to be hemodynamically similar to nicotine and cocaine.*

SOURCE: Oldendorf and Kitano 1965b, copyright 1965, *Neurology*

20

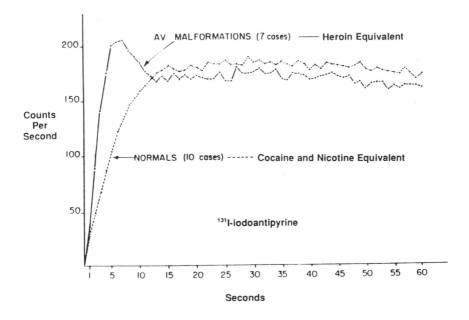

FIGURE 5. *These averaged curves show human brain content after IV* [131]*I-iodoantipyrine (8 to 20 μc), a lipophilic tracer. Time base starts at first appearance in head. The initially peaked curve probably would resemble incompletely cleared heroin. The unpeaked curve probably resembles cocaine and nicotine hemodynamically.*

SOURCE: Oldendorf and Kitano 1965b, copyright 1965, *Neurology*

microcirculation. The radioisotope being measured in this arteriovenous shunt rapidly leaves the brain. The remainder of the isotope passes through a capillary bed, and no peak is seen in the average normal subjects (dashed line).

In the rat model, iodoantipyrine, like cocaine, is cleared 100 percent during a single brain passage; heroin is about 65 percent cleared. These curves (figures 4 and 5) presumably closely resemble the human brain content following IV cocaine and approximate heroin given intravenously. The normal ^{131}I-iodoantipyrine curve shown in figure 4, with no initial peak, would be representative of the behavior of cocaine. The initially peaked curve shown in figure 5 should represent the curve expected from the incompletely cleared heroin.

21

When a drug that is almost completely cleared by brain is injected intravenously, its local concentration in brain some 15 seconds later is proportional to regional blood flow to that region. This regional distribution of blood flow ordinarily is unrelated to regional distribution of specific receptors.

Radiolabeled heroin and morphine have been injected intravenously into mature rats and then the amount of drug in total brain assessed 1 minute later (unpublished data). Approximately 50 times as much heroin distributed to brain relative to morphine. From this, one might expect heroin would be about 50 times more potent, mole for mole, as an analgesic than morphine. However, the usual relative analgesia attributed to these drugs is that heroin is 3 to 5 times as efficacious as morphine. One explanation of this unexpectedly low ratio is that the heroin probably is delivered to various regions of brain in proportion to blood flow, independent of receptor density.

Morphine, which is much more hydrophilic than heroin, is only about 1 percent cleared in a single rat brain passage but accumulates slowly in various regions in proportion to the local opiate receptor density. This may relate to morphine's clinically observed 10- to 15-minute delay before peak analgesia after IV injection.

Intranasal

From informal discussion with cocaine users, the stimulation after intranasal intake is more delayed than after IV injection. According to the hypothesis under discussion here, this stimulation delay should make intranasal cocaine slightly less addicting than IV cocaine. One also would expect other factors to enter into this, such as the relative simplicity of snorting vs. the paraphernalia required for an IV injection.

Ingestion

The major drug under consideration here is ethanol (alcohol). The partition coefficient (PC) of ethanol is ideal for a socially usable drug. Its olive oil:water PC is 0.04 (figure 6) (Oldendorf 1974). This means that ethanol achieves 25 times the concentration in water as in olive oil. If one assumed that olive oil is reasonably representative of human depot fat, then distribution of ethanol probably is predominantly to lean body mass. As such, obese drinkers can become intoxicated with little more ethanol than those of normal habitus.

If the PC of ethanol were one or two orders of magnitude larger, ethanol would tend to accumulate in depot fat and therefore require a much larger dose. Assuming its rate of metabolism would be unchanged, the effects of

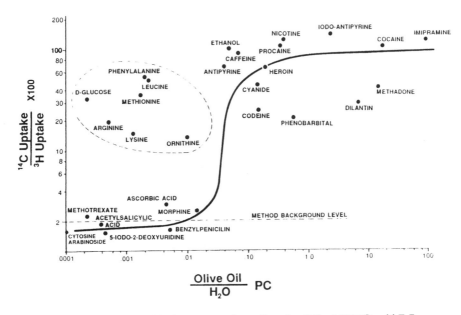

FIGURE 6. The relationship between olive oil:water PC at 37 °C, pH 7.5 (refined olive oil, Sigma, St. Louis) and single pass rat brain clearance following carotid injection. In addition to the drug's substantial clearance when its PC is greater than 0.05 in this system, there is another high uptake group having much lower PCs that lie above the average curve. They are encircled by a dashed line and are metabolized substances.

SOURCE: Oldendorf 1974, copyright 1974, Society for Experimental Biology and Medicine

ethanol would be considerably prolonged. Instead, the situation that exists is that a "social drinker" can drink during the evening, have a few hours of effect, and be sober by the next morning. The effects of alcohol ingestion are noted after perhaps 5 minutes. If one consumed alcohol in the evening and did not become intoxicated until the next morning, alcohol probably would largely cease to be a substance of abuse.

If the PC were one or two orders of magnitude lower, ethanol would equilibrate very slowly with brain through the BBB. As shown in figure 6, there seems to be a broad threshold at around 0.05 olive oil:water PC, above which the single pass clearance of a substance in the rat model is substantial. A drug such as ethanol has a PC just high enough to get into brain freely, yet not accumulate excessively in depot fat.

SUMMARY

Hemodynamic radioisotope studies of brain blood flow in humans have been correlated with the delivery of some common addictive drugs. Both lipophilic and hydrophilic tracers were used in the hemodynamic studies. Iodoantipyrine is lipophilic and is completely cleared by brain during a single brain circulatory passage, as are cocaine and nicotine. Iodohippurate is hydrophilic, so its brain clearance after IV injection resembles that of morphine.

The earlier studies performed in humans have been related here with recent studies of blood brain penetration of drugs of abuse. As presented, these separate studies are consistent with the proposed hypothesis that the interval between drug intake and perceived effect is a significant consideration when explaining severity of addiction. The shorter the time interval between drug intake and its perceived effect, the more severe the addiction appears to be. This relationship may explain differences in severity of addiction to the same drug taken by various routes of administration.

REFERENCES

Bradbury, M.W.B.; Patlak, C.S.; and Oldendorf, W.H. Analysis of brain uptake and loss of radiotracers after intracarotid injection. *Am J Physiol* 229(4):1110-1115, 1975.

Goldstein, A., and Kalant, H. Drug policy: Striking the right balance. *Science* 249:1513-1521, 1990.

Langer, R. New methods of drug delivery. *Science* 249:1527-1533, 1990.

Oldendorf, W.H. Measurement of the mean transit time of cerebral circulation by external detection of an intravenously injected radioisotope. *J Nucl Med* 3(5):382-398, 1962.

Oldendorf, W.H. Brain uptake of radiolabeled amino acids, amines, and hexoses after arterial injection. *Am J Physiol* 221(6):1629-1639, 1971.

Oldendorf, W.H. Lipid solubility and drug penetration of the blood brain barrier. *Proc Soc Exp Biol Med* 147:813-816, 1974.

Oldendorf, W.H. Clearance of radiolabeled substances by brain after arterial injection using a diffusible internal standard. In: Marks, N., and Rodnight, R., eds. *Research Methods in Neurochemistry*. Vol. V. New York: Plenum, 1981. pp. 91-112.

Oldendorf, W.H.; Braun, L.; and Cornford, E. pH dependence of blood-brain barrier permeability to lactate and nicotine. *Stroke* 10(5):577-581, 1979.

Oldendorf, W.H.; Hyman, S.; Braun, L.; and Oldendorf, S.Z. Blood-brain barrier: Penetration of morphine, codeine, heroin, and methadone after carotid injection. *Science* 178:984-986, 1972.

Oldendorf, W.H., and Kitano, M. Clinical measurement of brain uptake of radioisotope. *Arch Neurol* 9:574-585, 1963.

Oldendorf, W.H., and Kitano, M. Isotope study of brain blood turnover in vascular disease. *Arch Neurol* 12:30-38, 1965a.

Oldendorf, W.H., and Kitano, M. The symmetry of [131]I 4-iodoantipyrine uptake by brain after intravenous injection. *Neurology* 15(11):994-999, 1965b.

Oldendorf, W.H.; Kitano, M.; and Shimizu, S. Evaluation of a simple technique for abrupt intravenous injection of radioisotope. *J Nucl Med* 6:205-209, 1965b.

Oldendorf, W.H.; Kitano, M.; Shimizu, S.; and Oldendorf, S.Z. Hematocrit of the human cranial blood pool. *Circ Res* 17:532-539, 1965a.

Surgeon General, U.S. Public Health Service. *The Health Consequences of Smoking. Nicotine Addiction.* Department of Health and Human Services, Office of Smoking and Health. DHHS Pub. No. (CDC)88-8406. Washington, DC: Supt. of Docs., U.S. Govt. Print. Off., 1988.

AUTHOR

William H. Oldendorf, M.D.
Senior Medical Investigator
West Los Angeles VA Medical Center
B151C
Wilshire and Sawtelle Boulevards
Los Angeles, CA 90073

Professor of Neurology and Psychiatry
University of California, Los Angeles School of Medicine
Los Angeles, CA 90024

25

Neuroactive Peptides and Amino Acids at the Blood-Brain Barrier: Possible Implications for Drug Abuse

Berislav V. Zlokovic, J. Gordon McComb, Lynn Perlmutter, Martin H. Weiss, and Hugh Davson

INTRODUCTION

The blood-brain barrier (BBB) normally serves to isolate the brain, to a large degree, from compounds dissolved in blood plasma. However, the BBB must not be regarded as an absolute restriction to blood-borne molecules, but rather as a multiple regulatory brain unit(s) with highly developed transport, metabolic, and receptor-mediated functions (Oldendorf 1971; Davson 1976; Betz and Goldstein 1986; Pardridge 1988). These functions are of vital importance for regional homeostasis of the neural microenvironment and maintenance of normal local cell-to-cell communications within the brain. The BBB is described anatomically as a continuous cellular layer of the endothelial cells that are sealed by tight junctions (Brightman 1977). Several homeostatic BBB mechanisms are related to substances that act as neurotransmitters and/or neuromodulators in the brain and hormones at the periphery (Segal and Zlokovic 1990). This review is limited to the authors' observations with the vascular brain perfusion (VBP) model.

BBB TO NEUROACTIVE SUBSTANCES

The pioneering work of Oldendorf (1971) has shown that BBB restricts rapid penetration of monoamines (e.g., norepinephrine, dopamine, serotonin [5-HT]), amino acid neurotransmitters (e.g., glutamate, glycine, gamma aminobutyric acid [GABA]), and neuropeptides (e.g., enkephalins, thyrotropin-releasing hormone [TRH]) (Cornford et al. 1978), whereas some neuroactive drugs, such as amphetamine (Pardridge and Connor 1973) as well as cocaine and nicotine (Oldendorf 1981), can cross the BBB quite rapidly. Once in the brain, these drugs act on various neurotransmitter and neuropeptide systems to produce distinct psychostimulant and neurotoxic effects. A moderate BBB permeability to synthetic analogs of naturally occurring opioid peptides has been demonstrated by Rapoport and colleagues (1980). An enzymatic barrier with

26

a role in terminating actions of neurotransmitters (e.g., monoamines) also has been suggested (Harik, this volume). The hypothesis that the brain capillary receptor for peptide is a component of a BBB transport system has been formulated by Pardridge (1986), and specialized carrier-, receptor-, or absorption-mediated transcytosis mechanisms within the brain capillary endothelium have been shown for large peptides and proteins (e.g., insulin, insulin-like growth factor [IGF] I and II, transferrin, cationized albumin, and immunoglobulin G [IgG]) either by autoradiographic analysis of the in situ perfused brain or by capillary isolation methods (Pardridge 1988).

During recent years, the authors have developed a long-term (up to 20 minutes) VBP model in the guinea pig to investigate interactions of neuroactive substances at the blood-brain interface (Zlokovic et al. 1986). Investigations conducted with this technique suggested that extremely low initial brain extractions of neuropeptides (e.g., leucine-enkephalin [leu-enk], delta sleep-inducing peptide [DSIP], arginine-vasopressin [AVP]) and neurotransmitters (e.g., glutamic acid) may have resulted from relatively slow but specific uptake mechanisms at the luminal side of the BBB (Zlokovic 1990). The method has proven to be sensitive to measure discrete transient changes of impaired BBB permeability during chronic drug intoxication (Rakic et al. 1989) and in the brain affected by an autoimmune process (Zlokovic et al. 1989a).

VBP MODEL: TECHNICAL CONSIDERATIONS

The VBP model allows for experimental control of the concentration of test molecules and the composition of arterial inflow. In this preparation, brain perfusion is carried out through the right common carotid artery in the guinea pig, which is cannulated by fine polyethylene tubing connected to the extracorporeal perfusion circuit (Zlokovic et al. 1986). The contralateral carotid artery is ligated, and both jugular veins are cut to allow drainage of the perfusate. The perfusion medium is an artificial plasma and 20 percent sheep red blood cells. The surgical procedure in the guinea pig is reduced compared with the rat (Takasato et al. 1984) since the cauterization of the right superior thyroid, ophthalmic, and pterygopalatine artery is not required. The unique anatomy of the cerebral circulation in the guinea pig has not been found in any mammals other than cavoids (Bugge 1974). The forebrain supply relies largely on the external carotid artery, and the internal carotid artery normally does not exist. The blood flow in the internal ophthalmic artery is reversed under physiological conditions, due to five anastomotic new branches derived from the proximal part of the external carotid artery and the stapedial arterial system. The circle of Willis is complete, but communication between carotid and vertebral circulations is poor, resulting in the retrograde postcannulation pressure in the right common carotid artery between 10 and 15 mm Hg. The functional separation between artificial and vertebral circulations has been confirmed by isotope experiments (Zlokovic et al. 1988a). The molecules under study are protected from hydrolysis and, therefore, are presented to the blood-brain interface in the intact form.

During brain perfusion, jugular venous outflow can be collected for radioimmunoassay hormone analysis. Placement of an arterial carotid loop may be required when brain microdialysis is conducted simultaneously with vascular brain perfusion. The physiological (e.g., perfusion and arterial blood pressure, heart rate, respirations, electrocardiogram, electroencephalogram, cerebral blood flow, P_{CO_2}, acid-base status), biochemical (e.g., water, electrolyte, adenosine triphosphate, and lactate brain content) (Zlokovic et al. 1986), and morphological (e.g., brain immunogenicity, ultrastructural integrity of the neural tissue at the BBB and non-BBB regions) (figure 1) parameters remain normal in the perfused brain.

Biomathematical modeling of kinetic data from isotopic experiments relies on previously published treatments (Pardridge and Mietus 1982; Patlak et al. 1983; Smith et al. 1987). A novel computer-assisted microimaging of the perfused brain is based on immunohistochemical analysis of blood-borne peptide/protein.

NEUROPEPTIDES

The multiple time point/graphic analysis was used to estimate the unidirectional transfer rate constant, K_{in} (μL min^{-1} g^{-1}), for radiolabeled neuropeptides and inert polar molecules (figure 2). A time-dependent progressive linear brain uptake of leu-enk and TRH during the 20 minutes was significantly higher than for the inert polar molecules. Figure 2 shows that, during relatively short periods of 1 to 2 minutes, it is not possible to distinguish between the extraction for a given peptide from either those of inert polar molecules or those of other peptides. K_{in} values for neuropeptides, IgG, and inert polar molecules are given in table 1.

It has been demonstrated that K_{in} for the tracer estimated in the absence of potential inhibitors and/or competitors represents its maximal permeability surface area product (Smith et al. 1987). The cerebrovascular permeability constants for leu-enk, AVP, TRH, DSIP, cyclosporin A, and inert polar molecules have been correlated with their olive oil:water partition coefficients, or reciprocal values of the square root of their molecular weight (Zlokovic et al. 1990). This analysis indicated that lipophilicity and molecular weight are not good predictors for cerebrovascular permeability of small peptides.

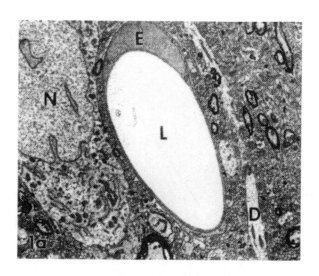

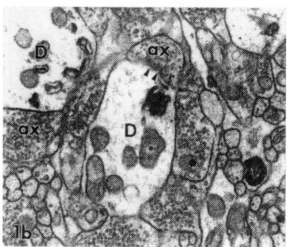

FIGURE 1. *Ultrastructural integrity of the ipsilateral supraoptic nucleus from guinea pig brain vascularly perfused for 10 minutes with the medium containing 20 percent sheep red blood cells suspended in artificial plasma. 1a. The capillary and cellular elements within the neuropil remain intact, retaining their appropriate morphological relationships. E, endothelial cell; L, capillary lumen; N, neuron; D, dendrite. Print magnification=X 7,000. 1b. Two dendrites cut in cross-section are contacted by several axon terminals (ax), and a synapse (arrowheads) is evident. Print magnification=X 31,000.*

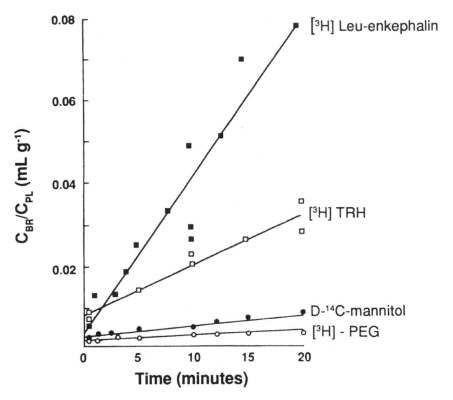

FIGURE 2. *Uptake of small neuropetides, D-mannitol, and polyethylene glycol (PEG) by the parietal cortex of perfused guinea pig brain*

NOTE: $K_{in}=[C_{BR}(T)/C_{PL}-V_i]/T$ where $C_{BR}(T)$ and C_{PL} are dpm per unit mass of brain and plasma, respectively, at perfusion time T; V_i is the initial volume of distribution (ordinate intercept).

SOURCE: Values are taken from Zlokovic et al. 1987, 1988a, and Rakic et al. 1989.

TABLE 1.   *Uptake of neuropeptides, IgG, and inert polar molecules at the luminal side of the BBB*

Tracer	K_{in} (μL min^{-1} g^{-1})	V_i (mL 100 g^{-1})
[^{3}H] Leu-enk	3.62±0.11	0.40±0.07
[^{3}H] AVP	2.78±0.04	0.27±0.04
[^{3}H] TRH	1.22±0.08	0.78±0.09
[^{125}I] DSIP	0.93±0.14	0.94±0.13
[^{125}I] IgG	0.58±0.05	0.29±0.03
[^{3}H] D-mannitol	0.24±0.04	0.35±0.07
[^{3}H] Dextran	0.05±0.01	0.31±0.02

NOTE: Values are means±SE of 7 to 12 perfused brains. K_{in} values are significantly different by analysis of variance (ANOVA). K_{in} and V_i values were graphically estimated in the parietal cortex using the equation given in figure 2. Molecular weight of dextran was 70,000.

SOURCE: Values are taken from Zlokovic et al. 1987, 1988a, 1988b, 1989a, 1989c, 1990.

The first interacting step of circulating neuropeptide at the BBB is the luminal site contact. The kinetics of radiolabeled peptide BBB uptake were examined in the presence of (1) fully saturated L-amino acid transporter, (2) aminopeptidase and amidase inhibitors, (3) unlabeled peptide, (4) peptide fragments, and (5) peptide receptor antagonists and agonists. These experiments failed to demonstrate cross-inhibition between neuropeptides and L-amino acids, confirming a hypothesis that peptide bond prevents utilization of amino acid BBB transporter (Zlokovic et al. 1983). It also has been difficult to demonstrate a carrier-mediated transport of amino acid residues released from peptides, which may suggest that the N-terminal enzymatic hydrolysis may not necessarily be the primary event during peptide interactions at the luminal BBB site. These findings have been supported by a lack of significant inhibition of leu-enk and AVP uptake in the presence of aminopeptidase inhibitors, bestatin, and bacitracin (Zlokovic et al. 1987, 1989b, 1990). The authors' earlier studies indicated that bacitracin reduced leu-enk brain uptake index (BUI) values to the level of intravascular markers, most likely by preventing actions of blood-borne aminopeptidases on the bolus (Zlokovic et al. 1985a). It has been shown that aminopeptidase rapidly degrades leu-enk in vitro (Pardridge and Mietus 1981), so the lack of this effect in the VBP model may suggest that the enzyme is situated at the abluminal site. It has been demonstrated that microvascular aminopeptidase M is a membrane-bound protein contributing to about 1 percent of the total brain "enkephalinase" activity, but its exact cellular location in the BBB has not been determined (Churchill et al. 1987).

The dose-dependent self-inhibition of K_{in} values was demonstrated for leu-enk and AVP, and Michaelis-Menten parameters are given in table 2. Table 2 shows that the K_m for leu-enk uptake is similar to the large neutral amino acids determined during brain perfusion in the rat (Smith et al. 1987), but the capacity of this system is about three orders of magnitude less. It would seem that leu-enk kinetic parameters compare best with the BBB transport mechanisms of purine bases and nucleotides, whereas the AVP system has K_m similar to the carrier-mediated transport system for thyroid hormones, but its capacity was about 35 times less (Pardridge 1988). The diffusion component, K_d, for both peptides was negligible. Leu-enk peptide fragments, Tyr-Gly, Tyr-Gly-Gly, and Gly-Gly-Phe-Leu (Zlokovic et al. 1987, 1989b), and AVP peptide fragments, AVP-(1-8), pressinoic acid, and [pGlu[4],Cyt[6]]AVP-(4-9) (Zlokovic et al. 1990), did not influence BBB uptake of their parent peptides. These results indicate saturable luminal BBB uptake of intact peptides, as well as the absence of significant saturable metabolism of the peptide fragments.

The specific σ-opioid receptor antagonist ally[2]-Tyr-AIB-Phe-OH, μ-opioid receptor agonist Tyr-D-Ala-Gly-Me-Phe-NH(CH$_2$)$_2$OH, and naloxone did not affect significantly uptake of [^{3}H]-leu-enk (Zlokovic et al. 1989b). On the other hand, the V_1-vasopressinergic receptor antagonist, TMeAVP

TABLE 2. *Kinetic parameters for leu-enk and AVP uptake at the luminal side of the BBB*

Peptide	K_m (μM)	V_{max} (pmol min^{-1} g^{-1})
Leu-enk	39±3.2	160±22
AVP	2±0.3	5.49±0.74

NOTE: Values are means±SE for 5 to 9 K_{in} observations in the parietal cortex. Michaelis-Menten parameters were estimated by fitting equation $K_{in}=V_{max}/(K_m+C_{PL})+K_d$ to the brain perfusion data with weighted nonlinear least squares. K_d values were not significantly different from zero.

SOURCE: Values are taken from Zlokovic et al. 1989b, 1990.

(1-β-mercapto-β,β,cyclopentamethylenepropionic acid,2-[O-methyl)tyrosine-vasopressin], but not the V_2-agonist, dDAVP (1-deamino-[8-D-arginine]-vasopressin), significantly inhibited AVP BBB uptake. The affinity of TMeAVP was about two times less than for the peptide (Zlokovic et al. 1990). The AVP BBB receptors may represent either a part of peptide BBB transport system, as demonstrated for insulin, IGF I and II, and transferrin (Pardridge 1986), or they can mediate hormone effects on the BBB. In the latter case, the cellular uptake of circulating peptide would be limited primarily to its binding at the blood-brain interface, similar to that observed for the in situ steroid hormone binding (Pardridge 1987).

The fact that small neuropeptides may be taken up intact at the luminal side of the BBB does not rule out the possibility that they may be subsequently metabolized in the adjacent compartments, such as the cytosolic endothelial space, abluminal surface of the BBB, and surrounding neuropil. This matter was investigated in more detail with AVP. High-performance liquid chromatography analysis of ipsilateral forebrain homogenates depleted from capillaries indicated that about 50 percent of the AVP remained in its intact form after 1 minute, whereas the percentage of the intact peptide progressively fell with time; after 10 and 15 minutes, the radioactivity was eluted primarily in the fraction corresponding to L-[^{3}H]-phenylalanine (Zlokovic et al. 1991a). This suggests that there is normally a time-dependent, progressive aminopeptidase degradation of circulating AVP once it has been transferred across the luminal BBB side; the possibility that AVP is a precursor of more potent centrally active fragments, such as [pGlu^4,Cyt^6]-AVP-(4-9), has been suggested (Burbach et al. 1983). On the other hand, thin-layer chromatography analysis of forebrain homogenates has shown that DSIP remained predominantly in intact form in the brain during the 10-minute period of perfusion, which is consistent with previously demonstrated resistance of this peptide to hydrolysis after crossing biological barriers (Banks et al. 1983).

Permeability of the special regions also has been examined by the VBP model and in the in situ isolated perfused choroid plexus of the sheep. Kinetic analysis revealed saturable AVP (Zlokovic et al. 1991b) and DSIP (Zlokovic et al. 1988b) uptake at the basolateral face of the choroid plexus with respective K_m values of about 30 and 5 nM. It is suggested that specific AVP uptake mechanisms in the choroid plexus can detect circulating hormone primarily by V_1-receptors. Saturable cellular uptake in the choroid plexus also has been found for leu-enk (Zlokovic et al. 1988c), but not for TRH (Zlokovic et al. 1985b). Selective permeability to blood-borne AVP has been demonstrated by immunohistochemical studies in the paraventricular nucleus (PVN) of the hypothalamus. In these experiments, brains were perfused with unlabeled AVP, and immunoreaction product was found to lightly stain only the perivascular space of the PVN, but not of the other BBB regions (B.V. Zlokovic, L. Perlmutter, J.G. McComb, and C. Segal, unpublished data). This pattern may be due either to selective permeability of PVN to the circulating AVP or to locally induced hormone release. Specific uptake mechanisms for AVP also have been described in the hypothalamo-pituitary axis and pineal gland (Zlokovic et al. 1991c), and it is suggested that AVP uptake in these regions represents hormone binding in situ primarily to the V_1-type receptors.

CIRCULATING NEUROACTIVE AMINO ACIDS

The BUI method indicated the presence of a low-capacity independent carrier system at the BBB, transporting two neurotransmitters, L-glutamic and L-aspartic acid (Oldendorf and Szabo 1976). Those studies were extended to determine Michaelis-Menten parameters for L-glutamic acid using the VBP model (Davson et al. 1990). Kinetic experiments revealed regional Michaelis constant between 3 and 5 µM and capacity that was three orders of magnitude lower than for neutral and basic amino acids. Regional unidirectional saturable influx of L-glutamic acid was inhibited by 72 to 94 percent in the presence of 0.5 mM L-aspartic acid. These results indicate that the carrier-mediated system for L-glutamic acid located at the luminal BBB side may be fully saturated at normal plasma concentrations of this amino acid. The physiological importance of this system and its relationship with N-methyl-D-aspartate (NMDA) receptors are under investigation. Unidirectional transfer rate constants for amino acid neurotransmitters and 5-HT are given in table 3. It can be seen that studied neurotransmitters exhibit significantly higher cerebrovascular permeability than N-methyl-α-aminoisobutyric acid (MeAIB), a model substrate for the A amino acid transport system (Zlokovic et al. 1986).

IMPLICATIONS FOR DRUG ABUSE

It has been shown that tricyclic antidepressants (e.g., amitriptyline, imipramine), which act as indirect adrenergic agonists, increase the diffusibility of water across the BBB (Prescorn et al. 1980). On the basis of these experiments, it has been suggested that there is a neuronal system acting in a humoral fashion to regulate the movement of substances across the BBB. The authors have explored this hypothesis by testing BBB permeability to inert polar molecules, leu-enk, AVP, glutamic acid, and GABA using the chronic amphetamine intoxication animal model. The VBP technique was employed to ensure control over peripheral factors (e.g., central hypertension) during tests of BBB functions. The behavioral syndrome—consisting of increased locomotor activity, stereotypy (continuous gnawing and sniffing of the cage floor and side bars), absence of normal exploratory and grooming behavior, and loss of weight—was developed in all animals treated with amphetamine for at least 14 days (Rakic et al. 1989). The effect of withdrawal was studied in animals that

TABLE 3. *Uptake of amino acid neurotransmitters, 5-HT, and MeAIB at the luminal side of the BBB*

Neurotransmitter	K_{in} (μL min^{-1} g^{-1})
L-[^{3}H] Glutamic acid	6.73$\pm$0.20
[^{3}H] Glycine	4.62$\pm$0.49
[^{3}H] GABA	1.09$\pm$0.20
5-[^{3}H] HT	1.02$\pm$0.35
[^{14}C] MeAIB	0.75$\pm$0.07

NOTE: Values are means$\pm$SE of 5 to 24 perfused brains. K_{in} values are significantly different by ANOVA, except for GABA and 5-HT. K_{in} values were graphically estimated using the equation given in figure 2.

SOURCE: Values for glutamic acid and MeAIB are taken from Davson et al. 1990 and Zlokovic et al. 1986.

had been treated with amphetamine for 20 days. The behavioral syndrome in these animals progressively subsided and was absent by 7 days. Figure 3 illustrates the changes in the ratio of cerebrovascular permeability constants for D-mannitol and PEG 4,000 simultaneously perfused in the guinea pig forebrain during the course of the induced amphetamine intoxication and recovery. It can be seen that ratio falls to about 1 after 14 days of treatment and stays about the same after the extension of treatment to 20 days. A spontaneous recovery of BBB to metabolically inert molecules was established 28 days after cessation of treatment. Opening of the BBB also was confirmed histologically by penetration of the fluorescent dye Lucifer yellow in animals treated with amphetamine for 14 days. A marked amphetamine-induced increase in leu-enk and AVP BBB uptake was shown after 20 days of amphetamine treatment. K_{in} values for both peptides exhibited similar time-dependent changes, suggesting an initial fourfold to fivefold increase in BBB uptake (figure 4). K_{in} vs. time curves may indicate no change in affinity but a significant increase of capacity of both peptide systems. It is noteworthy that only a modest increase in BBB permeability to TRH was measured. It also has been demonstrated that amphetamine significantly increases BBB uptake of glutamic acid and GABA (table 4).

Metaphit, an isothiocyanate analog of phencylidine (PCP) has been shown to induce audiogenic seizures (Debler et al. 1989). The authors have examined BBB permeability to glutamic acid in the guinea pig with metaphit-induced audiogenic seizures. A significant reduction of glutamic acid brain uptake was found in comparison with control animals. This finding is in contrast with an

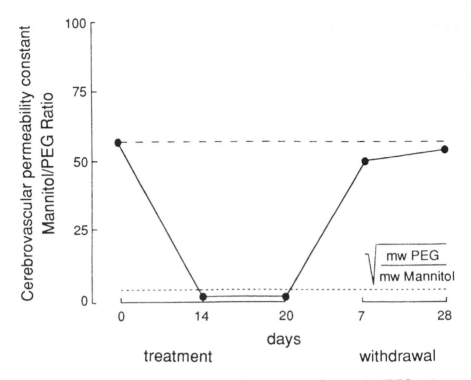

FIGURE 3. *Cerebrovascular permeability constant, P, mannitol/PEG ratio for vascularly perfused guinea pig forebrain during the course of chronic amphetamine intoxication after 14 and 20 days of treatment with D-amphetamine sulphate (i.p., 5 mg/kg daily), and 7 and 28 days after cessation of 20 days chronic treatment with amphetamine. Interrupted line represents $P_{mannitol}/P_{PEG}$ ratio obtained in control, nontreated animals; dashed line represents mannitol/PEG ratio of reciprocal values of the square root of molecular weight. Olive oil:water partition coefficient ratio of mannitol/PEG is 1:30. Values are means of 5 to 12 animals.*

SOURCE: Rakic et al. 1989, copyright 1989, Elsevier Science Publishers

increased cerebrovascular permeability to horseradish peroxidase observed in electrically induced seizures (Westergaard et al. 1978) and may suggest inhibition of specific uptake mechanism for the neurotransmitter. It has been proposed that metaphit may bind irreversibly to a site allosterically linked to NMDA receptor (Debler et al. 1989), and the authors' preliminary experiments demonstrated cross-inhibition between glutamic acid and NMDA BBB uptake.

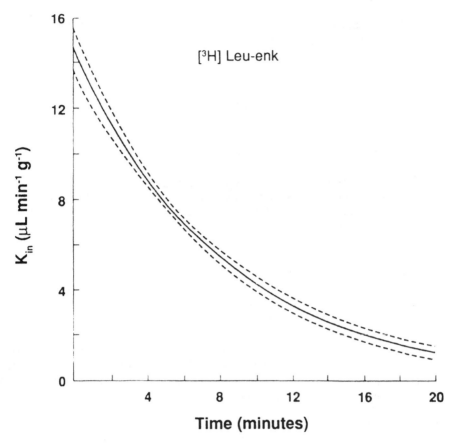

FIGURE 4. *Time-dependent changes of K_{in} leu-enk values in the forebrain of guinea pigs treated with amphetamine for 20 days as explained in figure 3. Curve is computed on the basis of 10 animals that were perfused at different times up to 20 minutes; interrupted lines are confidence bands.*

It has been demonstrated that tobacco smoking results in increased plasma AVP levels, and it has been suggested that some reinforcing and withdrawal effects of nicotine may depend on AVP psychoactive actions (Fuxe et al. 1989). The authors have shown that chronic 14-day treatment with nicotine administered to guinea pig by osmotic minipumps alters BBB permeability to AVP and hormone binding to non-BBB regions. An increased uptake was found in the caudate nucleus, as well as in capillary-depleted brain tissue and cerebral microvessels (M. Lipovac, B.V. Zlokovic, L. Perlmutter, and E. Barrone,

TABLE 4. *Uptake of L-glutamic acid and GABA by the parietal cortex in the guinea pig treated with amphetamine for 20 days*

$$C_{BR}/C_{PL} \text{ (mL g}^{-1})$$

Treatment	[^{3}H] Glutamic Acid	[^{3}H] GABA
Control	0.105±0.006 (9)	0.021±0.001 (5)
Amphetamine	0.151±0.008 (6)*	0.079±0.004 (4)*

NOTE: Values are means±SE (n); *p<0.001. C_{BR}/C_{PL} is the ratio of neurotransmitter radioactivity per unit mass of the brain and plasma measured during the 10-minute period of brain perfusion. Treatment with amphetamine is explained in figure 3.

unpublished data). Parallel preliminary ultrastructural examination of neurohypophysis has revealed fewer dense core vesicles than in control animals. As many of these vesicles contain AVP, this decrease is consistent with the reported increase in plasma AVP levels that accompanies chronic nicotine exposure. In addition, neurohypophyseal capillaries from nicotine-treated animals had prominent finger-like projections into the lumen, and the enclosure of axon terminals by pituicyte cytoplasm, a well-documented normal configuration of the region in times of low hormone demand (Hatton et al. 1984), was seen only in the control animals.

CONCLUSION

Cerebrovascular permeability to slowly penetrating neuropeptides (leu-enk, AVP, DSIP, TRH) and neurotransmitters (glutamic acid, glycine, GABA, 5-HT) is 5 to 120 times higher than for metabolically inert polar molecules. Olive oil:water partition coefficients and molecular weights are not good predictors of BBB permeability to small peptides. Neuropeptides do not use BBB amino acid transporters, and enzymatic hydrolysis may not necessarily be the primary event at the BBB. Specific uptake systems for leu-enk, AVP, DSIP, and glutamic acid have been demonstrated at the BBB and basolateral face of the choroid epithelium. There is no saturable brain uptake of peptide metabolites. Specific peptidergic receptors can mediate slow BBB uptake of circulating peptide and binding to non-BBB regions and the anterior pituitary. BBB postluminal step may result in transformation of peptide to its more potent neuroactive fragments. BBB restrictive properties, specific uptake mechanisms, and receptor sensitivity to neuroactive peptides and amino acids are influenced by behaviorally active drugs, such as tricyclic antidepressants, amphetamine, metaphit, and nicotine. The psychotropic drugs should no longer be assumed to cause their effects solely by altering neuron interactions. Therefore, therapeutic approaches in the treatment of addiction should complement restorative neurotransmitter and BBB therapy.

REFERENCES

Banks, W.A.; Kastin, A.J.; and Coy, D.H. Delta sleep-inducing peptide (DSIP) like material is absorbed by the gastrointestinal tract of the neonatal rat. *Life Sci* 33:1587-1597, 1983.

Betz, A.L., and Goldstein, G.W. Specialized properties and solute transport in brain capillaries. *Annu Rev Physiol* 48:241-250, 1986.

Brightman, M. Morphology of blood-brain interfaces. *Exp Eye Res* 25(Suppl):1-25, 1977.

Bugge, J. The cephalic arteries of hystriomorph rodents. *Symp Zool Soc (London)* 34:61-68, 1974.

Burbach, J.P.; Kovasc, G.L.; and de Wied, D. A major metabolite of arginine vasopressin in the brain is a highly potent neuropeptide. *Science* 221:1310-1312, 1983.

Churchill, L.; Bausback, N.H.; Gerritsen, M.E.; and Ward, P.E. Metabolism of opioid peptides by cerebral microvascular aminopeptidase M. *Biochim Biophys Acta* 923:35-41, 1987.

Cornford, E.M.; Braun, L.D.; Crane, P.D.; and Oldendorf, W.H. Blood-brain barrier restriction of peptides and the low uptake of enkephalins. *Endocrinology* 103:1297-1303, 1978.

Davson, H. The blood-brain barrier. *J Physiol* 225:1-28, 1976.

Davson, H.; Lipovac, M.N.; Mackic, J.B.; Preston, J.E.; Segal, M.B.; Tang, G.; and Zlokovic, B.V. Kinetics of L-glutamic acid uptake by the luminal side of the blood-brain barrier studied in an in situ perfused brain of the anaesthetized guinea pig. *J Physiol* 423:36P, 1990.

Debler, E.A.; Lipovac, M.N.; Lajtha, A.; Zlokovic, B.V.; Jacobson, A.E.; Rice, K.C.; and Reith, M.E.A. Metaphit, an isothiocyanate analog of PCP, induces audiogenic seizures in mice. *Eur J Pharmacol* 165:155-159, 1989.

Fuxe, K.; Anderson, K.; Eneroth, P.; Harfstrand, A.; and Agnati, L.F. Neuroendocrine actions of nicotine and exposure to cigarette smoke: Medical implications. *Psychoneuroendocrinology* 14:19-41, 1989.

Hatton, G.I.; Perlmutter, L.S.; Salm, A.K.; and Tweedle, C.D. Dynamic neuronal-glial interactions in hypothalamus and pituitary: Implications for control of hormone synthesis and release. *Peptides* 5:121-138, 1984.

Oldendorf, W.H. Brain uptake of radiolabeled amino acids, amines, and hexoses after arterial injection. *Am J Physiol* 221:1629-1639, 1971.

Oldendorf, W.H. Clearance of radiolabeled substances by brain after arterial injection using a diffusible internal standard. In: Marks, N., and Rodnight, R., eds. *Research Methods in Neurochemistry*. Vol 5. New York: Plenum, 1981. pp. 91-112.

Oldendorf, W.H., and Szabo, J. Amino acid assignment to one of three blood-brain barrier amino acid-carriers. *Am J Physiol* 230:372-376, 1976.

Pardridge, W.M. Receptor-mediated peptide transport through the blood-brain barrier. *Endocr Rev* 7:314-330, 1986.

Pardridge, W.M. Plasma protein-mediated transport of steroid and thyroid hormones. *Am J Physiol* 252:E157-E164, 1987.

Pardridge, W.M. Recent advances in blood-brain barrier transport. *Annu Rev Pharmacol Toxicol* 28:25-39, 1988.

Pardridge, W.M., and Connor, J.D. Saturable transport of amphetamine across the blood-brain barrier. *Experientia* 29:302-304, 1973.

Pardridge, W.M., and Mietus, L.J. Enkephalin and blood-brain barrier: Studies of binding and degradation in isolated brain microvessels. *Endocrinology* 109:1138-1143, 1981.

Pardridge, W.M., and Mietus, L.J. Kinetics of neutral amino acid transport through the blood-brain barrier of the newborn rabbit. *J Neurochem* 38:955-962, 1982.

Patlak, C.S.; Fentermacher, J.D.; and Blasberg, R.G. Graphical evaluation of blood-to-brain transfer constants from multiple-time uptake data. *J Cereb Blood Flow Metab* 3:1-7, 1983.

Prescorn, S.H.; Hartman, B.K.; Raichle, M.E.; Swanson, L.W.; and Clark, H.B. Central adrenergic regulation of cerebral microvascular permeability and blood flow: Pharmacologic evidence. In: Eisenberg, H.M., and Suddith, R.L., eds. *The Cerebral Microvasculature*. New York: Academic Press, 1980. pp. 127-138.

Rakic, L.M.; Zlokovic, B.V.; Davson, H.; Segal, M.B.; Begley, D.J.; Lipovac, M.N.; and Mitrovic, D.M. Chronic amphetamine intoxication and the blood-brain barrier permeability to inert polar molecules studied in the vascularly perfused guinea pig brain. *J Neurol Sci* 94:41-50, 1989.

Rapoport, S.I.; Klee, W.A.; Pettigrew, K.D.; and Ohno, K. Entry of opioid peptides into the central nervous system. *Science* 207:84-86, 1980.

Segal, M.B., and Zlokovic, B.V. *The Blood-Brain Barrier, Amino Acids and Peptides*. Norwell, MA: Kluwer Academic, 1990.

Smith, Q.R.; Momma, S.; Aoyagi, M.; and Rapoport, S.I. Kinetics of neutral amino acid transport from saline and plasma. *J Neurochem* 49:1651-1658, 1987.

Takasato, Y.; Rapoport, S.I.; and Smith, Q.R. An in situ brain perfusion technique to study cerebrovascular transport in the rat. *Am J Physiol* 247:H484-H493, 1984.

Westergaard, E.; Hertz, M.M.; and Bolwig, T.G. Increased permeability to horseradish peroxidase across cerebral vessels, evoked by electrically induced seizures in the rat. *Acta Neuropathol (Berlin)* 41:73-80, 1978.

Zlokovic, B.V. In vivo approaches for studying peptide interactions at the blood-brain barrier. *J Control Rel* 13:185-202, 1990.

Zlokovic, B.V.; Banks, W.A.; Kadi, El H.; Erchegyi, J.; McComb, J.G.; and Kastin, A.J. Blood-to-brain transport and metabolism of circulating vasopressin. *Soc Neurosci Abstr* 17:240, 1991a.

Zlokovic, B.V.; Begley, D.J.; and Chain, D.G. Blood-brain barrier permeability to dipeptides and their constituent amino acids. *Brain Res* 271:66-71, 1983.

Zlokovic, B.V.; Begley, D.J.; and Chain, D.G. Blood-brain barrier permeability to leucine-enkephalin, D-alanine²-D-leucine⁵-enkephalin and their N-terminal amino acid (tyrosine). *Brain Res* 336:125-132, 1985a.

Zlokovic, B.V.; Begley, D.J.; Djuricic, B.M.; and Mitrovic, D.M. Measurement of solute transport across the blood-brain barrier in the perfused guinea pig brain: Method and application to N-methyl-α-aminoisobutyric acid. *J Neurochem* 46:1444-1451, 1986.

Zlokovic, B.V.; Hyman, S.; McComb, J.G.; Lipovac, M.N.; Tang, G.; and Davson, H. Kinetics of arginine-vasopressin uptake at the blood-brain barrier. *Biochim Biophys Acta* 1025:191-198, 1990.

Zlokovic, B.V.; Hyman, S.; McComb, J.G.; Tang, G.; Rezai, A.; and Weiss, M.H. Vasopressin uptake by the hypothalamo-pituitary axis and pineal gland in guinea pigs. *Am J Physiol* 260:E633-E640, 1991c.

Zlokovic, B.V.; Lipovac, M.N.; Begley, D.J.; Davson, H.; and Rakic, L.M. Transport of leucine-enkephalin across the blood-brain barrier in the perfused guinea pig brain. *J Neurochem* 49:310-315, 1987.

Zlokovic, B.V.; Lipovac, M.N.; Begley, D.J.; Davson, H.; and Rakic, L.M. Slow penetration of thyrotropin-releasing hormone across the blood-brain barrier of an in situ perfused guinea pig brain. *J Neurochem* 51:252-257, 1988a.

Zlokovic, B.V.; Mackic, J.B.; Djuricic, B.; and Davson, H. Kinetic analysis of leucine-enkephalin cellular uptake at the luminal side of the blood-brain barrier of an in situ perfused guinea pig brain. *J Neurochem* 53:1333-1340, 1989b.

Zlokovic, B.V.; Segal, M.B.; Begley, D.J.; Davson, H.; and Rakic, L. Permeability of the blood-cerebrospinal fluid and blood-brain barriers to thyrotropin-releasing hormone. *Brain Res* 358:191-199, 1985b.

Zlokovic, B.V.; Segal, M.B.; Davson, H.; and Jankov, R.M. Passage of delta sleep-inducing peptide (DSIP) across the blood-cerebrospinal fluid barrier. *Peptides* 9:533-538, 1988b.

Zlokovic, B.V.; Segal, M.B.; Davson, H.; and Mitrovic, D.M. Unidirectional uptake of enkephalins at the blood-tissue interface of blood-cerebrospinal fluid barrier: A saturable mechanism. *Regul Pept* 20:33-45, 1988c.

Zlokovic, B.V.; Segal, M.B.; McComb, J.G.; Hyman, S.; Weiss, M.H.; and Davson, H. Kinetics of circulating vasopressin uptake by choroid plexus. *Am J Physiol* 260:F216-F224, 1991b.

Zlokovic, B.V.; Skundric, D.S.; Segal, M.B.; Colover, J.; Jankov, R.M.; Pejnovic, N.; Lackovic, J.; Mackic, J.; Lipovac, M.N.; Davson, H.; Kasp, E.; Dumonde, D.; and Rakic, L. Blood-brain barrier permeability changes during acute allergic encephalomyelitis induced in the guinea pig. *Metab Brain Dis* 4(1):33-40, 1989a.

Zlokovic, B.V.; Susic, V.; Davson, H.; Begley, D.J.; Jankov, R.M.; Mitrovic, D.M.; and Lipovac, M.N. Saturable mechanism of delta-sleep inducing peptide uptake at the blood-brain barrier of the vascularly perfused guinea pig brain. *Peptides* 10:249-254, 1989c.

ACKNOWLEDGMENTS

This work was supported by the Division of Neurosurgery, Children's Hospital of Los Angeles; the Wellcome Trust; the British Council Senior Fellowship (BVZ); and by funds provided by the Cigarette and Tobacco Surtax Fund of the State of California through the Tobacco-Related Disease Research Program of the University of California, grant 2RT 0071.

AUTHORS

Berislav V. Zlokovic, M.D., Ph.D.
Associate Professor of Neurosurgery, Physiology, and Biophysics

J. Gordon McComb, M.D.
Professor of Neurosurgery

Lynn Perlmutter, Ph.D.
Assistant Professor of Neurology

Martin H. Weiss, M.D.
Professor and Chairman of Neurosurgery

University of Southern California School of Medicine
RMR 407
2025 Zonal Avenue
Los Angeles, CA 90033

Hugh Davson, D.Sci.
Professor of Physiology
Sherrington School of Physiology
UMDS of Guy's & St. Thomas's Hospitals
London SE1 7EH
UNITED KINGDOM

MPTP Toxicity and the "Biochemical" Blood-Brain Barrier

Sami I. Harik

The discovery that 1-methyl-4-phenyl-1,2,3,6-tetrahydropyridine (MPTP) causes parkinsonism in humans (Davis et al. 1979; Langston et al. 1983) caused a major revolution in scientific research on the etiology, treatment, and prevention of Parkinson's disease (Snyder and D'Amato 1986; Singer et al. 1987; Kopin and Markey 1988). MPTP is now used to induce in nonhuman primates a clinical, pathological, and neurochemical condition, which is probably the best available experimental model of Parkinson's disease (Burns et al. 1983; Bankiewicz et al. 1986).

Although the mechanisms that underlie MPTP neurotoxicity are not entirely clear, investigations during the past few years have revealed several important points. First, MPTP is neurotoxic to humans and other primates when given parenterally in small doses, but chemists have synthesized MPTP in large quantities for years without taking unusually strict precautions and, with one exception (Langston and Ballard 1983), without evidence of neurotoxicity. Thus, MPTP neurotoxicity might not have been discovered had the unfortunate drug users not injected MPTP intravenously. It is likely that MPTP is detoxified by other organs when taken by other routes. Second, MPTP is not the ultimate neurotoxin. MPTP oxidation, mainly by the enzyme monoamine oxidase B (MAO-B), appears to be a necessary step for neurotoxicity since pretreatment of experimental animals with MAO-B inhibitors prevents MPTP neurotoxicity (Heikkila et al. 1984; Langston et al. 1984; Markey et al. 1984). MPTP oxidation to the intermediate metabolite 1-methyl-4-phenyl-2,3-dihydropyridinium ($MPDP^+$), and eventually to the neurotoxic culprit, 1-methyl-4-phenylpyridinium (MPP^+), is presumed to take place in the brain, primarily in glia (Uhl et al. 1985; Snyder and D'Amato 1986). The reason for considering glia as the main site for MPTP oxidation is that most of the MAO-B activity of the brain is thought to be in glia (Levitt et al. 1982; Westlund et al. 1985; Konradi et al. 1988). Third, $MPDP^+$ and MPP^+ are then exuded via an unknown mechanism into the extracellular space where they are selectively taken up by dopaminergic neurons that are equipped with the high-affinity dopamine uptake pump (Javitch et al. 1985). Concentration of MPP^+ by dopaminergic neurons may explain their

43

selective vulnerability. This view is supported by the finding that specific inhibitors of high-affinity dopamine uptake decrease MPTP neurotoxicity (Ricaurte et al. 1985). Fourth, MPP+ is further concentrated in mitochondria of dopaminergic neurons by an energy-dependent uptake process (Ramsay and Singer 1986), eventually causing metabolic failure by interfering with cellular respiration at Complex I (Nicklas et al. 1985; Ramsay et al. 1986, 1987).

However, this story has some loopholes and is dependent on several factors that are not universally accepted. For example, it is thought that MPTP permeates cell membranes easily in view of its lipophilicity, while MPP+ cannot cross the lipid bilayer of cell membranes because it is a polar, water-soluble compound. Systemic administration of MPP+ is not neurotoxic (Fuller and Hemrick-Luecke 1986; Johannessen et al. 1986) because of its inability to cross the blood-brain barrier (BBB) (Riachi et al. 1989). However, most scenarios of MPTP toxicity assume that MPP+ exudes easily out of astrocytes (Snyder and D'Amato 1986). This matter needs clarification and further examination.

A most intriguing aspect of MPTP neurotoxicity is that not all animals are equally susceptible. In fact, the most frequently used laboratory animals are quite resistant to MPTP neurotoxicity. Wistar and Sprague-Dawley rats are unaffected by MPTP in doses as high as 50 mg/kg/day given subcutaneously for several weeks (Harik et al. 1988). In contrast, as little as 0.2 mg/kg/day of MPTP given for 2 days to African Green monkeys causes dramatic clinical and biochemical parkinsonism and often results in death (Elsworth et al. 1987). The dramatic differences among mammals in their susceptibility to MPTP neurotoxicity drew attention to the biological bases that underlie these differences, not only because of their theoretical and heuristic value but also because of their possible immense practical implications in designing strategies for the treatment or prevention of Parkinson's disease. If MPTP toxicity has anything to do with Parkinson's disease, and if the ability of rats to withstand massive doses of MPTP can be transferred to humans, this would have major clinical significance.

Several possible explanations have been put forward for the differences among mammalian species, and even among strains of the same species, in their susceptibility to MPTP neurotoxicity. One explanation is related to neuromelanin. Humans and higher primates have more melanin in the substantia nigra than other mammals. It was hypothesized that MPTP and/or MPP+ bind to neuromelanin (D'Amato et al. 1986). Suggestions that aged animals and strains of mice with skin pigments are more sensitive to MPTP neurotoxicity than younger animals and albino strains were used to support the melanin hypothesis. The implications are that neuromelanin accumulates with age and that mouse or rat strains with dark skin have more melanin in their midbrain. There is no direct evidence to support either of these contentions. Furthermore, the melanin hypothesis does not explain why, after MPTP administration, the toxin and its metabolites accumulate primarily in the striatum (Johannessen et al. 1985), where there is no melanin. The melanin theory also ignores evidence suggesting that MPTP causes death of dopaminergic substantia nigra neurons by retrograde degeneration after massive destruction of their nerve endings in the striatum (Elsworth et al. 1987).

Another frequently used explanation for the differences in susceptibility to MPTP neurotoxicity among species and strains is the variation in brain MAO-B activity. CF1 albino mice, for example, were thought by Zimmer and Geneser (1987) to be less sensitive to MPTP than C57Bl mice because albino mice have lower MAO-B activity in their brains, and thus, MPP+ will not be formed in sufficient concentrations to cause neurotoxicity. However, biochemical assays show that MAO-B activity is similar among crude mitochondrial preparations of the brains of mice, rats, and humans, despite the major differences in their susceptibility to MPTP neurotoxicity (Kalaria et al. 1987, 1988; Kalaria and Harik 1987).

The author and colleagues' research group at Case Western Reserve University first addressed the question of the rat's resistance to systemic MPTP neurotoxicity by microinfusing MPTP directly into the substantia nigra of Wistar rats. One µmole of MPTP selectively destroyed the dopaminergic cell bodies of the pars compacta and caused near total depletion of dopamine and its metabolites in the ipsilateral striatum, without affecting nondopaminergic neurons in the pars reticulata of the substantia nigra or glial cells (Sayre et al. 1986; Harik et al. 1987). These experiments suggested that the unique resistance of Wistar rats to MPTP neurotoxicity is not due to resistance by dopaminergic neurons but is probably a reflection of insufficient MPP+ concentrations that accumulate in the rat substantia nigra.

Failure of MPTP metabolites to achieve toxic levels in the brains of Wistar rats can be due to detoxification of MPTP either in other organs or at the BBB. Indeed, Riachi and colleagues (1988) found that Wistar rats have a high capacity to detoxify and metabolize MPTP in the liver. To determine whether brain capillaries from different mammals can metabolize MPTP, isolated cerebral microvessels were assayed for their MAO activity. Large variations in MAO activity were found among mammals that were inversely related to their susceptibility to systemic MPTP neurotoxicity (Kalaria et al. 1987, 1988; Kalaria and Harik 1987). Initially this was demonstrated in humans (who are exquisitely sensitive to MPTP), Wistar rats (which are resistant to MPTP neurotoxicity), and albino mice (which are intermediate in their sensitivity to MPTP neurotoxicity). MAO was assessed by irreversible binding to [³H]pargyline and by oxidation of several substrates. Based on substrate specificity, on the ability of the selective MAO inhibitors (clorgyline and deprenyl) to block substrate oxidation, and on polyacrylamide gel electrophoresis studies, the vast majority of rat brain capillary MAO was of the B type (Kalaria et al. 1987; Kalaria and Harik 1987). The list of species was extended later to include rabbits, pigs, and guinea pigs. MAO specific activity was highest in brain microvessels of Wistar rats (Kalaria and Harik 1987). It was surprising that the MAO content of brain microvessels of Wistar rats was even higher than in the liver, the traditional tissue from which MAO is usually obtained. In fact, MAO activity was higher in brain microvessels of Wistar rats than in any other tissue that was ever investigated. This finding was even more surprising because immunocytochemical studies have failed to identify MAO activity in rat brain microvessels (Levitt et al. 1982). The reason(s) for this anomaly remains unknown.

On the other hand, human cerebral microvessels are almost devoid of MAO (Kalaria et al. 1987, 1988; Kalaria and Harik 1987). This is not because human brain microvessels were obtained at autopsy after a considerable postmortem delay. MAO is known to be quite resistant to the effects of postmortem autolysis (Mackay et al. 1978). Also, rat brain microvessels that were harvested from brains of rats that were decapitated many hours earlier did not show diminution in their MAO content (Kalaria et al. 1987). The author and colleagues now have extended this work to monkeys. Brain microvessels obtained from several types of monkeys were all as deficient in MAO activity as human brain microvessels (Riachi and Harik 1990).

In addition to studying the differences among animal species, we also investigated strains of the same species for differences in their susceptibility to MPTP neurotoxicity. Two strains of mice, CF1 albino and C57Bl, were first studied because of the known difference in their sensitivity to MPTP (Zimmer and Geneser 1987). The more sensitive strain had higher MAO activity in its brain, which was thought to account for the more facile conversion of MPTP to MPP+ (Zimmer and Geneser 1987). Riachi and Harik (1988) confirmed that the C57Bl mice are more sensitive to MPTP and also found that regional brain levels of MPTP and its metabolites were higher in the striata of C57Bl mice but not in their cerebral cortices or cerebella. When MAO activity was assayed in the cerebral cortices and striata of the two strains of mice, no significant differences were found in the striata but higher MAO activity was found in the cerebral cortices of C57Bl mice. More important, significantly higher MAO activity was found in isolated cerebral microvessels from CF1 albino mice than in cerebral microvessels of C57Bl mice (Riachi and Harik 1988). This, coupled with the finding that isolated brain microvessels from CF1 albino mice also were more capable of converting of MPTP to MPP+ in vitro than those from C57Bl mice, agreed well with the hypothesis that the higher activity of MAO in brain microvessels correlated inversely with the susceptibility of experimental animals to MPTP.

This work has now been extended to five rat strains (Riachi et al. 1991). It was found that not all rat strains are equally resistant to MPTP neurotoxicity. The differences were correlated among rat strains in their susceptibility to MPTP administered into the internal carotid artery in vivo, with MPTP oxidation by the cerebral cortex, striatum, and brain microvessels in vitro. The in vivo work was performed by assessing ipsilateral striatal depletion of dopamine and its metabolites 1 week after injecting MPTP directly into the cerebral arterial circulation. Dopamine depletion was found to be minimal in Sprague-Dawley and Wistar rats, but there was considerable dopamine depletion in the striata of the more sensitive rat strains that was MPTP dose-dependent. Differences in striatal dopamine depletion among these rat strains correlated best with differences in MAO activity in their isolated brain microvessels, but not with differences in MAO activity in either their striata or cerebral cortices (Riachi et al. 1991). These findings in the various rat strains are also consistent with the hypothesis that the resistance of Wistar and Sprague-Dawley rats to MPTP neurotoxicity is largely a property of their unique brain endothelium, which has high MAO-B activity.

A major portion of the MPTP that is systemically administered to experimental animals is sequestered and metabolized in peripheral organs, principally the liver. To ascribe the rat's resistance to systemic MPTP neurotoxicity to its unique BBB, it had to be shown that neurotoxicity does not occur even when MPTP is injected directly into the arterial circulation of the brain. In primates, internal carotid arterial administration of MPTP was shown to be a most effective means of inducing unilateral parkinsonism and nigrostriatal degeneration, even when given in doses that are not effective when administered systemically (Bankiewicz et al. 1986). Riachi and colleagues (1989) assessed the ability of MPTP, MPP+, and butanol to cross the BBB in rats by the indicator-fractionation method. As expected in view of their high lipid solubility, both MPTP and butanol are almost completely extracted by the brain on the first pass, but only minimal amounts of MPP+ cross from blood to brain. However, within seconds to minutes, butanol is rapidly washed out of the brain, while the [^{3}H] label of the MPTP tracer is retained for long periods. The retention of MPTP by the brain, at least in the early periods, was not due to its rapid metabolism by MAO because pargyline pretreatment did not affect MPTP retention by the brain (Riachi et al. 1989). However, 30 minutes after MPTP injection, brain retention of the [^{3}H] tracer was reduced significantly by pargyline treatment. Another finding of the pargyline pretreatment experiments is that a substantial amount of the MPTP that was taken by the brain was converted to

MPP+ even in the face of near total inhibition of MAO activity (Riachi et al. 1989). Other oxidative enzymes, such as the P450 enzyme system and the flavin-containing monoxygenases, were previously suspected of having a role in MPTP metabolism by other tissues (Weissman et al. 1985; Cashman and Ziegler 1986), but little is known about these enzyme systems in the brain or its microvessels. Also, pargyline pretreatment had no effect on the formation of the lactam metabolites of MPTP (Riachi et al. 1989) that were previously described by Arora and colleagues (1988).

Even when MPTP was administered into the internal carotid artery of Wistar rats, up to 5 mg of MPTP had relatively minor effects on dopamine levels in the ipsilateral striatum (Riachi et al. 1990, 1991). These minor effects were abolished after pargyline pretreatment. Larger doses of MPTP caused death from acute cardiorespiratory failure, and therefore larger doses of MPTP could not be studied. Riachi and coworkers (1990) calculated that between 15 and 20 percent of the MPTP dose was taken up by the ipsilateral cerebrum, which weighs about 0.7 g. This corresponds to more than 1 mg of MPTP/g of rat cerebrum. For comparison, injection of 2.5 mg of MPTP into the internal carotid artery of monkeys, which perfuses about 40 g of ipsilateral cerebrum, caused near complete depletion of striatal dopamine and major behavioral and motor abnormalities. Thus, the difference between rats and monkeys in their response to internal carotid MPTP injections is obvious. These experiments also provide crucial evidence that the resistance of Wistar rats to systemic MPTP toxicity is not simply due to failure of MPTP to reach the brain circulation because of sequestration and metabolism by peripheral organs but is indeed a reflection of true resistance to blood-borne MPTP. This, coupled with the selective degeneration of dopaminergic neurons when MPTP was infused directly into the rat substantia nigra (Sayre et al. 1986; Harik et al. 1987), strongly suggests that in the rat the blood-brain interface is a barrier to the entry of MPTP to the brain extracellular space where it can act on dopaminergic neurons.

If MPTP is taken up and retained by the rat brain but remains relatively ineffective in causing dopaminergic neurotoxicity, where is it going and how is it handled? The author and colleagues hypothesize that much of it is trapped within the brain endothelium. However, a high concentration of MPTP and MPP+ in rat brain endothelial cells may lead to their damage with consequent BBB dysfunction. In another study, Riachi and coworkers (1990) investigated in detail the effects on the BBB of MPTP given to rats via the internal carotid artery. They found that 5 hours, 1 day, or 1 week after the injection of MPTP into the internal carotid artery of Wistar rats there were no significant differences in the blood-to-brain transfer values for aminoisobutyric acid between the ipsilateral and contralateral cerebral hemispheres. Also, ultrastructural studies looking for evidence of BBB leakage of horseradish peroxidase after MPTP injections were unrewarding. These results indicate that rat brain endothelial cells are either insensitive to MPTP and its metabolites or that, if they are at all affected, such affection does not result in acute or chronic breaks in the integrity of the BBB. Thus, if MPTP and its metabolites are sequestered in rat brain endothelium, they must be within subcellular organelles and not available to brain endothelial mitochondria. It is also possible that polar metabolites of MPTP are being more efficiently dumped back into the circulation from rat brain endothelium. This would be consistent with the results of Johannessen and coworkers (1985), who showed higher levels of radioactivity in monkey brain than in rat brain at longer time intervals after [^{3}H]MPTP administration.

CONCLUSION

The major theme of this chapter is that brain endothelial cells are not simple "tiles" that line capillaries to prevent the extravasation of blood cells and large plasma proteins. The author and colleagues believe that brain capillary endothelial cells are highly sophisticated and complex and, in addition to their uniquely tight intercellular junctions that are credited with the "physical" attributes of the BBB, they have a variety of active enzyme systems that are capable of metabolizing lipid-soluble substances that can easily permeate the "physical" barrier. These enzymes, in addition to specialized subcellular organelles, can metabolize and sequester lipid-soluble toxins and prevent their entry into the brain. These enzyme systems constitute the basis of the *"biochemical" blood-brain barrier*, a concept first introduced by Bertler and colleagues in 1966.

REFERENCES

Arora, P.K.; Riachi, N.J.; Harik, S.I.; and Sayre, L.M. Chemical oxidation of 1-methyl-4-phenyl-1,2,3,6-tetrahydropyridine (MPTP) and its in vivo metabolism in rat brain and liver. *Biochem Biophys Res Commun* 152:1339-1347, 1988.

Bankiewicz, K.S.; Oldfield, E.H.; Chiueh, C.C.; Doppman, J.L.; Jacobowitz, D.M.; and Kopin, I.J. Hemiparkinsonism in monkeys after unilateral internal carotid artery infusion of 1-methyl-4-phenyl-1,2,3,6-tetrahydropyridine (MPTP). *Life Sci* 39:7-16, 1986.

Bertler, A.; Falck, B.; Owman, C.; and Rosengren, E. The localization of monoaminergic blood-brain barrier mechanisms. *Pharmacol Rev* 18:369-385, 1966.

Burns, R.S.; Chiueh, C.C.; Markey, S.P.; Ebert, M.H.; Jacobowitz, D.M.; and Kopin, I.J. A primate model of parkinsonism: Selective destruction of dopaminergic neurons in the pars compacta of the substantia nigra by

N-methyl-4-phenyl-1,2,3,6-tetrahydropyridine. *Proc Natl Acad Sci U S A* 80:4546-4550, 1983.

Cashman, J.R., and Ziegler, D.M. Contribution of N-oxidation to the metabolism of MPTP (1-methyl-4-phenyl-1,2,3,6-tetrahydro-pyridine) by various liver preparations. *Mol Pharmacol* 29:163-167, 1986.

D'Amato, R.J.; Lipman, Z.P.; and Snyder, S.H. Selectivity of the parkinsonian neurotoxin MPTP: Toxic metabolite MPP$^+$ binds to neuromelanin. *Science* 231:987-989, 1986.

Davis, G.C.; Williams, A.C.; Markey, S.P.; Ebert, M.H.; Caine, E.D.; Reichert, C.M.; and Kopin, I.J. Chronic parkinsonism secondary to intravenous injection of meperidine analogues. *Psychiatry Res* 1:249-254, 1979.

Elsworth, J.D.; Deutch, A.Y.; Redmond, D.E., Jr.; Sladek, J.R.; and Roth, R.H. Differential responsiveness to 1-methyl-4-phenyl-1,2,3,6-tetrahydropyridine toxicity in sub-regions of the primate substantia nigra and striatum. *Life Sci* 40:193-202, 1987.

Fuller, R.W., and Hemrick-Luecke, S.K. Depletion of norepinephrine in mouse heart by 1-methyl-4-phenyl-1,2,3,6-tetrahydropyridine (MPTP) mimicked by 1-methyl-4-phenyl-pyridinium (MPP$^+$) and not blocked by deprenyl. *Life Sci* 39:1645-1650, 1986.

Harik, S.I.; Riachi, N.J.; and LaManna, J.C. MPTP neurotoxicity and the "biochemical" blood-brain barrier. In: Hefti, F., and Weiner, W.J., eds. *Progress in Parkinson Research*. New York: Plenum, 1988. pp. 93-100.

Harik, S.I.; Schmidley, J.W.; Iacofano, L.A.; Blue, P.; Arora, P.K.; and Sayre, L.M. On the mechanisms underlying 1-methyl-4-phenyl-1,2,3,6-tetrahydropyridine neurotoxicity: The effect of perinigral infusion of 1-methyl-4-phenyl-1,2,3,6-tetrahydropyridine, its metabolite, and their analogues in the rat. *J Pharmacol Exp Ther* 242:669-676, 1987.

Heikkila, R.E.; Manzino, L.; Cabbat, F.S.; and Duvoisin, R.C. Protection against the dopaminergic neurotoxicity of 1-methyl-4-phenyl-1,2,5,6-tetrahydropyridine by monoamine oxidase inhibitors. *Nature* 311:467-469, 1984.

Javitch, J.A.; D'Amato, R.J.; Strittmatter, S.M.; and Snyder, S.H. Parkinsonism-inducing neurotoxin N-methyl-4-phenyl-1,2,3,6-tetrahydropyridine: Uptake of the metabolite N-methyl-4-phenylpyridine by dopamine neurons explains selective toxicity. *Proc Natl Acad Sci U S A* 82:2173-2177, 1985.

Johannessen, J.N.; Adams, J.D.; Schuller, H.M.; Bacon, J.P.; and Markey, S.P. 1-methyl-4-phenylpyridine (MPP$^+$) induces oxidative stress in the rodent. *Life Sci* 38:743-749, 1986.

Johannessen, J.N.; Chiueh, C.C.; Burns, R.S.; and Markey, S.P. Differences in the metabolism of MPTP in the rodent and primate. Parallel differences in sensitivity to its neurotoxic effect. *Life Sci* 36:219-224, 1985.

Kalaria, R.N., and Harik, S.I. Blood-brain barrier monoamine oxidase: Enzyme characterization in cerebral microvessels and other tissues from six mammalian species, including human. *J Neurochem* 49:856-864, 1987.

Kalaria, R.N.; Mitchell, M.J.; and Harik, S.I. Correlation of 1-methyl-4-phenyl-1,2,3,6-tetrahydropyridine neurotoxicity with blood-brain barrier monoamine oxidase activity. *Proc Natl Acad Sci U S A* 84:3521-3525, 1987.

Kalaria, R.N.; Mitchell, M.J.; and Harik, S.I. Monoamine oxidases of the human brain and liver. *Brain* 111:1441-1451, 1988.

Konradi, C.; Svoma, E.; Jellinger, K.; Riederer, P.; Denney, R.; and Thiebault, J. Topographic immunocytochemical mapping of monoamine oxidase-A, monoamine oxidase-B, and tyrosine-hydroxylase in human postmortem brain stem. *Neuroscience* 26:791-802, 1988.

Kopin, I.J., and Markey, S.P. MPTP toxicity: Implications for research in Parkinson's disease. *Annu Rev Neurosci* 11:81-96, 1988.

Langston, J.W., and Ballard, P.A. Parkinson's disease in a chemist working with 1-methyl-4-phenyl-1,2,3,6-tetrahydro-pyridine. *N Engl J Med* 309:10, 1983.

Langston, J.W.; Ballard, P.; Tetrud, J.W.; and Irwin, I. Chronic parkinsonism in humans due to a product of meperidine-analog synthesis. *Science* 219:979-980, 1983.

Langston, J.W.; Irwin, I.; Langston, E.B.; and Forno, L.S. Pargyline prevents MPTP-induced parkinsonism in primates. *Science* 225:1480-1482, 1984.

Levitt, P.; Pintar, J.E.; and Breakefield, X.O. Immunocyto-chemical demonstration of monoamine oxidase B in brain astrocytes and serotonergic neurons. *Proc Natl Acad Sci U S A* 79:6385-6389, 1982.

Mackay, A.V.P.; Davies, P.; Dewar, A.J.; and Yates, C.M. Regional distribution of enzymes associated with neurotransmission by monoamines, acetylcholine, and GABA in human brain. *J Neurochem* 30:827-839, 1978.

Markey, S.P.; Johannessen, J.N.; Chiueh, C.C.; Burns, R.S.; and Herkenham, M.A. Intraneuronal generation of a pyridinium metabolite may cause drug-induced parkinsonism. *Nature* 311:464-466, 1984.

Nicklas, W.J.; Vyas, I.; and Heikkila, R.E. Inhibition of NADH-linked oxidation in brain mitochondria by 1-methyl-4-phenyl-pyridine, a metabolite of the neurotoxin 1-methyl-4-phenyl-1,2,4,6-tetrahydropyridine. *Life Sci* 36:2503-2508, 1985.

Ramsay, R.R.; McKeown, K.A.; Johnson, E.A.; Booth, R.G.; and Singer, T.P. Inhibition of NADH oxidation by pyridine derivatives. *Biochem Biophys Res Commun* 146:53-60, 1987.

Ramsay, R.R.; Salach, J.I.; Dadgar, J.; and Singer, T.P. Inhibition of mitochondrial NADH dehydrogenase by pyridine derivatives and its possible relation to experimental and idiopathic parkinsonism. *Biochem Biophys Res Commun* 135:269-275, 1986.

Ramsay, R.R., and Singer, T.P. Energy-dependent uptake of N-methyl-4-phenyl-pyridinium, the neurotoxic metabolite of 1-methyl-4-phenyl-1,2,3,6-tetrahydropyridine, by mitochondria. *J Biol Chem* 262:7585-7587, 1986.

Riachi, N.J.; Behmand, R.A.; and Harik, S.I. Correlation of MPTP neurotoxicity in vivo with oxidation of MPTP by the brain and blood-brain barrier in vitro in five rat strains. *Brain Res* 555:19-24, 1991.

Riachi, N.J.; Dietrich, W.D.; and Harik, S.I. Effects of internal carotid administration of MPTP on rat brain and blood-brain barrier. *Brain Res* 533:6-14, 1990.

Riachi, N.J., and Harik, S.I. Strain differences in systemic 1-methyl-4-phenyl-1,2,3,6-tetrahydropyridine neurotoxicity in mice correlate best with monoamine oxidase activity at the blood-brain barrier. *Life Sci* 42:2359-2363, 1988.

Riachi, N.J., and Harik, S.I. Monoamine oxidase in the brain and cerebral microvessels of the Green African monkey. *Neurology* 40(Suppl 1):167, 1990.

Riachi, N.J.; Harik, S.I.; Kalaria, R.N.; and Sayre, L.M. On the mechanisms underlying 1-methyl-4-phenyl,1,2,3,6-tetrahydro-pyridine neurotoxicity. II. Susceptibility among mammalian species correlates with the toxin's metabolic patterns in brain microvessels and liver. *J Pharmacol Exp Ther* 244:443-448, 1988.

Riachi, N.J.; LaManna, J.C.; and Harik, S.I. Entry of 1-methyl-4-phenyl-1,2,3,6-tetrahydropyridine into the rat brain. *J Pharmacol Exp Ther* 249:744-748, 1989.

Ricaurte, G.A.; Langston, J.W.; DeLanney, L.W.; Irwin, I.; and Brooks, J.D. Dopamine uptake blockers protect against the dopamine-depleting effect of 1-methyl-4-phenyl-1,2,3,6-tetrahydropyridine (MPTP) in the mouse striatum. *Neurosci Lett* 59:259-264, 1985.

Sayre, L.M.; Arora, P.K.; Iacofano, L.A.; and Harik, S.I. Comparative toxicity of MPTP, MPP+, and 3,3-dimethyl-MPDP+ to dopaminergic neurons of the rat substantia nigra. *Eur J Pharmacol* 124:171-174, 1986.

Singer, T.P.; Castagnoli, N., Jr.; Ramsay, R.R.; and Trevor, A.J. Biochemical events in the development of parkinsonism induced by 1-methyl-4-phenyl-1,2,3,6-tetrahydropyridine. *Trends Biochem Sci* 12:266-270, 1987.

Snyder, S.H., and D'Amato, R.J. MPTP: A neurotoxin relevant to the pathophysiology of Parkinson's disease. *Neurology* 36:250-258, 1986.

Uhl, G.R.; Javitch, J.A.; and Snyder, S.H. Normal MPTP binding in parkinsonian substantia nigra: Evidence for extraneuronal toxin conversion in human brain. *Lancet* 1:956-957, 1985.

Weissman, J.; Trevor, A.; Chiba, K.; Peterson, L.A.; Caldera, P.; Castagnoli, N., Jr.; and Baillie, T. Metabolism of the nigrostriatal toxin 1-methyl-4-phenyl-1,2,3,6-tetrahydro-pyridine by liver homogenate fractions. *J Med Chem* 28:997-1001, 1985.

Westlund, K.N.; Denney, R.M.; Kochersperger, M.; Rose, R.M.; and Abell, C.W. Distinct monoamine oxidase A and B populations in primate brain. *Science* 230:181-183, 1985.

Zimmer, J., and Geneser, F.A. Difference in monoamine oxidase B activity between C57 black and albino NMRI mouse strains may explain differential effects of the neurotoxin MPTP. *Neurosci Lett* 78:253-258, 1987.

ACKNOWLEDGMENTS

The work described in this chapter was supported by U.S. Public Health Service grant HL-35617 and by the David S. Ingalls Fund.

AUTHOR

Sami I. Harik, M.D.
Professor
Departments of Neurology and Neuroscience
Case Western Reserve University
2074 Abington Road
Cleveland, OH 44106

An Overview of the Multiple Functions of the Blood-Brain Barrier

A. Lorris Betz

INTRODUCTION

The existence of a permeability barrier between the blood and the brain has been known for more than a century; however, during the past two decades there has been a tremendous expansion in knowledge of the multiple functions of the blood-brain barrier (BBB). Besides forming a permeability barrier that limits the movement of some solutes between blood and brain, the BBB is now seen as a metabolically active tissue that facilitates and controls the brain uptake of certain solutes while helping to maintain homeostasis within the central nervous system (CNS). Current studies are stimulated not only by an interest in understanding the normal physiology of the barrier and the role that it plays in disease processes, but also by a desire to be able to manipulate barrier permeability and thereby control the delivery of pharmaceuticals to the brain.

This chapter serves as an overview of the functions of the BBB. For a more detailed discussion, the interested reader is referred to the other chapters in this monograph and to other sources in the literature (Betz et al. 1989; Bradbury 1979; Fenstermacher 1984; Fishman 1980; Goldstein and Betz 1986; Oldendorf 1982; Pardridge 1983; Rapoport 1976; Spector and Johanson 1989).

THE BBB AS AN IMPERMEABLE WALL

German scientist Paul Ehrlich was the first to describe the existence of a permeability barrier between the blood and the brain (Ehrlich 1885). Following the injection of a vital dye such as trypan blue into the bloodstream, he observed that virtually all organs of the body stained blue except for the brain. Whereas Ehrlich believed that the dye did not stain the brain because the brain lacked the ability to bind the dye, his associate, Edwin Goldmann, later disproved this hypothesis by showing that trypan blue, when injected into the cerebrospinal fluid (CSF), did indeed stain the brain (Goldmann 1909). This experiment also demonstrated the presence of a brain-blood barrier as well as a BBB and, in addition, showed that there was no permeability barrier between CSF and brain.

Although several investigators later hypothesized that the blood vessels in the brain were the site of the BBB (Krogh 1946; Spatz 1933), this view was not widely held. However, in the 1960s Reese and Karnovsky (1967) and Brightman and Reese (1969) repeated the Ehrlich/Goldmann experiments at the ultrastructural level using electron microscopy to observe the distribution of the protein tracer horseradish peroxidase following intravenous or intrathecal administration. These experiments conclusively identified the brain capillary endothelial cell as the site of the BBB as well as the brain-blood barrier. Of primary importance in the formation of a permeability barrier by these cells is the presence of continuous tight junctions that seal together the margins of the endothelial cells (figure 1). Furthermore, in contrast to endothelial cells in many other organs, brain capillary endothelial cells contain no direct transendothelial passageways such as fenestrations or channels (Brightman and Kadota, this volume; Broadwell, this volume). Recent ultrastructural studies suggest that there may be an endocytotic process that is capable of moving protein tracers from the blood to the brain through the lysosomal and/or Golgi compartments of the brain capillary endothelial cell (Broadwell, this volume); however, the flux mediated by this pathway is substantially less than the transvascular permeability observed in most other vascular beds.

The brain capillary endothelial cell forms a barrier even to molecules that are much smaller than the protein tracers typically used in ultrastructural studies. For example, the electron-dense ion lanthanum has been shown by electron microscopy to be excluded by the tight junctions of the brain capillary endothelial cells (Dorovini-Zis et al. 1983). A multitude of radiotracer experiments using small molecules such as sucrose and mannitol also demonstrate highly restricted brain uptake (Fenstermacher, this volume). Finally, electrical measurements across the wall of blood vessels on the surface of the frog brain (Crone and Olesen 1982) or rat brain (Butt et al. 1990) demonstrate a very significant barrier to the movement of ions since the resistance of the vessel wall is at least 1,500 to 2,000 $\Omega \cdot cm^2$.

Although the vast majority of the brain's microvasculature is endowed with these special features that result in the formation of a BBB, there are specific localized areas of the brain, such as the circumventricular organs, that lack a BBB (Gross and Weindl 1987). These brain nuclei are involved in the hormonal regulation of other organ systems and therefore must be able to respond to changes in the concentration of peptides and other substances in the blood. The absence of a BBB in these regions is accompanied by differences in the ultrastructure of the endothelial cells, including open junctions and fenestrations

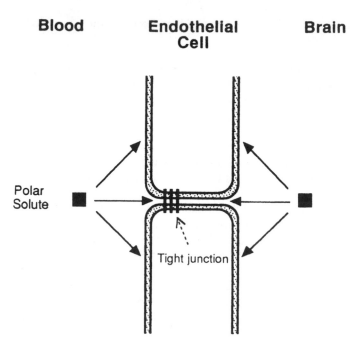

Blood   **Endothelial   Brain
                    Cell**

Polar
Solute

Tight junction

FIGURE 1.   *The BBB as an impermeable wall. The tight junctions and lipid
                  membrane of the brain capillary endothelial cell limit the diffusion
                  of polar solutes in both directions between the blood and the
                  brain.*

and increased distance between the endothelial cells and the surrounding
astrocytes (Laterra et al., this volume; Fenstermacher, this volume; Broadwell,
this volume). To help limit the brain uptake of substances through these leaky
brain regions, the ependymal cells that line the ventricular surface and normally
do not form a barrier are differentiated into barrier-forming cells in these
localized areas (Brightman et al. 1975). Although the signals that induce brain
capillary endothelial cells and special ependymal cells to form a barrier are not
known, recent studies point to the astrocyte as an important source for such an
inductive influence (Laterra et al., this volume).

THE BBB AS A SELECTIVE SIEVE

Clearly, the BBB cannot be absolute. The brain is dependent on the blood to
deliver metabolic substrates and remove metabolic wastes; therefore, the BBB
must facilitate the exchange of selected solutes. Lipid-soluble fuels and waste

products, such as O_2 and CO_2, readily cross the lipid bilayer membranes of the endothelial cell and, thus, encounter little difficulty in quickly exchanging between blood and brain (figure 2). Polar solutes such as glucose and amino acids, however, must depend on other mechanisms to facilitate their exchange. This is accomplished by the presence of specific, carrier-mediated transport proteins in the luminal and abluminal membranes of the brain capillary endothelial cell (figure 2).

The permeability of the BBB to lipid-soluble substances is not surprising in view of the large surface area of endothelial cell membrane (e.g., 100 cm^2/g brain in the rat [Bradbury 1979]) that separates the brain from the blood. In fact, the

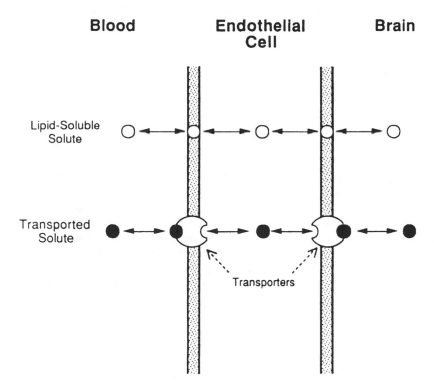

Blood   **Endothelial Cell**   **Brain**

FIGURE 2. *The BBB as a selective sieve. Lipid-soluble solutes can cross the BBB because they are able to penetrate the lipid bilayers of the endothelial cell. In addition, selected polar solutes can cross the BBB because specific, carrier-mediated transport systems are present in the endothelial cell membranes.*

relationship between the BBB permeability and the lipid solubility of a nontransported solute follows exactly the relationship predicted by studies with artificial lipid bilayers (Fenstermacher, this volume; Oldendorf, this volume). Thus, highly polar compounds such as mannitol penetrate the barrier very slowly, whereas lipid-soluble compounds such as butanol penetrate so rapidly that they are completely extracted from the blood by the brain during a single pass through the cerebral circulation. Uptake of very lipid-soluble compounds is so high that it is only limited by blood flow (Fenstermacher, this volume), and these substances are useful both clinically and experimentally for measuring the cerebral blood flow rate.

Seemingly small differences in lipid solubility can make a large difference in brain uptake. For example, the olive oil:water partition coefficient of heroin is only 10 times greater than that of morphine, yet the brain uptake of heroin is 30 times higher (Oldendorf 1982). This explains the greater speed with which heroin exerts its CNS effects compared with morphine, and it may contribute to its higher abuse potential (Oldendorf, this volume).

Although lipid-soluble compounds can enter the brain quite readily, most important metabolic substances are too polar to enter brain efficiently by simple diffusion. For these compounds, carrier-mediated transport systems are present to facilitate their brain uptake. The existence of carrier-mediated transport systems that operate across the BBB can be deduced on the basis of the selectivity that results from the binding of the solute to a recognition site on the carrier protein. Thus, carrier-mediated transport is saturable because the number of binding sites is limited; it is stereospecific because a specific structural arrangement of the solute is required for it to be recognized by the carrier; it can be competitively inhibited by structurally related compounds that compete for binding to the same carrier or noncompetitively by compounds that bind elsewhere on the carrier protein; and the rate of transport may be regulated by intracellular second messengers and/or by adding or removing carrier molecules from the membrane.

Because the brain uses glucose almost exclusively as a metabolic fuel, the BBB is richly endowed with glucose transporters, and this carrier system has been extensively studied (Betz et al. 1976; Lund-Andersen 1979; Pardridge 1983). The BBB glucose carrier recognizes D-glucose, D-galactose, D-mannose, and certain synthetic hexoses such as 2-deoxy-D-glucose and 3-O-methyl-D-glucose, but not L-glucose. Transport is half saturated at a plasma glucose concentration of 5 to 10 mM, which is within the normal physiologic range. BBB glucose transport is not energy dependent; therefore, it cannot move glucose against a concentration gradient. It is also symmetrical and transports glucose out of as well as into the brain. Thus, it is a facilitative-diffusion type of transporter that facilitates the equilibration of blood and brain glucose concentrations. In contrast to glucose transport in certain other cells, BBB glucose transport is not regulated by insulin. Recent studies of the quantity and distribution of glucose transporters in brain indicate a very rich endowment in brain capillary endothelial cells, consistent with their role in providing glucose for all the cells in the brain (Dick et al. 1984; Gerhart et al. 1989).

Another prominent transport system in the BBB enhances the brain uptake of large neutral amino acids, which are important precursors for neurotransmitter and protein synthesis. This carrier is similar to the L-system for amino acid transport described in other cells in that it has high affinity for large but not small neutral amino acids and is not sodium dependent (Betz and Goldstein 1978). In contrast to the glucose transporter for which glucose is the only naturally occurring substrate present in the blood at a significant concentration, the L-system amino acid carrier has affinity for at least 10 different amino acids that are present in the blood (Smith et al. 1987). Indeed, the carrier seems to be quite insensitive to the size of the hydrophobic side chain (Rapoport, this volume). The presence in blood of multiple substrates for the same carrier means that they compete with each other for transport into brain. Consequently, when the plasma concentration of one amino acid is increased, it can reduce the uptake of other amino acids, which may play a role in the neurologic damage that occurs in certain metabolic diseases such as phenylketonuria (Pardridge 1986).

It is now apparent that the BBB has many transport systems in addition to those for glucose and amino acids (table 1). Those with the greatest transport capacity were described first (metabolite transport systems), but as more sensitive techniques are developed to study BBB permeability, low-capacity transporters such as those for vitamins (Spector 1989), ions (see next section), and peptides (Zlokovic et al., this volume; Pardridge, this volume) have been detected. The peptide transport systems may involve a process of receptor-mediated endocytosis (Broadwell, this volume), a mechanism that is quite different from the carrier-mediated transport of small solutes.

THE BBB AS AN ACTIVE PUMP

Not all BBB transport systems operate equally well in both the blood-to-brain and brain-to-blood directions. For example, potassium is transported out of the brain by a saturable transport system that can be inhibited by ouabain (Bradbury and Stulcová 1970), whereas the flux of potassium from blood to brain is low (Hansen et al. 1977) and not inhibited by ouabain (Betz 1983). This asymmetrical transport of potassium is explained by the presence of the active

TABLE 1. *Transport systems that operate from blood to brain*

Transport System	Typical Substrate
Metabolites	
Hexose	Glucose
Large neutral amino acid	Phenylalanine
Basic amino acid	Lysine
Acidic amino acid	Glutamate
Monocarboxylic acid	Lactate
Amine	Choline
Purine	Adenine
Nucleoside	Adenosine
Saturated fatty acid	Octanoate
Micronutrients	
Thiamine	Thiamine
Pantothenic acid	Pantothenic acid
Biotin	Biotin
Vitamin B_6	Pyridoxal
Riboflavin	Riboflavin
Niacinamide	Niacinamide
Carnitine	Carnitine
Inositol	*Myo*-inositol
Electrolytes	
Sodium-chloride cotransport	Sodium chloride
Cation channel	Sodium, potassium
Heavy metal	Lead
Hormones	
Thyroid hormone	T_3
Vasopressin	Arginine vasopressin
Insulin	Insulin
Other Peptides	
Transferrin	Transferrin
Enkephalins	Leu-enkephalin

pump Na,K-ATPase on the abluminal but not the luminal side of the brain capillary endothelial cell (Betz et al. 1980). A similar asymmetry in the distribution of ion transporters is seen in fluid-transporting epithelial cells such as those in the choroid plexus. This cellular polarity forms the basis for their ability to actively secrete ions and water (Betz and Goldstein 1981). Other features that the brain capillary endothelium has in common with a typical epithelium (Betz 1985a; Crone 1986) include the presence of continuous tight junctions, a transcellular electrical resistance of approximately 2,000 Ω·cm^2 (Crone and Olesen 1982), a low hydraulic conductivity (Fenstermacher 1984), and a high mitochondrial content (Oldendorf et al. 1977), which is believed to be related to a high capacity for active transport. Since the brain capillary shares so many structural features in common with epithelia, it has been proposed that it functions like an epithelium as well (Betz 1985a; Crone 1986). If the BBB does indeed secrete fluid, this could be the explanation for the 10 to 30 percent of CSF that is produced from extrachoroidal sources (Milhorat et al. 1971), and it could account for the bulk flow of fluid through the brain's interstitial space (Szentistványi et al. 1984).

In addition to the presence of Na,K-ATPase on one side, fluid-secreting epithelial cells contain other sodium transporters on the opposite side that allow sodium to enter the cell (figure 3). Using intracarotid bolus injections to study single-pass sodium uptake, Betz (1983) observed two saturable sodium entry systems in the BBB. One is inhibited by furosemide, suggesting the presence of a Na-Cl cotransport system. The other is inhibited by amiloride, but its properties are not clearly identical to either the known amiloride-sensitive sodium channel or the Na/H exchanger. Specifically, Betz (1983) showed that the brain capillary sodium channel is highly sensitive to inhibition by amiloride as is the sodium channel in tight epithelia, but it is nonselective since amiloride also inhibits brain rubidium uptake. Recent studies confirm that brain sodium uptake can be inhibited by amiloride (Murphy and Johanson 1989) and that brain capillary endothelial cells contain an amiloride-sensitive cation channel that is permeable to both sodium and potassium (Vigne et al. 1989).

Active transport of ions across the brain capillary endothelium may play a role not only in fluid secretion but also in regulation of the potassium concentration of the brain's interstitial fluid (ISF). The potassium concentration of the CSF and ISF is held remarkably constant at approximately 3 mM despite acute or chronic changes in plasma potassium between 1.6 and 7 mM (Bradbury and Stulcová 1970; Jones and Keep 1987). The low permeability of the BBB to potassium in the blood-to-brain direction contributes to this potassium homeostasis (Hansen et al. 1977). However, potassium efflux (Bradbury and Stulcová 1970), mediated by Na,K-ATPase located on the abluminal side of the brain capillary endothelial cell (Betz 1986; Betz et al. 1980) and the apical side

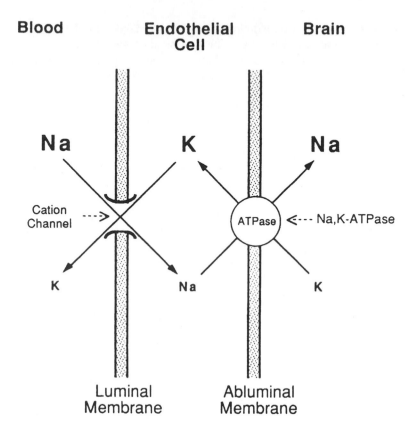

Blood   **Endothelial**   **Brain**
Cell

Na   **K**   **Na**

Cation Channel --->   ATPase <--- Na,K-ATPase

K   Na   K

Luminal   Abluminal
Membrane   Membrane

FIGURE 3. *The BBB as an active pump. Not all transport systems are evenly distributed between the luminal and abluminal membranes of the brain capillary endothelial cell. An asymmetric distribution of ion transporters and channels could provide the basis by which the BBB secretes fluid and helps maintain potassium homeostasis in brain.*

of the choroid plexus epithelial cell (Ernst et al. 1986), also plays a major role. Given that the total influx of potassium across the BBB is 10 times greater than across the blood-CSF barrier, the brain capillary is probably more important than the choroid plexus in brain potassium homeostasis (Bradbury 1979).

Astrocytic glial cells also are believed to play an important role in maintaining potassium homeostasis in brain (Bradbury 1979; Kimelberg and Norenberg 1989). This specialized glial cell has a large potassium conductance in its end-feet that allows it to quickly take up potassium from the surrounding fluid (Newman 1986). Localized uptake in an area where potassium is high is accompanied by the dumping of potassium in another area where its concentration is low. This type of spatial buffering of potassium is believed to be important for the second-to-second regulation of localized ISF potassium concentration (Kimelberg and Norenberg 1989), but it cannot by itself account for long-term global regulation of ISF potassium. For this, the brain capillary endothelial cell probably plays the primary role. One reason the brain capillary endothelial cell is so closely invested with glial foot processes may be to permit astrocytes and endothelial cells to work together to maintain potassium homeostasis.

The presence of other asymmetrically distributed transporters in the brain capillary endothelial cell (table 2) can be deduced by differences in transport rates in the blood-to-brain and brain-to-blood directions as explained above. Another approach is to study uptake by isolated brain capillaries in vitro. Since these structures have their abluminal membranes exposed to the incubation medium, transporters that are present on this side of the cell can be studied easily. Thus, those substances that are taken up by isolated capillaries, but that do not appreciably enter the brain from the blood, probably have transporters on the abluminal but not the luminal membrane of the endothelial cell. This approach has been used to demonstrate an asymmetry of A-system (Betz and Goldstein 1978) and ASC-system (Tayarani et al. 1987a) transporters for small neutral amino acids as well as transporters for taurine (Tayarani and Lefauconnier 1989) and monoamines (Hardebo and Owman 1980a). However, one must be aware that the isolated brain capillaries contain other cells, such as pericytes, that also might be transport sites.

TABLE 2. *Asymmetrically distributed BBB transport systems*

Transport System	Typical Substrate	Probable Location
Na,K-ATPase	Potassium	Abluminal
Sodium-chloride cotransport	Sodium chloride	Luminal
Cation channel	Sodium, potassium	Luminal
Sodium-hydrogen exchanger	Sodium, hydrogen	Abluminal
A-system for neutral amino acids	Glycine	Abluminal
ASC-system for neutral amino acids	Cysteine	Abluminal
β–amino acid	Taurine	Abluminal
Monoamine	Dopamine	Abluminal
Organic anion	p-Aminohippurate	Abluminal
Inorganic anion	Iodide	Abluminal
Prostaglandin	$PGF_{2\alpha}$	Abluminal

Finally, the presence of active transport out of the brain can be deduced by using transport inhibitors. When a substance is present under steady-state conditions at a lower concentration in the brain's ISF than in blood and a transport inhibitor increases the brain concentration, then the presence of an active efflux system can be deduced (Davson 1976). This approach has been used to demonstrate active BBB efflux systems for iodide (Davson and Hollingsworth 1973), prostaglandins (Bito et al. 1976), and organic acids such as p-aminohippurate (S.R. Ennis and A.L. Betz, unpublished results) and acid neurotransmitter metabolites (Aizenstein and Korf 1979).

THE BBB AS A METABOLIC BARRIER

The foregoing discussion emphasizes that the BBB is formed by a cell layer with different properties of the membranes on either side. These cells also have an intracellular cytoplasm and organelles containing specific enzymes that play an important role in BBB function (figure 4). One of the first demonstrations of the enzymatic BBB was made by Bertler and colleagues (1966), who observed intraendothelial histofluorescence of dopamine after intravascular administration of its precursor, L-3,4-dihydroxyphenylalanine (L-dopa). In later studies, they found that rat brain capillary endothelial cells were richly endowed in enzymes involved with neurotransmitter synthesis (e.g., aromatic amino acid decarboxylase) and degradation (e.g., monoamine oxidase [MAO]) (Hardebo and Owman 1980b). Since neurotransmitter precursors such as L-dopa can enter the endothelial cell from the blood via the L-system for large neutral amino acid transport, the subsequent intraendothelial metabolism provides an effective mechanism for preventing neurotransmitters from moving beyond the endothelial cell and into the brain. Neurotransmitter-degrading enzymes present in the endothelial cells also may play a role in inactivating neurotransmitters released during neuronal activity since, as discussed previously, transport systems for uptake of catecholamines by the endothelial cell appear to be present on the abluminal membrane.

Brain capillary endothelial cells contain many enzymes in addition to those involved with neurotransmitter metabolism (Mrsulja and Djuricic 1981). Besides the enzymes involved in energy metabolism (Mrsulja and Djuricic 1981), these cells also contain acid hydrolases typically found in lysosomes (Baranczyk-Kuzma et al. 1989) and aminopeptidase (Baranczyk-Kuzma and Audus 1987). Similar to other endothelial cells, they contain angiotensin-converting enzyme (Gimbrone et al. 1979), xanthine oxidase (Betz 1985b), and enzymes that protect cells from peroxidative damage such as superoxide dismutase, catalase, and glutathione peroxidase (Tayarani et al. 1987b).

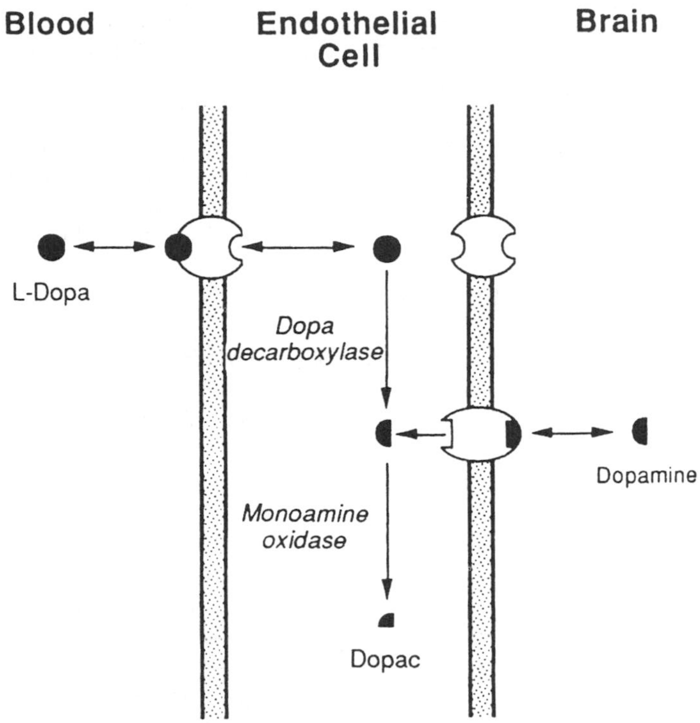

FIGURE 4. *The BBB as a metabolic barrier. Some molecules that enter the brain capillary endothelial cell are rapidly metabolized. This process not only helps control the brain uptake of potentially harmful chemicals present in the blood but also assists the brain in eliminating unwanted waste products. For example, the neurotransmitter precursor L-dopa enters the endothelial cell on the L-system amino acid transporter. It is then converted to dopamine by the enzyme dopa decarboxylase present in the endothelial cell. Dopamine is further degraded to 3,4-dihydroxyphenylacetic acid (dopac) by the enzyme monoamine oxidase. Dopamine also may be taken up from the brain and metabolized as a means of eliminating the neurotransmitter from the brain's ISF.*

MAO present in brain capillaries may serve to provide protection of the brain from circulating toxins (Harik, this volume; Takakura et al., this volume). Indeed, brain capillary endothelial cells are well equipped to handle circulating drugs and toxins since they contain drug-metabolizing enzyme systems such as cytochrome P-450-linked monooxygenases, epoxide hydrolase, NADPH:cytochrome P-450 reductase, and 1-napthol UDP-glucuronosyl transferase, which are typically found in the liver (Ghersi-Egea et al. 1988); they also contain a multidrug transport protein, P170 (Thiebaut et al. 1989).

REGULATION OF BBB FUNCTION

The availability of isolated brain capillaries as a model system for studying properties of the BBB has led to the discovery that brain capillary endothelial cells contain many neurotransmitter- and hormone-binding sites, as listed below.

β-Adrenergic	Insulin
α-Adrenergic	Transferrin
Dopamine	Vasoactive intestinal peptide
Histamine	Parathyroid hormone
Adenosine	Atrial natriuretic peptide
Muscarinic cholinergic	Vasopressin
Prostaglandin	Angiotensin II
Leukotriene C_4	Bradykinin

These receptors have been detected either by directly studying binding of radiolabeled ligands to the isolated capillaries or by observing changes in intracellular second messengers following exposure to agonists (figure 5). Beyond the changes in second messengers, however, little is known about the effects of hormones or neurotransmitters on endothelial cell function. The β-adrenergic receptors appear to be in some way involved with regulation of ion transport since ablation of adrenergic input to the cerebral microvasculature by lesioning the locus ceruleus leads to up-regulation of β-adrenergic receptors on the endothelial cells (Kalaria et al. 1989) and a down-regulation of their Na,K-ATPase activity (Harik 1986). Atrial natriuretic peptide (ANP) receptors also may play a role in ion transport regulation because ANP inhibits the amiloride-sensitive cation channel (Dóczi et al. 1990; Ibaragi et al. 1989). In vivo experiments have shown that corticosteroids reduce the passive permeability of the BBB (Betz and Coester 1990; Ziylan et al. 1988), and in vitro experiments suggest that cAMP, cGMP, and adenosine also may be involved in regulating barrier permeability (Horner et al., this volume). Finally, some receptors (e.g., those for insulin, transferrin, and vasopressin) may play a role in receptor-mediated transcytosis (Pardridge, this volume; Zlokovic et al., this volume) rather than regulating endothelial cell function.

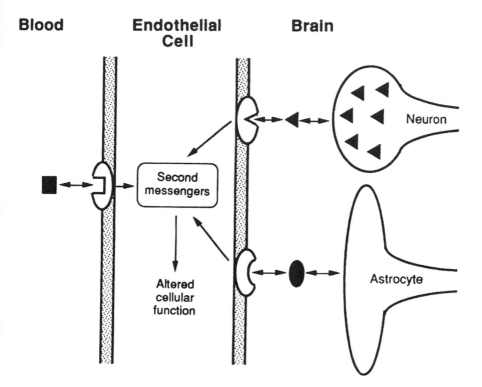

Blood **Endothelial Cell** **Brain**

Second messengers

Altered cellular function

Neuron

Astrocyte

FIGURE 5. *Regulation of BBB function. The brain capillary endothelial cell contains receptors for many hormones and neurotransmitters, substances that regulate BBB function through the production of various second messengers. Neurons and glia are probable sources for some of these regulatory factors, and others may be present in the blood.*

The endothelial cells also must contain other, as yet unidentified, receptors that allow them to respond to modulators present in brain and probably released by the astrocytes. As discussed elsewhere in this volume (Laterra et al., this volume; Horner et al., this volume), glial cells may be an important source of such signals since astrocytes or astrocyte-conditioned medium induce morphological and functional changes in brain capillary endothelial cells in tissue culture.

SUMMARY

The BBB formed by brain capillary endothelial cells is now recognized as more than an impermeable wall. It has specific transport systems that facilitate the uptake of important nutrients and hormones and active pumps that help to regulate the concentrations of ions and metabolites in the brain's ISF. Enzymes present in the endothelial cell metabolize neurotransmitters, drugs, and toxins before they can enter the brain and disrupt its function. Many of these properties are likely to be under regulation either by neurotransmitters and hormones released in the brain or by those present in the systemic circulation. As a result of this constellation of diverse functions, the brain capillary endothelial cell is able to efficiently supply the brain with the metabolites that it requires while contributing to the maintenance of the brain's ionic homeostasis and protecting it from circulating toxins.

REFERENCES

Aizenstein, M.L., and Korf, J. On the elimination of centrally formed 5-hydroxyindoleacetic acid by cerebrospinal fluid and urine. *J Neurochem* 32:1227-1233, 1979.

Baranczyk-Kuzma, A., and Audus, K.L. Characteristics of aminopeptidase activity from bovine brain microvessel endothelium. *J Cereb Blood Flow Metab* 7:801-805, 1987.

Baranczyk-Kuzma, A.; Raub, T.J.; and Audus, K.L. Demonstration of acid hydrolase acitivity in primary cultures of bovine brain microvessel endothelium. *J Cereb Blood Flow Metab* 9:280-289, 1989.

Bertler, A.; Falck, B.; Owman, C.; and Rosengern, E. The localization of mono-aminergic blood-barrier mechanisms. *Pharmacol Rev* 18:369-385, 1966.

Betz, A.L. Sodium transport from blood to brain: Inhibition by furosemide and amiloride. *J Neurochem* 41:1158-1164, 1983.

Betz, A.L. Epithelial properties of brain capillary endothelium. *Fed Proc* 44:2614-2615, 1985a.

Betz, A.L. Identification of hypoxanthine transport and xanthine oxidase activity in brain capillaries. *J Neurochem* 44:574-579, 1985b.

Betz, A.L. Transport of ions across the blood-brain barrier. *Fed Proc* 45:2050-2054, 1986.

Betz, A.L., and Coester, H.C. Effect of steroids on edema and sodium uptake of the brain during focal ischemia in rats. *Stroke* 21:1199-1204, 1990.

Betz, A.L.; Firth, J.A.; and Goldstein, G.W. Polarity of the blood-brain barrier: Distribution of enzymes between the luminal and antiluminal membranes of brain capillary endothelial cells. *Brain Res* 192:17-28, 1980.

Betz, A.L.; Gilboe, D.D.; and Drewes, L.R. The characteristics of glucose transport across the blood-brain barrier and its relation to glucose metabolism. In: Levi, G.; Battistin, L.; and Lajtha, A., eds. *Advances in Experimental Medicine and Biology.* New York: Plenum, 1976. pp. 133-149.

Betz, A.L., and Goldstein, G.W. Polarity of the blood-brain barrier: Neutral amino acid transport into isolated brain capillaries. *Science* 202:225-227, 1978.

Betz, A.L., and Goldstein, G.W. The basis for active transport at the blood-brain barrier. In: Eisenberg, H.M., and Suddith, R.L., eds. *Advances in Experimental Medicine and Biology.* New York: Plenum, 1981. pp. 5-16.

Betz, A.L.; Goldstein, G.W.; and Katzman, R. Blood-brain-cerebrospinal fluid barriers. In: Siegel, G.J.; Agranoff, B.; Albers, R.W.; and Molinoff, P., eds. *Basic Neurochemistry.* New York: Raven Press, 1989. pp. 591-606.

Bito, L.Z.; Davson, H.; and Hollingsworth, J. Facilitated transport of prostaglandins across the blood-cerebrospinal fluid and blood-brain barriers. *J Physiol* 256:273-285, 1976.

Bradbury, M. *The Concept of a Blood-Brain Barrier.* New York: Wiley, 1979.

Bradbury, M.W.B., and Stulcová, B. Efflux mechanism contributing to the stability of the potassium concentration in cerebrospinal fluid. *J Physiol* 208:415-430, 1970.

Brightman, M.W.; Prescott, L.; and Reese, T.S. Intercellular junctions of special ependyma. In: Knigge, K.M.; Scott, D.E.; Kobayashi, H.; and Ishii, S., eds. *Brain-Endocrine Interaction II.* Basel, Switzerland: Karger, 1975. pp. 146-165.

Brightman, M.W., and Reese, T.S. Junctions between intimately apposed cell membranes in the vertebrate brain. *J Cell Biol* 40:648-677, 1969.

Butt, A.M.; Jones, H.C.; and Abbott, N.J. Electrical resistance across the blood-brain barrier in anaesthetised rats: A developmental study. *J Physiol* 429:46-62, 1990.

Crone, C. The blood-brain barrier as a tight epithelium: Where is information lacking? *Ann N Y Acad Sci* 481:174-185, 1986.

Crone, C., and Olesen, S.P. Electrical resistance of brain microvascular endothelium. *Brain Res* 241:49-55, 1982.

Davson, H. The blood-brain barrier. *J Physiol* 255:1-28, 1976.

Davson, H., and Hollingsworth, J.R. Active transport of ^{131}I across the blood-brain barrier. *J Physiol* 233:327-347, 1973.

Dick, A.P.K.; Harik, S.I.; Klip, A.; and Walker, D.M. Identification and characterization of the glucose transporter of the blood-brain barrier by cytochalasin B binding and immunological reactivity. *Proc Natl Acad Sci U S A* 81:7233-7237, 1984.

Dóczi, T.; Joó, F.; and Bodosi, M. Central neuroendocrine control of the brain water, electrolyte, and volume homeostasis. *Acta Neurochir Suppl* 47:122-126, 1990.

Dorovini-Zis, K.; Sato, M.; Goping, G.; Rapoport, S.; and Brightman, M. Ionic lanthanum passage across cerebral endothelium exposed to hyperosmotic arabinose. *Acta Neuropathol* 60:49-60, 1983.

Ehrlich, P. *Das Sauerstoff-Bedurfnis des Organismus. Eine Farbenanalytische Studie.* Berlin: Hirschwald, 1885.

Ernst, S.A.; Palacios, J.R.; and Siegel, G.J. Immunocytochemical localization of Na^+,K^+-ATPase catalytic polypeptide in mouse choroid plexus. *J Histochem Cytochem* 34:189-195, 1986.

Fenstermacher, J.D. Volume regulation of the central nervous system. In: Staub, N.C., and Taylor, A.E., eds. *Edema.* New York: Raven Press, 1984. pp. 383-404.

Fishman, R.A. *Cerebrospinal Fluid in Diseases of the Nervous System.* Philadelphia: W.B. Saunders, 1980.

Gerhart, D.Z.; LeVasseur, R.J.; Broderius, M.A.; and Drewes, L.R. Glucose transporter localization in brain using light and electron immunocytochemistry. *J Neurosci Res* 22:464-472, 1989.

Ghersi-Egea, J.F.; Minn, A.; and Siest, G. A new aspect of the protective functions of the blood-brain barrier: Activities of four drug-metabolizing enzymes in isolated rat brain microvessels. *Life Sci* 42:2515-2523, 1988.

Gimbrone, M.A., Jr.; Majeau, G.R.; Atkinson, W.J.; Sadler, W.; and Cruise, S.A. Angiotensin-converting enzyme activity in isolated brain microvessels. *Life Sci* 25:1075-1084, 1979.

Goldmann, E. Die äussere und innere Sekretion des gesunden und kranken Organismus im Lichte der "vitalen Färbung." *Beitr Klin Chirurg* 64:192-265, 1909.

Goldstein, G.W., and Betz, A.L. The blood-brain barrier. *Sci Am* 254:74-83, 1986.

Gross, P.M., and Weindl, A. Peering through the windows of the brain. *J Cereb Blood Flow Metab* 7:663-672, 1987.

Hansen, A.J.; Lund-Andersen, H.; and Crone, C. K^+-permeability of the blood-brain barrier, investigated by aid of a K^+-sensitive microelectrode. *Acta Physiol Scand* 101:438-445, 1977.

Hardebo, J.E., and Owman, C. Barrier mechanisms for neurotransmitter monoamines and their precursors at the blood-brain interface. *Ann Neurol* 8:1-11, 1980b.

Hardebo, J.E., and Owman, C.H. Characterization of the in vitro uptake of monoamines into brain microvessels. *Acta Physiol Scand* 108:223-229, 1980a.

Harik, S.I. Blood-brain barrier sodium/potassium pump: Modulation by central noradrenergic innervation. *Proc Natl Acad Sci U S A* 83:4067-4070, 1986.

Ibaragi, M.-A.; Niwa, M.; and Ozaki, M. Atrial natriuretic peptide modulates amiloride-sensitive Na^+ transport across the blood-brain barrier. *J Neurochem* 53:1802-1806, 1989.

Jones, H.C., and Keep, R.C. The control of potassium concentration in the cerebrospinal fluid and brain interstitial fluid of developing rats. *J Physiol* 383:441-453, 1987.

Kalaria, R.N.; Stockmeier, C.A.; and Harik, S.I. Brain microvessels are innervated by locus ceruleus noradrenergic neurons. *Neurosci Lett* 97:203-208, 1989.

Kimelberg, H.K., and Norenberg, M.D. Astrocytes. *Sci Am* 260:66-76, 1989.

Krogh, A. The active and passive exchanges of inorganic ions through the surfaces of living cells and through membranes generally. *Proc R Soc Land [Biol]* 133:140-200, 1946.

Lund-Andersen, H. Transport of glucose from blood to brain. *Physiol Rev* 59:305-352, 1979.

Milhorat, T.H.; Hammock, M.K.; Rall, D.P.; and Levin, V.A. Cerebrospinal fluid production by the choroid plexus and brain. *Science* 173:330-332, 1971.

Mrsulja, B.B., and Djuricic, B.M. Biochemical characteristics of cerebral capillaries. In: Eisenberg, H.M., and Suddith, R.L., eds. *Advances in Experimental Medicine and Biology.* New York: Plenum, 1981. pp. 29-43.

Murphy, V.A., and Johanson, C.E. Acidosis, acetazolamide, and amiloride: Effects on ^{22}Na transfer across the blood-brain and blood-CSF barriers. *J Neurochem* 52:1058-1063, 1989.

Newman, E.A. High-potassium conductance in astrocyte endfeet. *Science* 233:453-454, 1986.

Oldendorf, W.H. Some clinical aspects of the blood-brain barrier. *Hosp Prac* 17:143-164, 1982.

Oldendorf, W.H.; Cornford, M.E.; and Brown, W.J. The large apparent work capacity of the blood-brain barrier: A study of the mitochondrial content of capillary endothelial cells in brain and other tissues of the rat. *Ann Neurol* 1:409-417, 1977.

Pardridge, W.M. Brain metabolism: A perspective from the blood-brain barrier. *Physiol Rev* 63:1481-1535, 1983.

Pardridge, W.M. Potential effects of the dipeptide sweetener aspartame on the brain. In: Wurtman, R.J., and Wurtman, J.J., eds. *Nutrition and the Brain.* New York: Raven Press, 1986. pp. 199-241.

Rapoport, S.I. *Blood-Brain Barrier in Physiology and Medicine.* New York: Raven Press, 1976.

Reese, T.S., and Karnovsky, M.J. Fine structural localization of a blood-brain barrier to exogenous peroxidase. *J Cell Biol* 34:207-217, 1967.

Smith, Q.R.; Momma, S.; Aoyagi, M.; and Rapoport, S.I. Kinetics of neutral amino acid transport across the blood-brain barrier. *J Neurochem* 49:1651-1658, 1987.

Spatz, H. Die Bedeutung der vitalen Färbung für die Lehre vom Stoffaustausch zwischen dem Zentralnervensystem und dem übrigen Körper. *Arch Psychiatrie* 101:267-358, 1933.

Spector, R. Micronutrient homeostasis in mammalian brain and cerebrospinal fluid. *J Neurochem* 53:1667-1674, 1989.

Spector, R., and Johanson, C.E. The mammalian choroid plexus. *Sci Am* 261:68-74, 1989.

Szentistványi, I.; Patlak, C.S.; Ellis, R.A.; and Cserr, H.F. Drainage of interstitial fluid from different regions of rat brain. *Am J Physiol* 246:F835-F844, 1984.

Tayarani, I.; Chaudiere, J.; Lefauconnier, J.-M.; and Bourre, J.-M. Enzymatic protection against peroxidative damage in isolated brain capillaries. *J Neurochem* 48:1399-1402, 1987b.

Tayarani, I., and Lefauconnier, J.-M. Sodium-dependent high-affinity uptake of taurine by isolated rat brain capillaries. *Biochim Biophys Acta* 985:168-172, 1989.

Tayarani, I.; Lefauconnier, J.-M.; Roux, F.; and Bourre, J.-M. Evidence for analanine, serine, and cysteine system of transport in isolated brain capillaries. *J Cereb Blood Flow Metab* 7:585-591, 1987a.

Thiebaut, F.; Tsuruo, T.; Hamada, H.; Gottesman, M.M.; Pastan, I.; and Willingham, M.C. Immunohistochemical localization in normal tissues of different epitopes in the multidrug transport protein P170: Evidence for localization in brain capillaries and crossreactivity of one antibody with a muscle protein. *J Histochem Cytochem* 37:159-164, 1989.

Vigne, P.; Champigny, G.; Marsault, R.; Barbry, P.; Frelin, C.; and Lazdunski, M. A new type of amiloride-sensitive cationic channel in endothelial cells of brain microvessels. *J Biol Chem* 264:7663-7668, 1989.

Ziylan, Y.Z.; Lefauconnier, J.M.; Bernard, G.; and Bourre, J.M. Effect of dexamethasone on transport of α-aminoisobutyric acid and sucrose across the blood-brain barrier. *J Neurochem* 51:1338-1342, 1988.

ACKNOWLEDGMENT

This work was supported in part by National Institutes of Health grant NS-23870.

AUTHOR

A. Lorris Betz, M.D., Ph.D.
Professor
Departments of Pediatrics, Surgery (Neurosurgery), and Neurology
University of Michigan
D3227 Medical Professional Building
Ann Arbor, MI 48109-0718

Formation and Differentiation of Brain Capillaries

John Laterra, Johannes E.A. Wolff, Christopher Guerin, and Gary W. Goldstein

INTRODUCTION

The blood-brain barrier (BBB), by regulating the exchange of substances from blood to brain, maintains an interstitial microenvironment optimal for neuronal function (Goldstein and Betz 1986a). Barrier function and dysfunction have important implications for brain physiology, pathophysiology, and therapy (Goldstein and Betz 1986b). An intact barrier may exclude potentially beneficial therapeutic agents. Barrier dysfunction associated with tumors, inflammation, trauma, and certain toxins may result in considerable morbidity from vasogenic brain edema and alterations in neuronal environments.

The BBB was first described by Paul Ehrlich (1885), who observed that certain vital dyes injected intravenously were specifically excluded from brain parenchyma. Detailed anatomic studies have since localized the BBB to capillary endothelial cells (Brightman and Reese 1969; Reese and Karnovsky 1967). These specialized endothelial cell functions appear gradually during development with the morphogenesis of leaky vessels to complete barrier expression in mature vessels. Recent studies described in this chapter indicate that both brain microvessel morphogenesis and barrier expression may be regulated by astrocytic cells. This chapter reviews evidence from the authors' laboratory and several other laboratories supporting this view. The hypothesis is presented that the earliest steps in brain capillary morphogenesis and the subsequent development of BBB properties are influenced by two distinct astrocytic "signals." The authors believe the predominant signal is dependent on the degree of astrocyte differentiation or activation.

BARRIER DEVELOPMENT IN VIVO

The brain is vascularized by sprouting vessels from the superficial perineural vascular plexus (Bar and Wolff 1972), which is primarily sinusoidal and lined by a fenestrated endothelium characteristic of nonbarrier vessels. In contrast, the

73

vascular sprouts penetrating brain parenchyma are composed of nonfenestrated endothelial cells. With continued development, a mature capillary-astrocytic complex is ultimately generated, consisting of endothelia, pericytes, and basement membrane ensheathed by astrocytic foot processes. Endothelial cells within this complex develop an array of barrier-specific properties, including a continuous network of complex tight junctions, specific glucose and amino acid transport systems, reduced vesicular density, and increased mitochondrial density (Goldstein and Betz 1986a; Betz, this volume). The most significant feature that distinguishes these from peripheral capillaries is their intimate association with perivascular astrocytes, and the expression of barrier coincides temporally with astrocytic ensheathement (Evans et al. 1974; Stewart and Hayakawa 1987). Thus, the phenotypic specialization of the brain capillary endothelium appears to be dependent on its unique relationship with the surrounding brain parenchyma or, more specifically, with the ensheathing perivascular astrocytes.

Svendgaard and colleagues (1975) were the first to ask experimentally if barrier characteristics of newly formed vessels are determined by inductive properties of the perivascular tissue. They assessed the development of barrier in vessels investing either iris tissue transplanted to caudal diencephalon or brain stem transplanted to the anterior chamber of the eye in rats. Vessels within central nervous system (CNS) tissue transplanted to eye expressed dopa-decarboxylase activity and limited the diffusion of 6-hydroxy-dopamine, two barrier properties. In contrast, vessels within iris transplanted to CNS lacked both properties. It was concluded that CNS parenchyma induces endothelial cells to express BBB features, although the researchers could not be sure that the vessels found within the transplants were host derived. These findings were confirmed by the classic chimeric transplant studies of Stewart and Wiley (1981), which demonstrated that vessels formed in similar transplants were, in fact, host derived. More recently, Risau and colleagues (1986) demonstrated that implantation of embryonic mouse brain onto the chick chorioallantoic membrane induces a barrier-specific, 74-kilodalton endothelial antigen. This experiment showed that the brain-derived signals inducing endothelial expression of barrier are conserved between species.

The CNS-derived tissues used in the transplant experiments described above contained neurons, oligodendroglia, and astrocytes. Of these cellular components, astrocytes are the most likely candidate for inducing the BBB due to their intimate association with brain microvessels. Direct experimental evidence for this hypothesis has been provided by Janzer and Raff (1987). They showed that microvessels from rabbit iris or chick chorioallantoic membrane form a barrier to the diffusion of vital dye after growing into an

74

aggregate of rat brain astrocytes. Controls using meningeal fibroblasts instead of astrocytes lacked barrier. Guerin and colleagues (1990) recently obtained evidence from human pathological specimens that extends the relevance of these findings to humans. They compared vascular permeability and endothelial expression of the brain-type glucose transporter in a series of human brain tumors using contrast-enhanced imaging and immunohistochemistry. Despite the absence of normal neuronal elements, vessels deep within both low-grade and anaplastic astrocytomas frequently stained with glucose transporter antibodies (figure 1). The expression of this barrier property diminished with increasing tumor grade. Interestingly, vessels in six of nine anaplastic astrocytomas were highly permeable but continued to express glucose transporter (figure 2). The independent expression of these two barrier properties suggests that distinct mechanisms may be responsible for their induction or maintenance.

BARRIER DEVELOPMENT IN VITRO

The expression of BBB properties by microvascular endothelial cells isolated from the CNS have been examined in several in vitro culture systems. Early investigations from the authors' laboratory established that bovine brain and retinal microvascular endothelial cells can be reliably cultured and used as a model for study of the BBB. Using freeze fracture analysis, Goldstein and colleagues (1984) demonstrated that monolayer endothelial cultures develop tight junctions (figure 3) that exclude the diffusion of intermediate-size molecules such as albumin and HRP and partially exclude smaller molecules such as monosaccharides (Bowman et al. 1983). Similar to their effects in vivo, hyperosmotic agents reversibly opened the tight junctions in vitro (Dorovini-Zis et al. 1987). Despite these findings, cultured endothelial cells were found to rapidly cease expressing several other BBB properties such as γ-glutamyl-transpeptidase and barrier function to small polar molecules and ions. Although various technical reasons might have been responsible for these deficiencies, this also may signify that an appropriate inductive environment is required for the expression of this specialized endothelial phenotype.

DeBault and Cancilla (1980) examined the presence of the barrier marker γ-glutamyl-transpeptidase in a brain-derived endothelial cell line (ME-2), cultured in the presence or absence of C_6 glioma cells. ME-2 cells lack this enzyme when cultured alone but were found to develop histochemical evidence of the enzyme after 72 to 96 hours in coculture with C_6 cells. The frequently cited conclusion that C_6 astroglial cells induce the expression of γ-glutamyl-transpeptidase in endothelial cells is complicated by the fact that cultured C_6 cells constitutively express high levels of γ-glutamyl-transpeptidase and

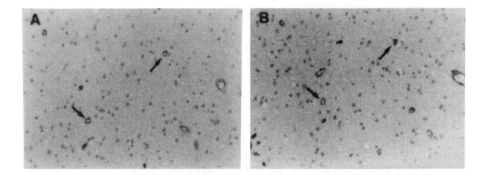

FIGURE 1.   *Low-grade human astrocytoma stained with (A) the endothelial vascular marker Ulex europis lectin I and (B) rabbit antihuman glucose transporter type I. Positive staining is evidenced by the horseradish peroxidase (HRP) reaction product that appears black. All vessels react positively with antiglucose transporter antibody.*

SOURCE: Guerin et al. 1990, copyright 1990, *Annals of Neurology*

messenger RNA (unpublished observations from the authors' laboratory). The possibility that endothelial-glial contact results in transfer of enzyme to endothelial cells rather than induction was not addressed. Shivers and coworkers (1988) qualitatively described the induction of interendothelial tight junctions by astrocyte-conditioned media. Using quantitative freeze fracture analysis of cultured cells, Tao-Cheng and coworkers (1987) demonstrated that astrocytes, but not fibroblasts, markedly enhanced the number and complexity of interendothelial tight junctions. In contrast to the findings of Shivers and coworkers (1988), astrocyte-endothelial contact was required. Dehouck and colleagues (1990) recently described the development of BBB properties in bovine brain microvascular endothelial cells grown on one side of a permeable membrane containing astrocytes on the other side. These cultures formed a monolayer with high electrical resistance and selectively restricted the diffusion of inulin and sucrose, but not leucine, consistent with the presence of complex interendothelial tight junctions and a functioning large neutral amino acid transport system. However, a receptor-mediated basis for the selective passage of leucine across the monolayer was not specifically demonstrated. Interestingly, large vessel bovine endothelial cells under identical conditions failed to develop these properties, suggesting that endothelial cells from different tissues vary in their ability to respond to astrocytic influences. Whether these differences

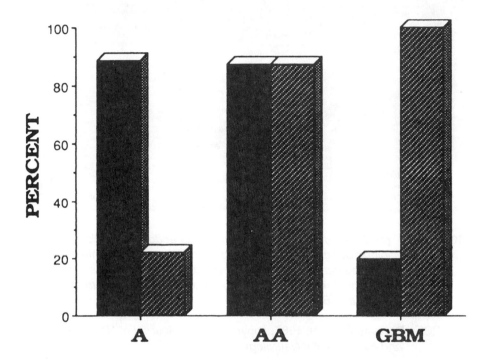

FIGURE 2. *Frequency of glucose transporter positivity and contrast enhancement as a function of tumor type. A: low-grade astrocytoma (n=9); AA: anaplastic astrocytoma (n=9); GBM: glioblastoma multiforme (n=10). Essentially all vessels of normal cerebrum (nonenhancing by definition) are known to be transporter positive. Low-grade astrocytomas and glioblastomas demonstrate an inverse relationship between transporter expression and contrast enhancement. The majority of anaplastic astrocytomas are transporter positive despite increased vascular permeability.*

SOURCE: Guerin et al. 1990, copyright 1990, *Annals of Neurology*

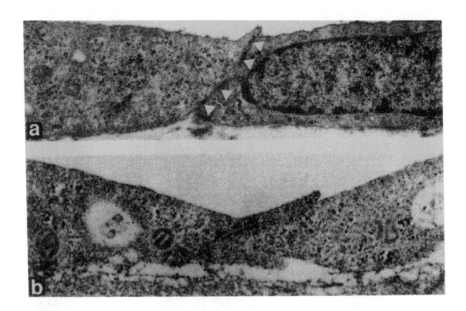

FIGURE 3. *(a) Cultured bovine brain microvessel endothelial cells are joined by tight junctional complexes (arrows) and contain few cytoplasmic vesicles and thin apical cytoplasmic folds. (b) Interendothelial tight junctions have a typical pentalaminar structure. Bar=0.1 microns.*

SOURCE: Dorovini-Zis et al. 1987, copyright 1987, *Journal of Neuropathology and Experimental Neurology*

result from in vivo events before endothelial isolation or from differences in the response of these cells to culture conditions is not known.

VESSEL FORMATION IN VIVO

The organization of endothelial cells into microvessels is a precondition to BBB expression in vivo. It has long been realized that capillaries form in developing neural tissue in close association with primitive glia (Bar and Wolff 1972). Ling and Stone (1988) demonstrated that the ingrowth of retinal microvessels is temporally and spatially coordinated with the migration of astrocytes from optic nerve into the retina. Furthermore, Schnitzer (1987) demonstrated in both monkey and horse that capillaries are restricted to retinal regions populated by astrocytes. These observations suggest that astrocytes influence vessel formation prior to inducing barrier formation.

78

VESSEL FORMATION IN VITRO

The authors' laboratory recently has focused on defining the cellular and biochemical determinants of early events in brain capillary formation. Microvascular endothelial cells grown as monolayers acquire cobblestoned morphologies that more closely resemble endothelial cells lining large vessels than those forming capillaries (figure 4). These distinct morphologies likely result from specific patterns of endothelial-endothelial and endothelial-matrix interaction determined, in part, by endothelial responses to environmental cues.

Experimental evidence for astrocyte induction of capillary formation thus far has been missing. To approach this problem, Laterra and colleagues (1990) recently developed an in vitro model of brain capillary formation in which astrocytes isolated from newborn rats induce bovine retinal microvascular endothelial (BRE) cells to reorganize into capillary-like structures. Cells of the C_6 line, which have astroglial properties, also induced this morphological change (figure 5). These astroglial-induced, capillary-like structures mimic in vivo cerebral capillaries by light microscopic criteria of size and shape, the accumulation of the basement membrane-associated protein laminin at endothelial-astroglial interfaces, and the "ensheathement" of the reorganized endothelial cells by astroglia. This "angiogenic" interaction shows CNS specificity since a fibroblastic normal rat kidney cell line did not induce BRE cell reorganization, and bovine adrenal microvascular endothelial cells failed to differentiate when cocultured with astroglia.

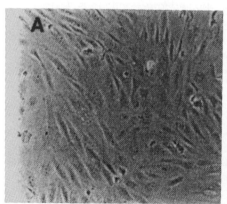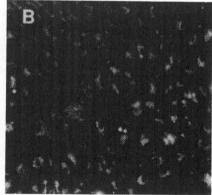

FIGURE 4. *(A) Cultured bovine retinal microvessel endothelial cells form a cobblestoned monolayer. (B) The endothelial character of these cells is demonstrated by staining with DiI-acyl-LDL.*

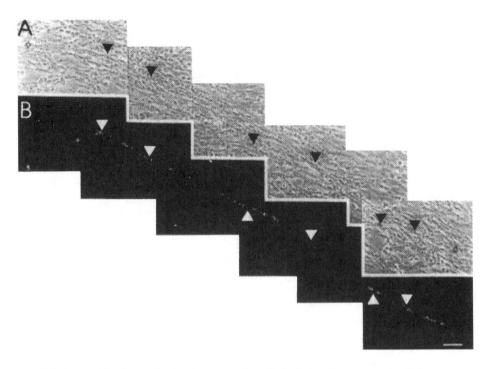

FIGURE 5. *Bovine retinal microvessel endothelial cells reorganize into capillary-like structures when cocultured with C_6 astroglial cells. Composite phase contrast (A) and fluorescence (B) photomicrographs were constructed from contiguous fields. (A) Numerous endothelial cells are organized into a 1.3-mm-long structure surrounded by C_6 cells. (B) DiI-acyl-LDL staining distinguishes endothelial cells from surrounding astroglia. This fluorescent marker accumulates around endothelial cell nuclei, some of which are indicated by arrows. Bar=50 microns.*

SOURCE: Laterra et al. 1990, copyright 1990, Wiley-Liss

Laterra and coworkers (1990) used this in vitro model to explore the molecular basis of astrocyte-endothelial interactions relevant to CNS microvessel formation. BRE cells were grown separated from astroglia by a porous membrane to distinguish between the effects of diffusible and nondiffusible inducers. Capillary-like structures failed to develop in the absence of direct heterologous cell-cell interactions. Likewise, neither astroglial-conditioned media nor coculture-conditioned media induced capillary-like structure formation in solo endothelial cell cultures. Although it is difficult to rule out a very labile diffusible substance that functions over extremely short distances, the findings are most consistent with induction by either a nondiffusible inducer or direct astroglia-endothelial contact.

The effects of transcription and translation inhibition on these morphogenic events were examined (table 1). Endothelial-astroglial cocultures were exposed to inhibitors for 15 hours immediately before the expected time of endothelial reorganization. Capillary-like structure formation was inhibited 50 to 70 percent in a concentration-dependent fashion by cycloheximide (0.01-0.1 μg/mL), puromycin (0.1-0.25 μg/mL), and actinomycin-D (0.01-.025 μg/mL). These results demonstrated a requirement for transcriptional events but did not identify either cell type as the necessary and sufficient site of inhibitory action. The effects of steroid hormones that are physiologically and therapeutically relevant agents that regulate gene transcription also were examined (table 1). Glucocorticoids are known to increase astroglial differentiation (Freshney 1984); to enhance BBB function, especially in diseases associated with blood vessel proliferation (i.e., brain tumors) (Long et al. 1966); and to be antiangiogenic in peripheral tissues (Folkman and Ingber 1987). Dexamethasone at 10^{-8} M inhibited astrocyte-induced, capillary-like structure formation by 70 to 100 percent. Inhibition was concentration dependent and receptor mediated. Both astroglial and BRE cells have glucocorticoid receptors, so the target cell for this effect was not immediately clear. The nonglucocorticoid progesterone, at 10^{-8} and 10^{-6} M, inhibited capillary-like structure formation by 30 and 60 percent, respectively. Astroglial, but not BRE, cells were found to have progesterone receptors, indicating that inhibition by progesterone most likely occurs by altering astroglial function. The nonglucocorticoid steroids— cholesterol, hydroxyprogesterone, and tetrahydrocortisol—failed to inhibit astrocyte-induced, capillary-like structure formation. These data demonstrate

TABLE 1. *Inhibition of astroglial-induced, in vitro angiogenesis*

Drug	Concentration	Percent Inhibition
Dexamethasone	10^{-8} M	80
Hydrocortisone	10^{-8} M	40
Progesterone	10^{-8} M	35
Tetrahydrocortisone	10^{-8} M	0
17 α-hydroxyprogesterone	10^{-8} M	5
Cycloheximide	0.1 μg/mL	80
Actinomycin-D	0.025 μg/mL	70

that "angiogenic" astrocyte-endothelial interactions may be mediated and manipulated by alterations in gene expression. Furthermore, as evidenced by the site of action of progesterone, the astrocyte may be a selective target for these molecular events.

Additional evidence that astrocytic functions are altered by these inhibitors was obtained by studying another model of in vitro angiogenesis. Endothelial cells reorganize into capillary-like forms in vitro in response to various well-defined extracellular matrices (Ingber and Folkman 1989; Kubota et al. 1988). Matrigel, extracellular matrix material derived from the Engelbreth-Holm-Swarm sarcoma, induces BRE cells to form capillary-like structures that morphologically mimic astrocyte-induced structures (Kubota et al. 1988). This response occurs in the absence of astrocytes within 12 hours of plating BRE cells on Matrigel-coated surfaces. Comparisons of BRE cell behavior in response to either Matrigel or astrocytes under various experimental conditions allowed the authors to distinguish between astrocyte-independent and astrocyte-dependent events (Laterra and Goldstein, in press; Wolff et al., in press). Neither cycloheximide, actinomycin-D, dexamethasone, nor progesterone were found to affect Matrigel-induced, capillary-like structure formation. Therefore, the endogenous endothelial processes associated with reorganization into capillary-like structures (e.g., migration, generation of homologous endothelial-endothelial adhesions, cytoskeletal changes, cell shape changes) may occur without RNA or protein synthesis and are unaffected by steroids. Based on these results, the authors propose that astrocytes produce signals that initiate an endogenous endothelial morphogenic program resulting in endothelial organization into capillaries. The activity of these astrocytic "angiogenic" signals are under pretranslational control and may be modulated by steroids.

CONCLUSION

The in vivo and in vitro experimental evidence presented in this chapter implicates perivascular astrocytes in the regulation of two brain microvascular endothelial cell functions, microvessel morphogenesis and the generation of the BBB phenotype. These two processes appear to be mutually exclusive. For instance, developing brain, cerebral inflammatory disease, and brain tumors are associated with neovascularization and incomplete BBB function. These states are characterized by the presence of proliferating, undifferentiated, or reactive astrocytes. This is in contrast to the quiescent, differentiated astrocytes of the normal adult brain in which angiogenesis is minimal and the BBB is intact. Taken together, these observations suggest that proliferating/ reactive astrocytes generate "signals" that enhance vessel growth. On the other hand, quiescent/differentiated astrocytes appear to lack these angiogenic signals and instead may induce microvascular endothelial cells to differentiate

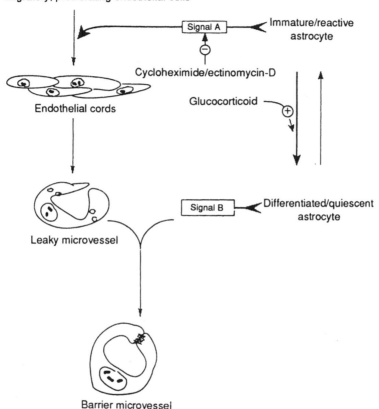

Migratory, proliferating endothelial cells

Signal A — Immature/reactive astrocyte

Cycloheximide/ectinomycin-D

Endothelial cords

Glucocorticoid

Leaky microvessel

Signal B — Differentiated/quiescent astrocyte

Barrier microvessel

FIGURE 6. *Model of angiogenic and barrier-inducing astrocyte-endothelial interactions. Immature, poorly differentiated, and reactive astrocytes influence endothelial cells to form new vessels. Differentiated quiescent astrocytes influence already established microvessels to express the BBB phenotype. Angiogenic astrocyte-endothelial interactions require RNA and protein synthesis. Glucocorticoids inhibit astroglial-induced angiogenesis and enhance barrier expression by altering astrocytic functions.*

and express barrier. Astrocyte-derived "angiogenic" signals are likely to differ from those that enhance barrier, and agents that modify astrocytes (e.g., steroids) have the potential to influence which signal predominates (figure 6). Elucidation of the nature of these signals should provide novel approaches to the modulation of brain vessel behavior and BBB expression.

REFERENCES

Bar, T.H., and Wolff, J.R. The formation of capillary basement membranes during internal vascularization of the rat's cerebral cortex. *Z Zelforsch* 133:231-248, 1972.

Bowman, P.D.; Ennis, R.R.; Rarey, K.E.; Betz, A.L.; and Goldstein, G.W. Brain microvessel endothelial cells in tissue culture: A model for study of BBB permeability. *Ann Neurol* 14:396-402, 1983.

Brightman, M.W., and Reese, T.S. Junctions between intimately apposed cell membranes in the vertebrate brain. *J Cell Biol* 40:648-677, 1969.

DeBault, L.E., and Cancilla, P.A. Gamma-glutamyl transpeptidase in isolated brain endothelial cells: Induction by glial cells in vitro. *Science* 207:653-655, 1980.

Dehouck, M.-P.; Meresse, S.; Delorme, P.; Fruchart, J.-C.; and Cecchelli, R. An easier, reproducible, and mass-production method to study the BBB in vitro. *J Neurochem* 54:1798-1801, 1990.

Dorovini-Zis, K.; Bowman, P.D.; Betz, A.L.; and Goldstein, G.W. Hyperosmotic urea reversibly opens the tight junctions between brain capillary endothelial cells in cell culture. *J Neuropathol Exp Neurol* 46(2):130-140, 1987.

Ehrlich, P. *Das Sauerstoff-Bedurfnis des Organismus: Eine Farbenanalytische Studie*. Berlin: Hirschwald, 1885.

Evans, C.A.N.; Reynolds, J.M.; Reynolds, M.L.; Saunders, N.R.; and Segal, M.B. The development of a BBB mechanism in foetal sheep. *J Physiol* 238:371-386, 1974.

Folkman, J., and Ingber, D.E. Angiostatic steroids. Method of discovery and mechanism of action. *Ann Surg* 206(993):374-383, 1987.

Freshney, R.I. Effects of glucocorticoids on glioma cells in culture. *Exp Cell Biol* 52:286-292, 1984.

Goldstein, G.W., and Betz, A.L. The BBB. *Sci Am* 254:74-83, 1986a.

Goldstein, G.W., and Betz, A.L. Blood vessels and the BBB. In: Asbury, A.K.; McKhann, G.M.; and McDonald, W.I., eds. *Diseases of the Nervous System*. Philadelphia: W.B. Saunders, 1986b. pp. 172-184.

Goldstein, G.W.; Betz, A.L.; and Bowman, P.D. Use of isolated brain capillaries and cultured endothelial cells to study the BBB. *Fed Proc* 43:191-195, 1984.

Guerin, C.; Laterra, J.; Hruban, R.H.; Brem, H.; Drewes, L.R.; and Goldstein, G.W. The glucose transporter and BBB of human brain tumors. *Ann Neurol* 28:758-765, 1990.

Ingber, D.E., and Folkman, J. Mechanochemical switching between growth and differentiation during fibroblast growth factor-stimulated angiogenesis in vitro: Role of extracellular matrix. *J Cell Biol* 109:317-330, 1989.

Janzer, R.C., and Raff, M.C. Astrocytes induce blood-brain barrier properties in endothelial cells. *Nature* 325:253-257, 1987.

Kubota, Y.; Kleinman, H.K.; Martin, G.R.; and Lawley, T.J. Role of laminin and basement membrane in the morphological differentiation of human endothelial cells into capillary-like structures. *J Cell Biol* 107:1589-1598, 1988.

Laterra, J., and Goldstein, G.W. Astroglial-induced in vitro angiogenesis: Requirements for RNA and protein synthesis. *J Neurochem*, in press.

Laterra, J.; Guerin, C.; and Goldstein, G.W. Astrocytes induce neural microvascular endothelial cells to form capillary-like structures in vitro. *J Cell Physiol* 144:204-215, 1990.

Ling, T., and Stone, J. The development of astrocyte in the cat retina: Evidence of migration from the optic nerve. *Dev Brain Res* 44:73-85, 1988.

Long, D.M.; Hartmann, J.F.; and French, L.A. The response of human cerebral edema to glucosteroid administration. An electron microscopic study. *Neurology* 16:521-528, 1966.

Reese, T.S., and Karnovsky, M.J. Fine structural localization of a BBB to exogenous peroxidase. *J Cell Biol* 34:207-217, 1967.

Risau, W.; Hallmann, R.; Albrecht, U.; and Henke-Fahle, S. Brain induces the expression of an early cell surface marker for BBB-specific endothelium. *EMBO J* 5:3179-3183, 1986.

Schnitzer, J. Retinal astrocytes: Their restriction to vascularized parts of mammalian retina. *Neurosci Lett* 78:29-34, 1987.

Shivers, R.R.; Arthur, F.E.; and Bowman, P.D. Induction of gap junctions and brain endothelium-like tight junctions in cultured bovine endothelial cells: Local control of cell specialization. *J Submicrosc Cytol Pathol* 20(1):1-14, 1988.

Stewart, P.A., and Hayakawa, E.M. Interendothelial junctional changes underlie the developmental "tightening" of the BBB. *Dev Brain Res* 32:271-281, 1987.

Stewart, P.A., and Wiley, M.J. Developing nervous tissue induces formation of blood-brain barrier characteristics in invading endothelial cells: A study using quail-chick transplantation chimeras. *Dev Biol* 84:183-192, 1981.

Svendgaard, N.; Björklund, A.; Hardebo, J.E.; and Stenevi, U. Axonal degeneration associated with a defective BBB in cerebral implants. *Nature* 255:334-337, 1975.

Tao-Cheng, J.-H.; Nagy, Z.; and Brightman, M.W. Tight junctions of brain endothelium in vitro are enhanced by astroglia. *J Neurosci* 7:3293-3299, 1987.

Wolff, J.E.A.; Laterra, J.; and Goldstein, G.W. Steroid inhibition of microvessel morphogenesis in vitro: Receptor-mediation and astroglial-dependence. *J Neurochem*, in press.

ACKNOWLEDGMENTS

This work was supported by National Institutes of Health research grants ES-02380 and EY-03772 (GWG) and by a grant from the Juvenile Diabetes Foundation International (JL). J. Laterra is a Clinical Investigator Development Awardee of the National Institute of Neurological Disorders and Stroke (NS-01329). C. Guerin is a National Research Service Awardee (CA-09574). J. Wolff is funded by the Dr. Mildred Scheel Foundation for Cancer Research, F.R.G.

AUTHORS

John Laterra, M.D., Ph.D.
Assistant Professor
Department of Neurology
The Johns Hopkins University School of Medicine
Assistant Professor
The Kennedy Institute

Johannes E.A. Wolff, M.D.
Research Fellow
The Kennedy Institute

Christopher Guerin, M.D.
Research Fellow
Departments of Neurosurgery and Oncology
The Johns Hopkins University School of Medicine
Research Fellow
The Kennedy Institute

Gary W. Goldstein, M.D.
Professor
Departments of Neurology and Pediatrics
The Johns Hopkins University School of Medicine
President
The Kennedy Institute

707 North Broadway
Baltimore, MD 21205

Nonpermeable and Permeable Vessels of the Brain

Milton W. Brightman and Yoshiaki Kadota

INTRODUCTION

The moment-to-moment regulation of interstitial fluid (IF) composition within the central nervous system (CNS) is made possible by certain structural peculiarities of the CNS vessels' endothelium. This endothelium, enclosed almost in its entirety by an astroglial sheath, comprises a continuous, sealed cell layer that circulating, hydrophilic molecules first encounter before they can reach the surface of any other cell within the CNS. The morphological substrate of the selective exclusion of solutes as small as ions is the circumferential belts of tight junctions between the endothelial cells (Reese and Karnovsky 1967) and endocytotic vesicles that incorporate circulating protein but, except for certain ligands, do not transfer protein across the cells (Broadwell 1989). The consequence of this physical blood-brain barrier (BBB) is to enable the endothelial cell, by excluding or selectively transferring solutes, to exert control over what may be allowed to reach even its immediate astroglial neighbor and neuronal cells.

However, there are seven small circumscribed areas at the ependymal border around the cerebral ventricles, the capillaries of which do not constitute a barrier but are, instead, passively permeable to hydrophilic solutes. It is the epithelium that caps these vessels and that blocks the exchange of large molecules between blood and cerebrospinal fluid. This chapter stresses the similarity of the capillary structure in these circumventricular organs (CVOs) to those of certain transplants in brain and to vessels of brain tumors. A consideration of these permeable vessels also provides the basis for describing the routes taken by molecules that have gained access to the IF compartment.

The aspects of brain vessels considered in this chapter are (1) the interactions between endothelium and astroglia in determining their structural effects on the BBB; (2) fenestrated vessels, the vessels of the brain that lie outside the barrier; (3) whether there is neurovascular specificity in neuroendocrine systems; and (4) the barrier in peripheral tissues grafted to the brain.

ENDOTHELIAL-ASTROGLIAL INTERACTIONS

Barrier Site

When the glycoprotein horseradish peroxidase (HRP) is administered intravascularly, it is prevented from moving between the blood and the IF of the CNS by zonular tight junctions that occlude the extracellular cleft between adjacent endothelial cells and by the paucity of endocytotic pits (Reese and Karnovsky 1967).

Until 1967 the site of the barrier to the passive migration of large hydrophilic molecules across the cerebral capillary was ascribed either to the capillary or to its enveloping astroglial sheath. The concept of the barrier was brought into question when electron micrographs of mammalian CNS tissue depicted an extremely high cellularity that left little extracellular room in which tracer molecules could accumulate in sufficient amounts to become visually detectable. There was purported to be no distinctive cellular barrier, either endothelial or astroglial, but rather a penetrable but very small IF or indicator space. That the lack of an appreciable IF space did not account for an illusory barrier was demonstrated in the tailed amphibian, the mudpuppy (*Necturus maculosus*). The cerebral capillaries of this amphibian are simple hairpin loops surrounded by a connective tissue-containing perivascular space large enough to accommodate HRP infused into its cerebral ventricles. However, when the protein was injected intravascularly, it was prevented by the endothelium from reaching the perivascular space. The failure to enter the IF was the outcome of an endothelial barrier and not the absence of an appreciable IF space (Bodenheimer and Brightman 1968).

The impermeable endothelium of the "barrier" blood vessels throughout the CNS can be rendered permeable by opening its tight junctions or by momentarily inducing the microinvagination of the endothelial cell membrane to form a transient, vesiculo-tubular, transcellular channel. The reversible opening of the BBB has been achieved by administering in vivo hyperosmotic solutions of saccharides (Rapoport et al. 1972). The mechanism of breaching the barrier is still controversial. Patent, HRP-filled endothelial junctions have been demonstrated in mammals treated with hyperosmotic solutions (Brightman et al. 1973), and comparable experiments in lower forms also open the BBB; but the junctions appear to remain tightly closed, and there is a proliferation of vesiculotubular profiles in the endothelial cytoplasm (Farrell and Shivers 1984). The interpretation of such profiles as transcellular channels in normal endothelium (Hashimoto 1972) and in perturbed endothelium (Lossinsky et al. 1979) has been convincingly refuted (Balin et al. 1987).

Dissemination of Exogenous Protein Through Interstitial Fluid

Once the proteins cross the cerebral capillary, there is no structural impediment to their flow through the IF clefts of the cerebral parenchyma (Brightman 1977). However, the extracellular dissemination of the larger ferritin molecule (Brightman 1965), the apoferritin shell being ~445 kD, is not as extensive as the smaller, 40-kD HRP molecule (Brightman et al. 1970) following the perfusion of these molecules through the cerebral ventricles.

The rapidity with which HRP is dispersed from the ventricles and subarachnoid space throughout the perivascular channels of the brain has been convincingly demonstrated to be the result of the pulsatile activity of the heart (Rennels et al. 1985). Because this rapid dissemination is confined to perivascular channels and does not include the IF clefts around neurons and glial cells, it has been suggested that the pulsatile action is a means of clearing molecules such as HRP from the brain rather than spreading an appreciable amount of such charged macromolecules to the surface of brain cells (Brightman 1989).

The fraction of HRP that penetrates the 20 nm-wide perineuronal and periglial clefts at some distance from its original point of entry, the permeable vessels of CVOs or peripheral tissue graft, may be so small that it cannot be detected even with the sensitive tetramethylbenzidine method. A telltale sign that the glycoprotein has infiltrated the extensive network of the comparatively larger *perivascular* clefts is the uptake of the exogenous HRP by perivascular pericytes. Unlike the endothelial cells, the farflung pericytes do not form a continuous cell layer, but their ubiquity and labeling by HRP indicate that the protein had traveled along the perivascular clefts for considerable distances. The inference that pericyte labeling connotes the spread of HRP through the perivascular clefts of the IF compartment is, of course, based on the reasonable premise that the endothelium under the pericytes has an intact blood-IF barrier. There is normally no, or very little, transendothelial migration of circulating protein, but a small rupture of the endothelium could supplement the HRP flowing along the periendothelial clefts from a CVO, a tumor, or a graft of peripheral tissue in the brain.

Whether HRP enters the IF compartment from the blood or from the cerebral ventricles, the astroglia does not prevent the protein from reaching the cell processes of neurons or the abluminal face of the endothelium. The plaque-like gap junctions tethering astrocytes to each other are, unlike zonular tight junctions between endothelial cells, discontinuous and cicumventable by HRP (Brightman and Reese 1969). Although the perivascular astrocyte does not prevent HRP from flowing into the IF, its ubiquity as a periendothelial investment suggests that it could contribute to the composition of the IF and may influence the function of the endothelium. However, the size of the molecule, as well as its coulombic charge, determines how far it will move through the IF. In contrast to HRP (40 kD), gamma globulin G (160 kD) injected into peripheral blood does cross the permeable vessels of a graft on the surface of the brain, but it penetrates the IF of the underlying brain for a distance of only about 1 mm in 1-month-old grafts (Wakai et al. 1986).

Effect of Astrocytes on Endothelial Cell Membrane

The first experimental intimation that brain cells were involved with the formation of the endothelial barrier came with the highly significant observations that peripheral, permeable vessels become impermeable where they invade brain tissue (Stewart and Wiley 1981). Embryonic avian brain, before it had become vascularized and when it was placed on the chorioallantois, was penetrated by vessels from this organ. On entering the piece of embryonic brain, the vessels from the chorioallantois were no longer permeable to circulating Evans blue-albumin complex. Something within the brain tissue had converted once-permeable vessels into barrier vessels.

The identity of the CNS component responsible for the conversion from permeable to impermeable vessels was made by in vivo and in vitro approaches. When astrocytes grown in cell culture were aggregated and implanted into the iris of the rodent eye, iris vessels, normally permeable to Evans blue-albumin, became impermeable when the vessels entered the astrocyte aggregate (Janzer and Raff 1987). In another approach, the cell membranes of bovine brain endothelial cells, maintained in solo cultures, were assessed in replicas of freeze-fractured cell membranes (Tao-Cheng et al. 1987). As in other cell types, the tight junctions of the endothelial cells were characterized by strands or ridges within the lipid bilayer of the fractured plasma membrane. However, instead of forming complex, interconnecting strands several rows wide, the ridges were discontinuous, fragmentary, and relatively few in number. Moreover, unlike tight junctions of brain barrier vessels, many gap junctions were distributed among the tight junction strands (Tao-Cheng et al. 1987). When the brain endothelial cells were cocultured with primary cultures of rat astrocytes, the junctions became enhanced: The constituent strands became longer and more continuous, there were more rows of strands, many of the rows were connected, and there were few gap junctions among the strands. The astrocytes had "normalized" the endothelial tight junctions (Tao-Cheng et al. 1987). In similar cocultures, the *induction* of strand development in brain endothelium by astrocytes also has been described but without a decrement in gap junctions (Arthur et al. 1987).

The inference that the barrier attributes of brain endothelium are imposed by astrocytes has been further reinforced by in vitro experiments. A relatively high electrical resistance (R) has been attained across a monolayer of brain endothelium that is maintained in culture with astroglia or its conditioned medium. The R between the lumen and perivascular fluid of anuran pial vessels is about 1,800 Ω•cm^2 in vivo (Crone and Olesen 1982). Until recently, attempts to increase the R, beyond 50 to 100 Ω•cm^2, across brain endothelium grown in coculture with astroglia or its conditioned medium have been unsuccessful. One successful method has been to select and clone endothelial cells from capillaries, in contrast to venules, where the barrier may be incomplete. If the cloned endothelial cells are grown on one side of a collagen-coated filter and astrocytes are grown on the opposite side, a continuous, barrier-type of endothelial layer is obtained (Meresse et al. 1989) with an average R of 600 Ω•cm^2 across the two cell layers (Dehouck et al. 1990). A second method, which also yields a comparable or higher R, requires the continuous exposure of brain endothelial cells to astrocyte-conditioned medium, stimulation of adenylyl cyclase, and the immunological removal of pericytes from the cultures (Rubin et al., in press). The exciting prospects offered by these in vitro preparations are not only the rapid and simple electrical assay of agents that might affect the barrier but also new glimpses of how monocytes, endothelial cells, and astrocytes might interact under immunologically defined conditions.

As strong as the accumulating evidence is that the astrocyte affects the structure of the endothelial cell and its permeability toward large, hydrophilic molecules, there are several reasons for doubting this relationship. (1) The cerebral endothelium of some elasmobranchs, such as the shark and dogfish, has open junctions and is permeable to HRP, whereas its perivascular astroglia forms the impermeable layer (Brightman et al. 1971; Bundgaard and Cserr 1981). Either these particular perivascular astrocytes ensure that the endothelial junctions remain open rather than closed, or the open junctional configuration is an inherent one, independent of the adjacent astrocyte. Similarly, the closed tight junction may be inherent to mammalian cerebral endothelium and independent of astrocytes. (2) Dissociated, cloned brain endothelial cells in vitro can form a continuous layer with an R of 157 to 783 Ω•cm^2 in the absence of astrocytes (Rutten et al. 1987). (3) Astrocytes of the hypothalamic median eminence and the astrocyte-like cells, the pituicytes of the neural lobe of the pituitary gland, are neighbors of an endothelium that is not tight but rather fenestrated and permeable to HRP. Therefore, it is still conceivable that the in situ development of barrier characteristics is inherent to the cerebral endothelium and independent of the astrocyte.

Influence of Endothelium on Astrocyte Cell Membrane

Just as astrocytes influence the membrane structure of brain endothelium, so does the endothelium modulate the internal structure of the astrocyte cell membrane. Viewed in freeze-fracture replicas, the plasma membrane of the perivascular astrocyte contains numerous, randomly dispersed orthogonal aggregates of intramembranous particles or assemblies (Dermietzel 1973; Landis and Reese 1974; Anders and Brightman 1979).

In vitro primary cultures of brain cells enriched with astrocytes contain assemblies that are greatly reduced in number but that, as in their in vivo situation, are randomly dispersed (figure 1). In the company of brain endothelial cells or fibroblasts, the assemblies aggregate, and a few become aligned in rows (figure 2) similar to those in situ where the plasma membrane of two astrocytes abut one another (Tao-Cheng et al. 1990). Some of the randomness is converted into an orderly arrangement of the particles when brain endothelial cells and fibroblasts are in vitro neighbors of astrocytes. It is not surprising that the effect also is exerted by fibroblasts because the fibroblast-like cells constituting the pia-arachnoid, in addition to the endothelium of the brain, subtend astrocytic end-feet rich in assemblies, some of which are in orderly array.

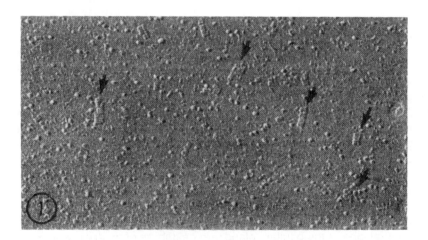

FIGURE 1.   *Solo primary culture of astrocytes at 18th day in vitro. Assemblies (arrows) are randomly scattered within the lipid bilayer of the cell membrane. X 105,000*

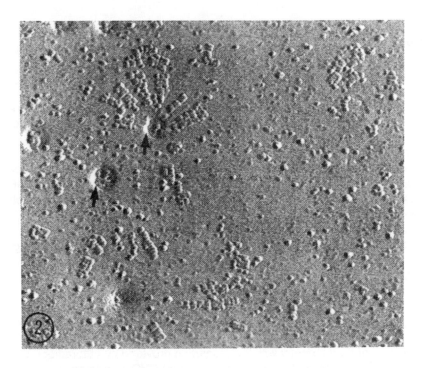

FIGURE 2.   *Primary astroglial culture, 10 days old, was grown on a cover slip and placed facing brain endothelial cells for 7 days. Assemblies have aggregated and form orderly trains of particles radiating from caveolae (arrows). X 105,000*

The function of the assembly is not known. It is doubtful that the assemblies are involved with active transport across the astrocytes' cell membrane (Gotow and Hashimoto 1988). It is more likely that they are associated with potassium channels (Newman 1985). The high concentration of assemblies in the Müller cell end-foot that faces the vitreous of the frog eye closely matches the sites of high K^+ conductance (Newman 1985). Whether potassium channels of astrocytes, like assemblies, can aggregate and become aligned, whether this redispersal into rows ensures a highly localized withdrawal of K^+ from the IF, and the significance of such a focal "spatial buffering" of potassium are not known.

FENESTRATED BLOOD VESSELS

Circumventricular Organs

The BBB is focally circumvented at discrete sites that have a neuroendocrine function and that are situated around the lateral, III, and IV cerebral ventricles (Weindl 1973; Klara and Brizee 1975). These CVOs, except for the subcommissural organ, do not have a BBB. They are characterized by a connective tissue space enclosing fenestrated, permeable capillaries capped by an impermeable epithelium (Hashimoto and Hama 1968; Brightman 1968). The epithelial cells of one such CVO, the choroid plexus, are linked to each other by zonular tight junctions impermeable to HRP (Brightman 1968), although they are permeable to a smaller solute, lanthanum salt (Bouldin and Krigman 1975). At other CVOs, such as the median eminence, the tight epithelium consists of specialized ependymal cells, the tanycytes (Weindl 1973), that also block the passive, extracellular flow of HRP between perivascular space and the cerebrospinal fluid of the ventricles.

The permeability of the CVOs to a small, neutral amino acid, alpha-amino isobutyric acid, has been measured by quantitative autoradiography. The correlation of morphometry with the resolution provided by autoradiography has permitted the blood flow and permeability of CVO subregions to be delineated in terms of the arrangement, structure, and density of their microvessels (Shaver et al. 1990a, 1990b). A consistent pattern has been emerging. For example, in the subfornical organ the rostral region is supplied by barrier vessels, whereas the caudal region receives fenestrated vessels highly permeable to the amino acid. The possible correlation within the CVOs of regional permeability and blood flow with the presence of neuroendocrine axons has led to an interesting and reasonable speculation. The hypothesis is that the density of permeable vessels is concordant with a localized, high metabolic activity that subserves complex neuroendocrine functions (Shaver et al. 1990b).

NEUROVASCULAR SPECIFICITY?

The permeable, fenestrated capillaries of the CVO, unlike the barrier vessels of the adjacent brain in most species, are surrounded by two basal laminae with an intervening space containing extracellular matrix, which includes collagen and basal lamina material (figures 3 through 5). In CVOs, such as the median eminence of the hypothalamus and the neural lobe (NL) of the pituitary gland, this perivascular space is bordered by the terminals of magnocellular, neurosecretory axons (NSAs) that in turn are enveloped by astrocyte-like cells, the pituicytes. The NSAs from the magnocellular

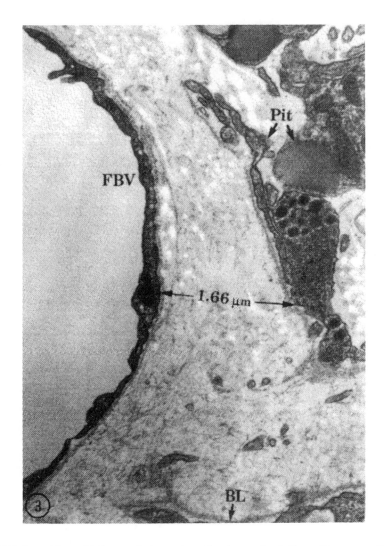

FIGURE 3. *Neural lobe graft 4 weeks after transplantation. Regenerating NSA terminal, containing small vesicles and about nine neurosecretory vesicles, is 1.66 μm from a fenestrated vessel (FBV). The terminal is separated from the FBV by a process, presumably a pituicyte (Pit), subtended by basal lamina (BL). Pituicytes often have lipid droplets. X 29,000*

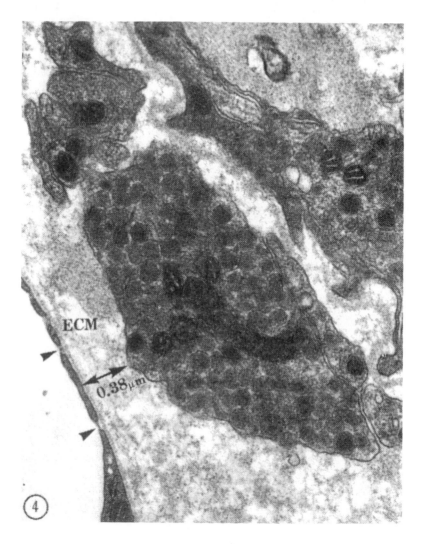

FIGURE 4.   *Pineal graft 2 weeks after transplantation. Regenerating NSA is 0.38 μm from capillary with fenestrae (arrowheads). Axon and capillary lie in extracellular matrix (ECM). X 42,100*

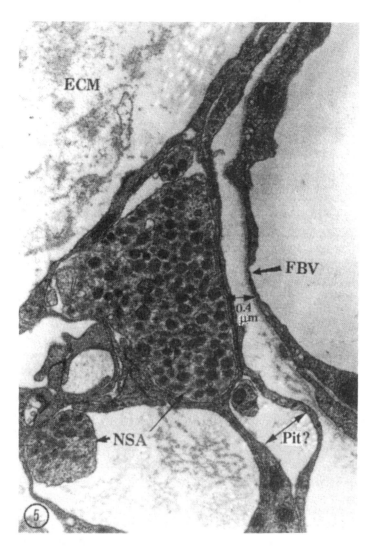

FIGURE 5. *Adrenal medulla graft, 2 weeks old. Shortest separation of NSA from fenestrated capillary (FBV) is 0.4 µm, but two thin cell processes (Pit) intervene. The processes, having no BL, may be fibroblasts. NSA and FBV lie in ECM. X 20,500*

neurosecretory cells of the hypothalamic supraoptic and paraventricular nuclei thus terminate as neurovascular endings.

The question posed by the lead author of this chapter is whether a regenerating NSA becomes as closely associated with the fenestrated endothelium of other CVOs or of endocrine glands as it does with the fenestrated vessels of its own CVO target. To answer the question, fragments of NL (figure 3), pieces of another CVO, the pineal gland (figure 4), and fragments of a peripheral endocrine gland, the adrenal medulla (figure 5), were inserted into the lateral retrochiasmatic area (Kadota et al. 1990). Through this area, NSAs from both nuclei course as a compact bundle on their way to the NL (Palkovits 1984). The area is anterior to the median eminence and is supplied by very few, if any, fenestrated vessels; thus, any such vessels next to or within graft tissue would have been introduced by the transplants. The act of inserting the grafts inevitably damages some of the NSAs, and it was expected that collateral sprouts from adjacent, intact NSAs would be in a position to terminate on nearby, fenestrated vessels. A few such NSAs did penetrate each type of graft to terminate as closely on the fenestrated vessels of the pineal and adrenal medulla as they did on similar vessels of the NL transplants. There appeared to be no specificity with respect to the closeness of association between NSAs and fenestrated capillaries (figures 3 through 5) (Kadota et al. 1990).

However, there may be a chemotactic specificity between the regrowing NSAs and either the fenestrated capillaries or the pituicytes. By 2 to 4 weeks after transplantation, the NL grafts consisted primarily of fenestrated vessels, pituicytes, redundant basal lamina, fibroblasts, and collagen, with the NSAs within the NL grafts having degenerated. Although the results were not statistically significant, there was a consistent tendency for more NSAs, more fenestrated capillaries, and more NSA-capillary associations to be included in the NL grafts than in either the pineal or adrenal ones (Kadota et al. 1990). At present, the pituicyte is suspected of being the source of the purported chemoattractant and not only may provide a tropic factor or directional guidance to ingrowing axons and vessels but also might be trophically "axonogenic" and vasogenic as well. If there is a vasogenic factor, like purported adrenal and pineal factors, it might induce the formation of fenestrae within the regenerating capillary endothelium.

THE BARRIER IN GRAFTS OF PERIPHERAL TISSUE TO BRAIN

Tissue Grafts

It is certain that the solid grafts of CVO and endocrine tissue contained some of their intrinsic, fenestrated blood vessels. As will be shown, it is also likely that the parenchymal cells of the grafts must have influenced the structure and permeability of regenerating vessels growing into the transplants. By means of this influence, the ingrowing capillaries came to resemble the intrinsic ones normally supplying the grafted tissue.

A discrete, invasive means of circumventing the passive BBB is by creating a nonendocrine, CVO-like structure in the form of a graft of peripheral tissue to the ventricular surface of the brain. This focal circumvention can be accomplished by transplanting solid tissues or by implanting pure populations of cell lines. Allografts consisting of fragments of (Rosenstein and Brightman 1983) or whole (Tsubaki et al. 1987) superior cervical ganglia, when placed into the fourth ventricle of rodents, survive indefinitely. These periventricular grafts are permeable to exogenous protein (Rosenstein and Brightman 1983) and, as measured by quantitative autoradiography, to a small amino acid as well (Tsubaki et al. 1987).

The same bypass can be accomplished with isografts of skeletal muscle. Small pieces about 1 to 2 mm^2 are carefully inserted into the IV ventricle of mature rats. As with other tissues (Rosenstein and Brightman 1983; Tsubaki et al. 1987) it is essential to force the grafts against or into the choroid plexus. In such transplants of, for example, the superior cervical ganglion, vessels from both pia and choroid plexus rapidly enter and anastomose with the vessels of the graft (Tsubaki et al. 1987). Being skeletal muscle, the "milieu" imposes permeable features on the regenerating endothelium that enters the graft. Circulating HRP quickly crosses the permeable muscle type of capillaries within the transplant to enter the muscle's interstitial space. From here, the protein enters the IF of the contiguous brain, that is, the medulla oblongata and cerebellum (Wakai et al. 1986). The interstitial pathway taken by the protein is longitudinal, between the dorsal, long fiber tracts of the medulla, and may extend for about 0.6 to 1.0 mm (Wakai et al. 1986).

The muscle autografts survive indefinitely on the ependymal or pial surface but soon die if they are placed within the neural parenchyma. The transplants on the brain's surface endure because they become innervated by myelinated fibers that can form myoneural junctions (Wakai et al. 1986). Whereas most of the muscle cells do not become innervated and undergo fatty degeneration, some cells do receive innervation and survive. The source of the innervation is unknown. The grafts might receive branches from one of the nearby cranial nerves (e.g., the facial nerves). Another possible source of the myelinated axons might be branches of the superior cervical ganglion that innervates the pia. If so, then the IV ventricle, as a chamber for receiving grafts, can be compared with the anterior chamber of the eye. The insertion of intraocular grafts inevitably injures the iris and the nerves of the superior cervical ganglion supplying it. One result is that collateral sprouts from uninjured fibers or perhaps damaged but regenerating axons then innervate the graft.

In summary, transplants of peripheral neural or muscle tissue to the surface of the brain survive for longer periods than those inserted into the CNS parenchyma and are sites for the focal entry into the brain's IF of large, hydrophilic solutes, elsewhere excluded by the BBB.

Cell Implants

Grafts of solid pieces of peripheral tissue within the brain are supplied by vessels with the permeable characteristics of the grafts' original vessels. It is likely that surviving portions of the grafts' blood vessels regenerate and anastomose with the ingrowing endothelium of the adjacent brain (Stewart and Wiley 1981; Tsubaki et al. 1987). However, the new vessels in the graft are not necessarily derived, even in part, from vessels that had survived within the graft. Rather, the vessels in and around a transplant may arise solely from the intrinsic vessels of the surrounding brain.

Pure cultures of neoplastic cells, without any endothelial contaminant, when introduced into the brain substance, can induce brain endothelium to take on the permeability of the vessels once associated with the cells from which the tumor had been originally derived. A cell line, PC12, derived from a rat pheochromocytoma, consists of replicating adrenal chromaffin-like cells (Greene and Tischler 1976). When such dividing, naive, PC12 cells are treated with nerve growth factor, they differentiate—they stop dividing, emit neurites, and, like naive cells, are able to synthesize both catecholaminergic and cholinergic neurotransmitters (Greene and Tischler 1976). The growth factor must be continually replenished or the neurone-like cells revert to the mitotic naive state. A longer, apparently indefinite, differentiation has been attained by infecting naive PC12 cells with a retrovirus containing the Kirsten-ras oncogene (Noda et al. 1985).

When naive, mitotic PC12 cells are implanted into the brain of rats, some vessels within or adjacent to the implant may become fenestrated, such as those depicted in figures 3 through 5 (Jaeger 1987; Pappas and Sagen 1988). As do the cells of brain tumors, PC12 cells appear to elaborate and release something that induces the formation of fenestrae and, presumably, the associated tubulovesicular apparatus. It is the tubulovesicular complex, rather than the diaphragm-covered fenestrae, that transfers large, hydrophilic solutes from blood to IF (Coomber and Stewart 1988).

100

Brain Tumors

Fenestrated blood vessels supply not only CVOs but also normally developing brain (Bar and Wolff 1972) and tumors of the brain (Groothuis and Vick 1982). All these fenestrated vessels are structurally the same, are associated with a generous perivascular space, and are passively permeable to circulating molecules. In normal rat embryos at 11 to 12 days of gestation, fenestrated capillaries lie at the border between the periventricular, neuroepithelial cell layer and the rest of the parenchyma. By the 17th day of embryonic life, when neuroblasts are being formed, the fenestrae disappear, presumably because of a differentiating influence of neuroblasts and glial cells (Yoshida et al. 1988).

At least some of the vasculature supplying almost all brain tumors is fenestrated. Brain tumors that are induced by the intracerebral inoculation of virus (Vick 1980) or the administration of nitrosourea compounds (summarized by Groothuis and Vick 1982), as well as primary and metastatic gliomas in human brains (Hirano and Matsui 1975), all contain some vessels that are fenestrated. The number and location of fenestrated microvessels in experimentally induced and in spontaneously arising brain tumors are highly variable within individual tumors and between tumors (Groothuis and Vick 1982). Whereas these vessels are permeable to x-ray contrast media and chemotherapeutic agents, neighboring vessels within the tumor or near its border with normal brain are barrier vessels. Consequently, the BBB must be opened (e.g., osmotically [Neuwelt and Rapoport 1984]) to attain a greater entry of agents into brain tumors.

Necrotic brain tissue does not induce the formation of fenestrae in regenerating blood vessels. Presumably, a substance secreted by normal fetal brain cells or a variety of neoplastic cells brings about the development of fenestrae in growing, responsive endothelium. A substance in the form of a 30-kD protein is elaborated by malignant glioma cells in vitro (Bruce et al. 1987). The protein, which has been designated as a vascular permeability factor (VPF), rapidly augments the permeability of already permeable intradermal blood vessels. This property has been taken to suggest that a VPF also may cause the vasogenic edema often associated with brain tumors (Bruce et al. 1987). However, an increased permeability and the development of fenestrae in brain endothelium exposed to VPF have yet to be demonstrated.

It is conceivable that PC12 cells may secrete a substance that causes brain endothelial cells to become fenestrated. Counter to this notion is the observation that, in vitro, the presence of PC12 cells does not result in the development of fenestrae in adjacent endothelial cells (Tao-Cheng et al. 1989).

Moreover, the implantation of PC12 cells does not always result in tumor formation. On the contrary, if placed within the brain of otherwise normal adult rats, naive PC12 cells may cause the development of hemorrhagic cysts and disappear (Freed et al. 1986; Okuda et al. 1991). The hemorrhages suggest that the endothelial cells had been damaged by the naive PC12 cells, but endothelial cells are not damaged when cocultured with naive PC12 cells (J.H. Tao-Cheng, O. Okuda, L.S. Simpson, L. Chang, and M.W. Brightman, unpublished results). If ras-oncogene, differentiated PC12 cells are implanted into the brain opposite to the side that had received the naive cells, few if any small hemorrhages develop, and some of the PC12 cells persist for at least 8 weeks (Okuda et al. 1991).

Do PC12 cells, like other tumor cells, secrete a VPF that converts barrier, impermeable vessels into fenestrated, permeable ones? It may be that cerebral vessels have to be "primed" in some fashion before they can become responsive to factors that might be released from PC12 or glioma cells.

If PC12 cells were a rich source of a VPF, it may be informative to determine the conditions under which normal, barrier endothelium might be converted to the permeable, fenestrated type. It may be anticipated that PC12 cells, differentiated by either nerve growth factor or ras oncogene, may stop producing or releasing VPF and that the nearby capillaries would remain unfenestrated and impermeable to large hydrophilic molecules. However, the number of passages of PC12 cells maintained in vitro may result in a varying rate of fenestrae formation. Repeated cell passages also might diminish unpredictably the amount of VPF being elaborated by the cells. The resulting variability in the number of fenestrated vessels would make it difficult to ascertain whether differentiated PC12 cells no longer induce the creation of fenestrae. Nevertheless, the identification of the conditions under which brain endothelium can become responsive to secreted permeability factors might yield further insight into the modulation of endothelial permeability to hydrophilic substances.

CONCLUSIONS

There is strong evidence obtained from in vivo and in vitro experiments that the structural and functional barriers of CNS endothelium are influenced by astrocytes. New in vitro, methodological variations have yielded a confluent, endothelial cell layer with a high R, provided that astrocytes or their secreted products are present. However, cloned brain endothelial cells also may exhibit a high R in the absence of astroglia, and in some species, brain endothelium is permeable to large solutes, whereas its astrocytic sheath acts as a barrier between blood and brain IF. Therefore, the possibility remains that the barrier properties of endothelium may be an intrinsic, inherent property independent of astrocytes.

CVOs, grafts to the brain of muscle or endocrine tissue, and brain tumors all have some vessels that are fenestrated and permeable. These vessels enable circulating protein to bypass the BBB. Whether developing or regenerating blood vessels become fenestrated and permeable in response to factors secreted by certain cells, including tumor cells, has yet to be fully explored. While regenerating NSAs of one CVO, the pituitary gland's neural lobe, may nonspecifically regrow in vivo to grafted fenestrated vessels from a variety of sources, the axons may be specifically attracted to and maintained by the lobe's pituicytes. Further definition of how such permeable vessels are induced and how they affect the contents of the brain's IF may add to a perspective of how the properties of barrier vessels may be induced and maintained.

REFERENCES

Anders, J.J., and Brightman, M.W. Assemblies of particles in the cell membranes of developing, mature and reactive astrocytes. *J Neurocytol* 8:777-795, 1979.

Arthur, F.E.; Shivers, R.R.; and Bowman, P.D. Astrocyte-mediated induction of tight junctions in brain capillary endothelium: An efficient in vitro model. *Dev Brain Res* 36:155-159, 1987.

Balin, B.J.; Broadwell, R.D.; and Salcman, M. Tubular profiles do not form transendothelial channels through the blood-brain barrier. *J Neurocytol* 16:721-735, 1987.

Bar, T.H., and Wolff, J.R. The formation of capillary basement membranes during internal vascularization of the rat's cerbral cortex. *Z Zellforsch* 133:231-248, 1972.

Bodenheimer, T.S., and Brightman, M.W. A blood-brain barrier to peroxidase in capillaries surrounded by perivascular spaces. *Am J Anat* 122:249-267, 1968.

Bouldin, T.W., and Krigman, M.R. Differential permeability of cerebral capillary and choroid plexus to lanthanum ion. *Brain Res* 99:444-448, 1975.

Brightman, M.W. The distribution within the brain of ferritin injected into cerebrospinal fluid compartments, part 2 (parenchymal distribution). *Am J Anat* 117:193-220, 1965.

Brightman, M.W. The intracerebral movement of proteins injected into blood and cerebrospinal fluid of mice. *Prog Brain Res* 29:19-37, 1968.

Brightman, M.W. Morphology of blood-brain barrier interfaces. *Exp Eye Res* 25:1-25, 1977.

Brightman, M.W. The anatomic basis of the blood-brain barrier. In: Neuwelt, E.A., ed. *Implications of the Blood-Brain Barrier and Its Manipulation.* Vol. 1. New York: Plenum, 1989. pp. 53-83.

Brightman, M.W.; Hori, M.; Rapoport, S.I.; Reese, T.S.; and Westergaard, E. Osmotic opening of tight junctions in cerebral endothelium. *J Comp Neurol* 152:317-326, 1973.

Brightman, M.W.; Klatzo, I.; Olsson, Y.; and Reese, T.S. The blood-brain barrier to proteins under normal and pathological conditions. *J Neurol Sci* 10:215-239, 1970.

Brightman, M.W., and Reese, T.S. Junctions between intimately apposed cell membranes in the vertebrate brain. *J Cell Biol* 40:648-677, 1969.

Brightman, M.W.; Reese, T.S.; Olsson, Y.; and Klatzo, I. Morphological aspects of the blood-brain barrier to peroxidase in elasmobranchs. *Prog Neuropathol* 1:146-161, 1971.

Broadwell, R.D. Transcytosis of macromolecules through the blood-brain barrier: A cell biological perspective and critical appraisal. *Acta Neuropathol* 79:117-128, 1989.

Bruce, J.N.; Criscuolo, G.R.; Merrill, M.J.; Moquin, R.R.; Blacklock, J.B.; and Oldfield, E.H. Vascular permeability induced by protein product of malignant brain tumors: Inhibition by dexamethasone. *J Neurosurg* 67:880-884, 1987.

Bundgaard, M., and Cserr, H.F. A glial blood-brain barrier in elasmobranchs. *Brain Res* 226:61-73, 1981.

Coomber, B.L., and Stewart, P.A. Three-dimensional reconstruction of vesicles in endothelium of blood-brain barrier versus highly permeable microvessels. *Anat Rec* 215:256-261, 1988.

Crone, C., and Olesen, S.P. Electrical resistance of brain microvascular endothelium. *Brain Res* 241:49-55, 1982.

Dehouck, M.P.; Meresse, S.; Delorme, P.; Fruchart, J-C.; and Cecchelli, R. An easier, reproducible, and mass-production method to study the blood-brain barrier in vitro. *J Neurochem* 54:1798-1801, 1990.

Dermietzel, R. Visualization by freeze-fracturing of regular structures in glial cell membranes. *Naturwissenschaften* 60:208-209, 1973.

Farrell, C.L., and Shivers, R.R. Capillary junctions of the rat are not affected by osmotic opening of the blood-brain barrier. *Acta Neuropathol* 63:179-189, 1984.

Freed, W.; Patel-Vaidya, U.; and Geller, H.M. Properties of PC12 pheochromocytoma cells transplanted to the adult rat brain. *Exp Brain Res* 63:557-566, 1986.

Gotow, T., and Hashimoto, P.H. Deep-etch structure of astrocytes at the superficial glia limitans, with special emphasis on the internal and external organization of their plasma membranes. *J Neurocytol* 17:399-413, 1988.

Greene, L.A., and Tischler, A.S. Establishment of a noradrenergic clonal line of rat adrenal pheochromocytoma cells which respond to nerve growth factor. *Proc Natl Acad Sci U S A* 73:2424-2428, 1976.

Groothuis, D.R., and Vick, N. Brain tumors and the blood-brain barrier. *Trends Neurosci* 5:232-235, 1982.

Hashimoto, P.H. Intracellular channels as a route for protein passage in the capillary endothelium of the shark brain. *Am J Anat* 134:41-58, 1972.

Hashimoto, P.H., and Hama, K. An electron microscope study on protein uptake into brain regions devoid of the blood-brain barrier. *Med J Osaka Univ* 18:331-346, 1968.

Hirano, A., and Matsui, T. Vascular structures in brain tumors. *Hum Pathol* 6:611-621, 1975.

Jaeger, C.B. Morphological and immunocytochemical characteristics of PC12 cell grafts in rat brain. *Ann N Y Acad Sci* 495:334-350, 1987.

Janzer, R.C., and Raff, M.C. Astrocytes induce blood-brain properties in endothelial cells. *Nature* (London) 325:253-257, 1987.

Kadota, Y.; Pettigrew, K.D.; and Brightman, M.W. Regrowth of damaged neurosecretory axons to fenestrated vessels of implanted perpheral tissues. *Synapse* 5:175-189, 1990.

Klara, P.M., and Brizee, K.R. The ultrastructural morphology of the squirrel monkey area postrema. *Cell Tissue Res* 160:315-326, 1975.

Landis, D.M., and Reese, T.S. Arrays of particles in freeze-fractured astrocytic membranes. *J Cell Biol* 60:316-320, 1974.

Lossinsky, A.S.; Garcia, G.H.; Iwanowski, L.; and Lightfoot, W.E. New ultrastructural evidence for a protein transport system in endothelial cells of gerbil brains. *Acta Neuropathol* 47:105-110, 1979.

Meresse, S.; Dehouck, M.P.; Delorme, P.M.; Bensaid, J.P.; Tauber, C.; Delbart, C.; Fruchart, J.C.; and Cecchelli, R. Bovine brain endothelial cells express tight junctions and monoamine oxidase activity in long-term culture. *J Neurochem* 53:1363-1371, 1989.

Neuwelt, E.A., and Rapoport, S.I. Modification of the blood-brain barrier in the chemotherapy of malignant brain tumors. *Federations Proc* 43:214-219, 1984.

Newman, E.A. Membrane physiology of retinal glial (Müller) cells. *J Neurosci* 5:2225-2239, 1985.

Noda, M.; Ko, M.; Ogura, A.; Liu, D.-G.; Amano, T.; Takano, T.; and Ikawa, Y. Sarcoma viruses carrying ras oncogenes induce differentiation-associated properties in a neuronal cell line. *Nature* 318:73-75, 1985.

Okuda, O.; Bressler, J.; Chang, L.; and Brightman, M.W. Viral Kirsten ras infection differentiates PC12 cells and enhances their survival upon implantation to brain. *Exp Neurol* 113:330-337, 1991.

Palkovits, M. Neuropeptides in the hypothalamo-hypophyseal system: Lateral retrochiasmatic area as a common gate for neuronal fibers toward the median eminence. *Peptides* 5(Suppl 1):35-39, 1984.

Pappas, G.D., and Sagen, J. Fine structural correlates of vascular permeability of chromaffin cell transplants in CNS pain modulatory regions. *Exp Neurol* 102:280-289, 1988.

Rapoport, S.I.; Hori, M.; and Klatzo, I. Testing of a hypothesis for osmotic opening of the blood-brain barrier. *Am J Physiol* 223:323-331, 1972.

Reese, T.S., and Karnovsky, M.J. Fine structural localization of a blood-brain barrier to exogenous peroxidase. *J Cell Biol* 34:207-217, 1967.

Rennels, M.L.; Gregory, T.F.; Blaumanis, O.R.; Fujimoto, K.; and Grady, P.A. Evidence for a paravascular fluid circulation in the mammalian central nervous system, provided by the rapid distribution of tracer protein throughout the brain from the subarachnoid space. *Brain Res* 326:47-63, 1985.

Rosenstein, J.M., and Brightman, M.W. Circumventing the blood-brain barrier with autonomic ganglion transplants. *Science* 221:879-881, 1983.

Rubin, L.L.; Barbu, K.; Bard, C.; Cannon, D.E.; Hall, H.; Horner, M.; Janatpour, C.; Liaw, C.; Manning, K.; Morales, J.; Porter, S.; Tanner, L.; Tomaselli, K.; and Yednock, T. Differentiation of brain endothelial cells in cell culture. In: Abbott, J.; Lieberman, E.M.; and Raff, M., eds. *Glial-Neuronal Interaction.* Vol. 633. New York: New York Academy of Sciences, in press.

Rutten, M.J.; Hoover, R.L.; and Karnovsky, M.J. Electrical resistance and macromolecular permeability of brain endothelial monolayer cultures. *Brain Res* 425:301-310, 1987.

Shaver, S.W.; Kadekaro, M.; and Gross, P.M. Differential rates of glucose metabolism across subregions of the subfornical organ in Brattleboro rats. *Regul Pept* 27:37-49, 1990a.

Shaver, S.W.; Sposito, N.M.; and Gross, P.M. Quantitative fine structure of capillaries in subregions of the rat subfornical organ. *J Comp Neurol* 294:145-152, 1990b.

Stewart, P.A., and Wiley, M.J. Developing nervous tissue induces formation of blood-brain characteristics in invading endothelial cells: A study using quail-chick transplantation chimeras. *Dev Biol* 84:183-192, 1981.

Tao-Cheng, J.-H.; Nagy, Z.; and Brightman, M.W. Tight junctions of brain endothelium in vitro are enhanced by astroglia. *J Neurosci* 7:3293-3299, 1987.

Tao-Cheng, J.-H.; Nagy, Z.; and Brightman, M.W. Astrocytic orthogonal arrays of intramembranous particle assemblies are modulated by brain endothelial cells in vitro. *J Neurocytol* 19:143-153, 1990.

Tao-Cheng, J.-H.; Okuda, O.; Chang, L.; and Brightman, M.W. Cellular interactions between brain endothelial and neuronal cells in vitro. *Soc Neurosci Abstr* 15:691A, 1989.

Tsubaki, S.I.; Brightman, M.W.; Nakagawa, H.N.; Owens, E.; and Blasberg, R.G. Local blood flow and vascular permeability of autonomic ganglion transplants in the brain. *Brain Res* 424:71-83, 1987.

Vick, N.A. Brain tumor microvasculature. In: Weiss, L.; Gilbert, H.A.; and Posner, J.B., eds. *Brain Metastases.* Boston: G.K. Hall, 1980. pp. 115-133.

Wakai, S.; Meiselman, S.E.; and Brightman, M.W. Focal circumvention of blood-brain barrier with grafts of muscle, skin and autonomic ganglia. *Brain Res* 386:209-222, 1986.

Weindl, A. Neuroendocrine aspects of circumventricular organs. In: Ganong, W.F., and Martini, L., eds. *Frontiers in Neuroendocrinology.* New York: Oxford Press, 1973. pp. 3-32.

Yoshida, Y.; Yamada, M.; Wakabayashi, K.; and Ikuta, F. Endothelial fenestrae in the rat fetal cerebrum. *Dev Brain Res* 44:211-219, 1988.

AUTHORS

Milton W. Brightman, Ph.D.
Section Head
Laboratory of Neurobiology
National Institute of Neurological Disorders and Stroke
National Institutes of Health
Building 36, Room 2A-29
9000 Rockville Pike
Bethesda, MD 20892

Yoshiaki Kadota, M.D.
Neurosurgeon
Department of Neurosurgery
Juntendo University School of Medicine
Tokyo
JAPAN

The Blood-Brain Barrier Is Not a "Barrier" for Many Drugs

Joseph D. Fenstermacher

INTRODUCTION

Because there is little or no movement of solute between blood and brain through the intercellular clefts of the capillaries, drugs and other compounds enter most brain areas by passing through the endothelial cells (the exceptions to this are the choroid plexus and circumventricular organs, where rapid transfer may occur by way of the intercellular junctions and/or transendothelial fenestrations). To some extent, all solutes move across the blood-brain barrier (BBB) by dissolving in the endothelial cell membranes and diffusing through them and the endothelial cytoplasm. In addition, blood-brain transfer of some solutes is facilitated by specific membrane transporters or carriers or is set, in part, by other processes.

More than 90 years ago, Overton (1900) demonstrated that the permeability of cell membranes depends on the lipid solubility and diffusability of the penetrating solute. More recently, Orbach and Finkelstein (1980) have shown that the permeability of planar lipid (lecithin) bilayer membranes to nonelectrolytes is in agreement with Overton's rule; that is, permeability was proportional to the hexadecane:water partition coefficient times diffusion coefficient (PcDc). (Incidentally, as pointed out by Orbach and Finkelstein, lipid solubility can be approximated by solubility in many nonpolar organic solvents, including hexadecane, olive oil, ethyl ether, and octanol.) This suggests that BBB permeability also might follow Overton's rule.

OVERTON'S RULE AND THE BLOOD-BRAIN BARRIER

To show that solute permeation through the BBB fits Overton's rule, good experimental estimates of blood-brain transfer constants are needed. Transfer constants are determined by intravenously administering the material of interest and subsequently measuring its time course in blood and uptake by brain. From these data, one or more of three unidirectional transfer constants—the

108

extraction fraction (E), the influx rate constant (K_1), and the efflux rate constant (k_2)—is calculated. If the rate of cerebral blood flow is known and the experiments have been carefully designed and rigorously executed, then a permeability-surface area (PS) product can be calculated from E, K_1, or k_2 and used as an indicator of BBB "permeability" (Fenstermacher et al. 1986).

With respect to the lipid solubility part of Overton's rule, several respectable experimental studies have indicated a linear correlation between PS product and either olive oil:water or octanol:water Pc for cerebral capillaries (Cornford et al. 1982; Levin 1980; Oldendorf 1974; Rapoport et al. 1979). The applicability of Overton's rule per se to the BBB has been examined in several reviews (Fenstermacher 1983, 1989; Fenstermacher and Rapoport 1984). In these reviews, blood-to-brain transfer constants were determined from published reports for 11 or more physiological substances, and PS products were calculated from these constants. Plots of PS product vs. the product of the octanol:water PcDc yielded a linear relation over a 10,000-fold range. In agreement with Overton's rule, the slope was one (1.0) on a log-log scale. Recently, this relationship has been extended for the BBB to cover 23 physiological compounds, 76 measurements, and a millionfold range (J.D. Fenstermacher and C.S. Patlak, manuscript in preparation).

Figure 1 is an example of such a plot with data for 11 compounds and 41 measurements (1 to 10 different measurements per compound); the slope of the parallel lines enveloping the points is one. Transfer of these substances across the BBB, therefore, seems to follow Overton's rule. Incidentally, the major cause of the variation in the PcDc product is the partition coefficient, and a log-lot plot of PS vs. Pc for these same data also yields a linear plot with a slope of one.

The good agreement between BBB permeability and Overton's rule implies that the cerebral capillary wall functions like an aporous membrane. That is, the aqueous channels through the BBB, if present, are so small that most compounds cannot pass through them. This is consistent with earlier reports that suggest the effective pore radius or slit width of the BBB is around 0.7 nm (Fenstermacher and Johnson 1966; Paulson et al. 1977), but it conflicts with the more recent estimates of an effective pore radius of 8 nm for frog cerebral capillaries (Crone 1984) and for confluent monolayers of cerebral endothelial cells (van Bree et al. 1988). An effective pore radius of 8 nm, however, seems unduly large since aqueous channels of such size would yield a PS product for sucrose, a relatively impermeable solute, twentyfold greater than measured (figure 1) if these pores comprise as little as 0.001 percent of the BBB surface area (Dorovini-Zis et al. 1983).

109

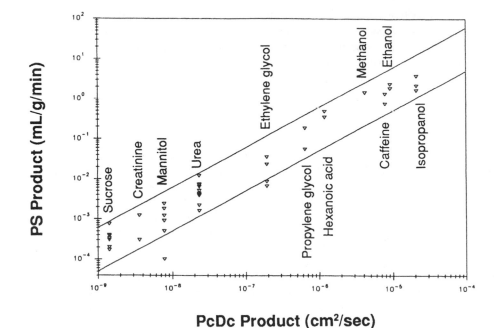

FIGURE 1. *Log-lot plot of PS product vs. octanol:water PcDc product for 11 physiological compounds. The PS products are from Fenstermacher (1983, 1989) and Fenstermacher and Rapoport (1984). Two or more PS values are plotted for 10 of these 11 compounds because two or more separate measurements of K_1 or E were found. The parallel diagonal lines enclose or envelop 38 of the 41 points and have a slope of one. The vertical spread of the envelope is 10 mL/g/min (one order of magnitude of PS).*

The influx of a highly permeable compound is almost completely limited by the rate of blood flow or, more precisely, the product of the rate of blood flow (F) and the distribution volume of the exchangeable material in the blood (V_f). For most of the studies providing data for the present (figure 1) and the published PS vs. PcDc plots (Fenstermacher 1983, 1989; Fenstermacher and Rapoport 1984), the animals were anesthetized with pentobarbital, and the forebrain or part of the forebrain was sampled. In the case of highly permeable solutes, the blood flow-exchangeable volume product (FV_f) is around 1 mL/g/min. When E or extraction is greater than 95 percent, then tissue influx is considered to be flow-limited, and the PS/FV_f ratio is equal to or greater than 3.0 according to the single capillary model and the Renkin-Crone equation (Crone 1965; Fenstermacher et al. 1986; Renkin 1959). If FV_f is therefore assumed to be around 1.0 mL/g/min, then PS should be greater than 3.0 mL/g/min for a substance whose rate of influx across the BBB is set virtually completely by blood flow. As indicated in figure 2, this condition would be expected to hold when the PcDc product $>2x10^{-5}$ cm^2/sec or the octanol:water Pc>1.2 (PS vs. Pc plot not shown).

The influx of a relatively impermeable solute is virtually completely set by its PS product at the BBB. For the permeability-limited case, the extraction fraction is less than 0.2, and $PS/FV_f<0.2$ (Fenstermacher et al. 1986). Since $FV_f=0.5$ mL/g/min for relatively impermeable solutes because they mainly distribute in plasma, then PS should be less than 0.1 mL/g/min, which occurs when the PcDc product $<6x10^{-7}$ cm^2/sec (figure 2) or the octanol:water Pc$<5x10^{-2}$ (graph not shown).

For solutes with PS products between 0.1 and 3.0 mL/g/min, influx depends strongly on both PS and FV_f. In this situation, PcDc products would be expected to be around $6x10^{-7}$ to $2x10^{-5}$ cm^2/sec (octanol:water Pc between 0.05 and 1.2). This "area" lies between the PS-limiting and FV_f-limiting domains in figure 2.

Carrier systems or transporters facilitate the transfer of several compounds across the BBB. For example, the fluxes of D-glucose and L-phenylalanine across the BBB are enhanced by the glucose transporter, GLUT-1, and the large neutral amino acid carrier, respectively. The measured PS products of such compounds would be considerably higher than those predicted on the basis of their PcDc products and the relationship shown in figure 2 if the transporter-mediated flow accounts for a major portion of the flux. As previously indicated (Fenstermacher 1983), the PS product of D-glucose is 50 to 100 times higher than that predicted by the PS vs. PcDc plot and that of L-glucose, whose transcapillary flux is not facilitated, and the PS product of L-phenylalanine is about 10 times greater than predicted. Incidentally, this analysis indicates the usefulness of PS vs. PcDc plots in assessing the relative importance of simple diffusional (lipid-mediated) and carrier-mediated flows of solutes across the BBB.

DRUG INFLUX ACROSS THE BBB

Acceptable estimates of transfer rate constants and PcDc products have been found not only for the physiological compounds indicated above (figure 1) but

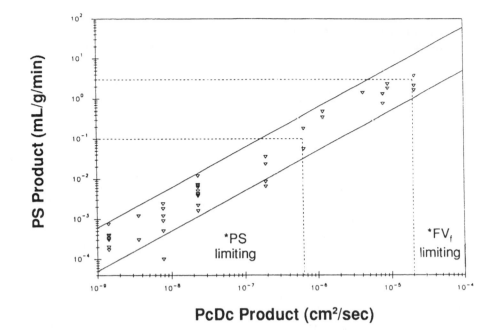

FIGURE 2. *This graph is identical to figure 1 except the names of the compounds have been deleted and dashed lines have been added marking the putative permeability (PS)-limiting and blood flow (FV_f)-limiting domains. These domains are defined as PS<0.10 mL/g/min and PS>3.0 mL/g/min, respectively.*

also for 22 drugs; subsequently, the PS products of these drugs have been calculated and tabulated (Fenstermacher 1989). The PS and PcDc products of these 22 drugs and the relationship between PS and PcDc, shown in figure 2, indicate several points.

First, the experimentally derived PS products of most of these drugs are less than the PS products estimated from their partition and diffusion coefficients. That is, the experimental PS products were around or below the lower diagonal line in figures 1 and 2. Figure 3 shows this relationship for a representative set of 12 of these 22 drugs. Since none of the experimental PS products were above the upper diagonal line, carrier- or transporter-mediated flux does not appear to be involved with the blood-to-brain transfer of any of these drugs.

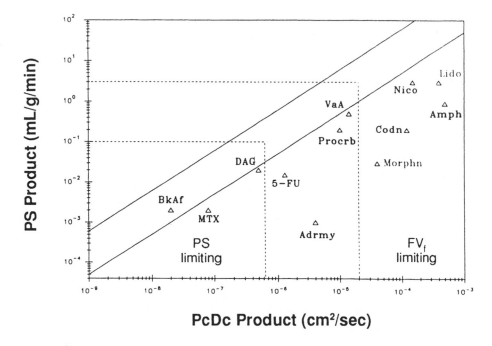

FIGURE 3. *This graph is similar to figure 2. The 41 PS products in figures 1 and 2 have been dropped, and PS products for 12 representative drugs have been plotted. These values have been taken from Fenstermacher (1989). The drugs' names and abbreviations are Baker's antifol (BkAf), methotrexate (MTX), dianhydrogalactitol (DAG), 5-fluorouracil (5-FU), Adriamycin (Adrmy), procarbazine (Procrb), valproic acid (VaA), morphine (Morphn), codeine (Codn), nicotine (Nico), amphetamine (Amph), and lidocaine (Lido).*

Second, the lipid solubility is very low for only three of these drugs—BkAf, MTX, and DAG—and their PcDc products place them in the "PS-limiting" domain (figure 3). In other words, the BBB would be expected to limit markedly the influx of only 3 of these 22 drugs. Incidentally, the experimental PS product of BkAf falls within the envelope formed by the parallel diagonal lines in figure 3; it may be one of the few drugs in this set whose rate of influx depends almost entirely on its ability to dissolve in and diffuse through the BBB. For DAG, MTX, and most of the other drugs, different processes may be important in setting their rates of influx across the BBB.

Third, the PcDc products of 13 of these 22 drugs are greater than 2×10^{-5} cm^2/sec, which roughly corresponds to an octanol:water Pc greater than 2; therefore, in accordance with the preceding suggestion, the rates of influx of these drugs would be anticipated to be set mainly by the rate of blood flow or FV_f (figure 3). The PS products of five drugs with PcDc products between 2×10^{-5} and 1×10^{-3} cm^2/sec are indicated in figure 3; the data for three other drugs in this group, BCNU, propranolol, and phenobarbital, are not presented in figure 3. The PcDc products of the five remaining drugs in this set—phenytoin, vincristine, pyrimethamine, diazepam, and CCNU—are equal to or greater than 3×10^{-3} cm^2/sec. The PS products of these five drugs ranged from 0.006 (vincristine) to >3 (diazepam) mL/g/min and are not plotted in figure 3. The PS products of flow-limited solutes at the BBB will be around 2 to 3 mL/g/min because higher values cannot be accurately determined when $PS>3FV_f$ (Fenstermacher 1989). The drugs with measured PS products in this range are nicotine, lidocaine, and diazepam; thus, the major process in setting the influx rate of these three drugs is the rate of delivery of exchangeable drug to the microvessels. The PS products for the remaining 10 drugs in the FV_f-limiting group lie considerably below the lower line of the diagonal envelope in figure 3, and processes other than blood flow and dissolving and diffusing through the BBB are likely to be important in setting influx.

Fourth, the remaining 6 of these 22 drugs are moderately lipid soluble (0.08<Pc<1.0) and have PcDc products between 8×10^{-7} and 2×10^{-6} cm^2/sec. According to figure 2, the influx rate of these drugs would be expected to depend on both PS and FV_f, and their PS products should be between 0.1 and 1.2 mL/g/min. The data for four of the six drugs in the moderately lipid-soluble group are given in figure 3. The measured PS products of these six drugs are either somewhat below the lower diagonal line of the envelope (valproic acid, procarbazine, tegafur [Ftorafur], and 5-fluorouracil) or 1 to 2 orders of magnitude below this line (dibromodulcitol and doxorubicin hydrochloride [Adriamycin]). This suggests that distributional processes other than passage through the BBB and blood flow affect the influx of these six drugs and, especially, strongly affect that of Adriamycin. Incidentally, the experimentally measured PS products for two additional "drugs" with PcDc products in this range, caffeine and ethanol, fit within the diagonal envelope (figure 1); and their rates of influx appear to depend on PS and FV_f in accordance with the equation for the single capillary model (Renkin 1959; Crone 1965) and Overton's rule.

As is apparently true for many physiological materials, the measured PS products at the BBB of six drugs fit Overton's rule as set forth in figures 1 and 2. These six drugs are ethanol and caffeine (figure 1), nicotine, lidocaine, and BkAf (figure 3) plus diazepam. The PS products of two other drugs, DAG and valproic acid (figure 3), appear to fit Overton's rule fairly closely. The measured PS products of the remaining drugs in this group, most of which are moderately to highly lipid soluble, are less than would be predicted from Overton's rule (figure 3). Instead of questioning the broad applicability of Overton's rule to drug permeation through the BBB, two other possibilities are worthy of consideration: (1) the incorrect measurement of transfer constants and PS products and (2) the involvement of other physiological and pharmacological processes.

MEASUREMENT PROBLEMS

Since the PS products of 16 of these drugs were low relative to their lipid solubility and diffusability, their transfer constants may have been underestimated. Low transfer constants are obtained when the amount of drug that has influxed into the brain is underevaluated and/or when the driving force for influx, the concentration-time integral of exchangeable drug within the perfused capillaries, is overestimated (Fenstermacher et al. 1986).

Underestimation of drug influx arises most commonly from not properly accounting for drug efflux during the course of the experiment. With some techniques, it is assumed that all drug that has entered the brain during the experiment is still there at the time of tissue sampling. For a permeable drug that does not instantly and virtually completely bind within the capillaries and parenchyma, drug efflux may be appreciable after only a few seconds. With these approaches and such drugs, tissue samples must be obtained within 5 to 15 seconds after drug administration. For other techniques, tissue is sampled several times, a compartmental model is assumed, and influx and efflux rate constants are estimated by compartmental analysis. The results obtained are model-specific and depend strongly on accurate and extensive sampling of tissue and blood. With such approaches, erroneous values of K_1 are obtained readily and often for drugs with complicated distribution kinetics.

The concentration-time integral within the capillaries can be overestimated easily with drugs that bind to plasma proteins and/or interact with blood cells. The transfer constants should be determined on the basis of drug concentration in the fluid (blood or infusate) flowing into the capillaries. The value obtained will then be correct with respect to this part of the calculation of E or K_1, but the accurate evaluation of PS from these transfer constants requires additional data plus a more complex model and equation than the single capillary model and the Renkin-Crone equation (Pardridge and Landaw 1984; Robinson and Rapoport 1986). Further analysis of this problem is beyond the scope of this review, and plasma protein binding and blood cell interaction are discussed only in a simple, qualitative sense below.

OTHER PROCESSES INVOLVED WITH BLOOD-BRAIN TRANSFER

Over the past decade, various observations have indicated several processes that may be involved in limiting or lowering blood-to-brain transfer of drugs. In addition to plasma protein binding and red cell interaction, these processes include metabolism within the endothelial cell and transfer from the endothelial cell back into the blood.

Many drugs bind to plasma proteins (Cornford et al. 1983, 1985; Dubey et al. 1989; Hamberger et al. 1987; Pardridge et al. 1983; Rapoport et al. 1979). More than half of the 22 drugs mentioned above bind to plasma proteins; incorrect accounting for this can lead to sizable (more than 1,000-fold) overestimation of the drug's effective concentration-time integral. In recent years, several groups have produced evidence that some drugs rapidly dissociate from plasma proteins and are available for blood-to-brain exchange. For example, using the brain uptake index technique, Pardridge and colleagues (1983) have shown that propranolol and lidocaine dissociate from plasma proteins during a single capillary passage and enter brain tissue, and Hamberger and colleagues (1987) have observed that some of the progabide bound to plasma proteins and contained in red blood cells exchanges across the BBB. Clearly, binding to plasma proteins and availability for exchange across cerebral capillaries is a complicated and variable process for many drugs, and careful examination of this is necessary to understand blood-to-brain transfer. The same thing holds for drug uptake and release from blood cells.

Ghersi-Egea and colleagues (1988) have reported measurable levels of four drug-metabolizing enzymes in microsomal fractions from endothelial cells obtained from rat brain microvessels. These enzymes are cytochrome P-450-linked monooxygenases, epoxide hydrolase, NADPH:cytochrome P-450 reductase, and 1-naphthol NDP-glucuronosyl transferase. Lipophilic xenobiotics are substrates for these enzymes. Other studies also have indicated the presence of dopa-decarboxylase and monoamine oxidase in cerebral capillaries (Kalaria et al. 1988; Wade and Katzman 1975a). The capacity of these systems to reduce the penetration of their substrate drugs has not been examined in vivo; and the fate of these metabolites have not been determined, with the exception of L-dopa and the dopa-decarboxylase-monoamine oxidase system (Wade and Katzman 1975a, 1975b).

Brain capillaries recently have been shown to express or contain P-glycoprotein (Pgp or P-170), the multidrug resistant (MDR) transporter that mediates the efflux of various natural-product drugs (e.g., vincristine and Adriamycin) from drug-resistant cultured tumor cells (Cordon-Cardo et al. 1989; Thiebaut et al. 1989). The blood-to-brain transfer of these drugs is notoriously slow and may be limited by the MDR transporter moving them from endothelial cells back into blood.

The distribution of drugs between blood and brain involves several different processes. Some of these processes (e.g., cerebral blood flow and local BBB permeability) are known to vary among brain areas. In addition, local variations in some of these other disposition processes—for instance, monoamine oxidase activity (Kalaria et al. 1988)—have been suggested. Drug influx almost certainly varies widely among brain areas because of these dissimilarities.

CONCLUSION

The BBB does not restrict the entry of many addictive drugs, including alcohol, nicotine, and caffeine. In fact, the initial distribution of such drugs in the brain is likely to reflect blood flow, whereas the later phase(s) of distribution strongly depends on the fate of the drug within the brain parenchyma (e.g., metabolism and receptor binding). The somewhat lower influx rates of such drugs as codeine and phenobarbital may be more the result of plasma protein binding and blood cell interaction than of modest BBB permeability. Thus, for many drugs, the BBB is not much of a "barrier," and this aspect of their blood-brain distribution contributes to their popularity in this impatient age and disenchanted society.

REFERENCES

Cordon-Cardo, C.; O'Brien, J.P.; Casals, D.; Rittman-Grauer, L.; Biedler, J.L.; Melamed, M.R.; and Bertino, J.R. Multidrug-resistance gene (P-glycoprotein) is expressed by endothelial cells at blood-brain barrier sites. *Proc Natl Acad Sci U S A* 86:695-698, 1989.

Cornford, E.M.; Braun, L.D.; Oldendorf, W.H.; and Hill, M.A. Comparison of lipid-mediated blood-brain barrier penetrability in neonates and adults. *Am J Physiol* 243:C161-C168, 1982.

Cornford, E.M.; Diep, C.P.; and Pardridge, W.M. Blood-brain transport at valproic acid. *J Neurochem* 44:1541-1550, 1985.

Cornford, E.M.; Pardridge, W.M.; Braun, L.D.; Oldendorf, W.H.; and Hill, M.A. Increased blood-brain barrier transport of protein-bound anticonvulsant drugs in the newborn. *J Cereb Blood Flow Metab* 3:280-286, 1983.

Crone, C. The permeability of brain capillaries to non-electrolytes. *Acta Physiol Scand* 64:407-417, 1965.

Crone, C. Lack of selectivity to small ions in paracellular pathways in cerebral and muscle capillaries of the frog. *J Physiol* 353:317-337, 1984.

Dorovini-Zis, K.; Sato, M.; Goping, G.; Rapoport, S.; and Brightman, M. Ionic lanthanum passage across cerebral endothelium exposed to hyperosmotic arabinose. *Acta Neuropathol (Berl)* 60:49-60, 1983.

Dubey, R.K.; McAllister, C.B.; Inoue, M.; and Wilkinson, G.R. Plasma binding and transport of diazepam across the blood-brain barrier. *J Clin Invest* 84:1155-1159, 1989.

Fenstermacher, J.D. Drug transfer across the blood-brain barrier. In: Breimer, D.D., and Speiser, P., eds. *Topics in Pharmaceutical Science 1983.* Amsterdam: Elsevier, 1983. pp. 143-154.

Fenstermacher, J.D. The pharmacology of the blood-brain barrier. In: Neuwelt, E., ed. *Implications of the Blood-Brain Barrier and Its Manipulation.* Vol. 1. New York: Plenum, 1989. pp. 137-155.

Fenstermacher, J.D.; Blasberg, R.G.; and Patlak, C.S. Methods for quantifying the transport of drugs across brain barrier systems. In: Goldman, I.D., ed. *Membrane Transport Antineoplastic Agents: The International Encyclopedia of Pharmacology and Therapeutics.* Oxford, England: Pergamon, 1986. pp. 113-146.

Fenstermacher, J.D., and Johnson, J.A. Filtration and reflection coefficients of the rabbit blood-brain barrier. *Am J Physiol* 211:341-346, 1966.

Fenstermacher, J.D., and Rapoport, S.I. The blood-brain barrier. In: Renkin, E.M., and Michel, C.C., eds. *Handbook of Physiology: The Microcirculation.* Bethesda, MD: American Physiological Society, 1984. pp. 969-1000.

Ghersi-Egea, J.-F.; Minn, A.; and Siest, G. A new aspect of the protective functions of the blood-brain barrier: Activities of four drug-metabolizing enzymes in isolated rat brain microvessels. *Life Sci* 42:2515-2523, 1988.

Hamberger, C.; Urien, S.; Essassi, D.; Grimaldi, B.; Barre, J.; Taiclet, A.; Thenet, J.P.; and Tillement, J.P. Effect of erythrocytes and plasma protein binding on the transport of progabide and SL 75102 through the rat blood-brain barrier. *Biochem Pharmacol* 36:2641-2645, 1987.

Kalaria, R.N.; Mitchell, M.J.; and Harik, S.I. Monoamine oxidase of the human brain and liver. *Brain* 111:1441-1451, 1988.

Levin, V.A. Relationship of octanol/water partition coefficient and molecular weight to rat brain capillary permeability. *J Med Chem* 23:682-684, 1980.

Oldendorf, W.H. Lipid solubility and drug penetration of the blood-brain barrier. *Proc Soc Exp Biol Med* 147:813-816, 1974.

Orbach, E., and Finkelstein, A. The nonelectrolyte permeability of planar lipid bilayer membranes. *J Gen Physiol* 75:427-436, 1980.

Overton, E. Studien uber die Aufnahme der Anilin farben durch die lebende Zelle. *Jahrbach Wissenschattlich Botanik* 34:669-701, 1900.

Pardridge, W.M., and Landaw, E. Tracer kinetic model of blood-brain barrier transport of plasma-protein ligands. Empiric testing of the free hormone hypothesis. *J Clin Invest* 74:745-752, 1984.

Pardridge, W.M.; Sakiyama, R.; and Fierer, G. Transport of propranolol and lidocaine through the rat blood-brain barrier. Primary role of globulin-bound drug. *J Clin Invest* 71:900-908, 1983.

Paulson, O.B.; Hertz, M.H.; Bolwig, T.G.; and Lassen, N.A. Filtration and diffusion of water across the blood-brain barrier. *Microvasc Res* 13:113-124, 1977.

Rapoport, S.I.; Ohno, K.; and Pettigrew, K.D. Drug entry into brain. *Brain Res* 172:354-359, 1979.

Renkin, E.M. Transport of potassium-42 from blood to tissue in isolated mammalian skeletal muscles. *Am J Physiol* 197:1205-1210, 1959.

Robinson, P.J., and Rapoport, S.I. Kinetics of protein binding determine rates of uptake of drugs by brain. *Am J Physiol* 251:R1212-R1215, 1986.

Thiebaut, F.; Tsuruo, T.; Hamada, H.; Gottesman, M.A.; Pastan, I.; and Willingham, M.C. Immunohistochemical localization in normal tissue of different epitopes in the multidrug transport protein P170: Evidence for localizing in brain capillaries and crossreactivity of one antibody with a muscle protein. *J Histochem Cytochem* 37:159-164, 1989.

van Bree, J.B.M.M.; deBoer, A.G.; Danhof, M.; Ginsel, L.A.; and Breimer, D.D. Characterization of an "in vitro" blood-brain barrier: Effects of molecular size and lipophilicity on cerebrovascular endothelial transport rates of drugs. *J Pharmacol Exp Ther* 247:1233-1239, 1988.

Wade, L.A., and Katzman, R. Rat brain regional uptake and decarboxylation of L-dopa following carotid injection. *Am J Physiol* 228:352-359, 1975a.

Wade, L.A., and Katzman, R. Synthetic amino acids and the nature of L-dopa transport at the blood-brain barrier. *J Neurochem* 25:837-842, 1975b.

ACKNOWLEDGMENT

Preparation of this chapter was supported in part by National Institutes of Health grants NS-21157, NS-26004, and HL-35791.

AUTHOR

Joseph D. Fenstermacher, Ph.D.
Professor
Department of Neurological Surgery
State University of New York at Stony Brook
Health Science Center, T12-080
Stony Brook, NY 11794-8122

Drug Delivery to the Brain: Barrier Modification and Drug Modification Methodologies

Stanley I. Rapoport

INTRODUCTION

Recent advances in the fields of pharmacology and molecular biology have led to a greater understanding of disease processes, allowing development of new classes of therapeutic agents that can interact with specific intracellular and extracellular targets (Greig et al. 1990a; Pomponi et al. 1990). Several drugs, peptides, biological response modifiers, and monoclonal antibodies are available and have proven of value (1) in inhibiting a variety of malignant and infectious diseases; (2) in ameliorating neurotransmitter, enzyme, or growth imbalances in culture systems; or (3) in animal models using direct intracranial administration. However, therapeutic efficacy in vivo, particularly with regard to the central nervous system (CNS), frequently is diminished or prevented by the inability of the agent to reach and maintain active concentrations in the brain for an appropriate length of time. Frequently, the molecule is too large or has polar functional groups, so that its access to the brain target organ is limited by the blood-brain barrier (BBB).

The BBB is a system of layers of cells—at the cerebral capillary endothelium, the choroid plexus epithelium, and the arachnoid membranes—that are connected by tight junctions (zonulae occludens) and that together separate the brain and cerebrospinal fluid (CSF) from blood (Rapoport 1976). The junctions confer on each layer the properties of an extended cell membrane, as they limit paracellular exchange of water-soluble nonelectrolytes, ions, proteins, and peptides, forcing transcellular exchange. The cell membranes at each of the layers are lipoid in nature, so that the property that generally governs passive penetration of a drug into the brain, via these layers, is the extent of its lipid solubility, measured as the octanol:water partition coefficient.

Figure 1 illustrates that cerebrovascular permeability is roughly proportional to lipid solubility for nonelectrolytes whose molecular weights are less than 1,000

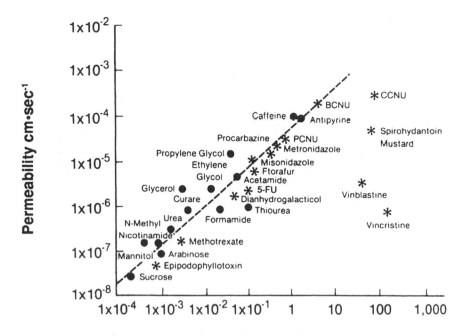

FIGURE 1. *Relation between cerebrovascular permeability and octanol:water partition coefficient of several agents (asterisk designates anticancer drug)*

SOURCES: Ohno et al. 1978; Greig et al. 1990a, 1990b

daltons, including anticancer drugs. The permeability coefficient, P cm•sec^{-1}, is defined by the following operational equation for unidirectional flux from blood to brain across cerebral capillaries and can be determined experimentally by appropriate quantitative techniques (e.g., Ohno et al. 1978; Takasato et al. 1984):

$$dC_{brain}/dt = PA\,fC_{plasma} \qquad (1)$$

C_{plasma} is the net plasma concentration at any time t after drug administration; C_{brain} is the brain parenchymal concentration (excluding intravascular material); A is the surface area of the capillary bed (about 180 cm^2•g brain^{-1} for gray matter); and f is the steady-state fraction of drug unbound and un-ionized in plasma. In equation 1, the ionized form of a dissociable drug, whose plasma fraction depends on plasma pH (see below), is ignored because its permeability at the BBB is about one-thousandth of the permeability of the un-ionized form (Rapoport 1976). Equation 1 holds following an intravenous (IV) bolus injection of a labeled drug, where it is not so long as to allow sufficient accumulation of drug in the brain to provide significant back-diffusion to blood (Ohno et al. 1978). However, to calculate the time-dependent concentration profile in the brain for any administration regimen one needs to know the extended plasma concentration profile; the concentration profile of the agent in CSF; and the exchange coefficients between blood and brain, between CSF and brain, and between extracellular and intracellular (or bound) brain compartments. Appropriate equations derived for a bolus injection, continuous IV infusion, and a step elevation in blood concentration of drugs have been derived (Rapoport et al. 1982).

Exceptions to the proportionality relation in figure 1 have been noted for several compounds. For example, the lipophilic anticancer vinca alkaloids vinblastine and vincristine are much less permeable than expected from their high octanol: water partition coefficients (Greig et al. 1990b). For such relatively large compounds (vincristine has a molecular weight of 825 daltons; vinblastine, 814 daltons), steric hindrance and molecular charge distribution also influence cerebrovascular permeability. The author suggests that the additive rules that govern bulk phase octanol:water partition coefficients (Hansch 1972) break down for large molecules in which distances between hydrophobic and ionic regions within the molecule become significant with respect to the distance of the membrane-water interface and of the thickness of the biological membrane (about 100 Å).

For organic acids, as well as for such bases as morphine, the extent of dissociation in blood may markedly influence access to the brain, as the un-ionized form usually has an octanol:water partition coefficient 1,000 times greater than the ionized form (Rapoport 1976). Thus, for morphine, a pK_a of 7.93 at 37 °C causes its rate of entry into the brain from blood to increase with metabolic alkalosis by as much as fourfold between a blood pH of 7.2 and 7.6 (Shulman et al. 1984).

Availability of a drug for entry into the brain depends not only on its plasma concentration profile (Rapoport et al. 1982) but also on the extent and kinetics of its binding with and release from plasma proteins and other plasma constituents (Robinson and Rapoport 1986). Equation 1 indicates that only unbound drug in plasma is available for entry into the brain. However, recent studies have challenged this "free drug hypothesis," at least with regard to some agents (Greig et al. 1990a). Experiments using palmitate, arachidonate, phenytoin, diazepam, and other benzodiazepines have demonstrated that these latter agents, unlike such others as bilirubin, erythrocin B, and phenobarbital, are not restrictively bound to plasma constituents and that their extraction from blood into brain is greater than predicted by their steady-state free plasma concentrations, fC_{plasma} (Rapoport 1983a; Cornford 1984; Levitan et al. 1984; Jones et al. 1988). The rates of release of these drugs (off-rates) from plasma protein are quite rapid, allowing them to be stripped and made available for diffusion into brain during the second or two that blood passes through brain capillaries (circulation time). Their extraction fraction (upper bound) is given as follows:

$$E = 1 - e^{-(1-\alpha)k_3' t} \qquad (2)$$

where E is the fraction of total drug that is extracted during passage of blood through brain; t is transit time of blood passing through brain capillaries; k_3' is effective rate constant for drug uptake into brain; and α is equilibrium fraction of total drug bound to protein in arterial plasma.

In addition to the proportionality between permeability and octanol:water partition that characterizes simple passive diffusion between blood and brain (figure 1), entry into the brain in some important cases depends on specific transport mechanisms at the BBB. For example, there are several facilitated, stereospecific, and saturable transport systems at cerebral capillaries for amino acids, peptides, small organic acids, and monosaccharides, whose affinity characteristics can be exploited to enhance drug entry into the brain (see below) (Rapoport 1976; Greig et al. 1987; Smith et al. 1989). Furthermore, receptor-mediated transfer of such proteins as transferrin and of such peptides as insulin at the cerebrovasculature has been demonstrated, as well as enhanced transcytosis of positively charged compared with neutral or negatively charged proteins and large polysaccharides (Fishman et al. 1987; Armstrong et al. 1989; Pardridge et al. 1990). Proteins also can gain access to the brain after first entering CSF at the choroid plexus (Felgenhauer 1974; Rapoport 1983b), and their rates of entry are greater if they are more positively charged (Griffin and Giffels 1982). Finally, enzymes existing at the cerebral capillaries can be inhibited to enhance entry of drugs sensitive to metabolism. Thus, administration of inhibitors of capillary dopa-decarboxylase enhances brain uptake of L-dopa in the treatment of Parkinson's disease (Sourkes 1981).

This chapter examines studies on enhancing drug entry into the brain, which were conducted, to a large extent, at the Laboratory of Neurosciences in Bethesda, MD. Two approaches are discussed, one based on the structure and vulnerability of the BBB to osmotic exposure, the other on drug modification with a view to enhance brain uptake by any of the following factors: prolonging half-life in blood, increasing lipid solubility to enhance passive diffusion according to the principle of figure 1, or enhancing transport of the drug via established carrier mechanisms for amino acids.

OSMOTIC OPENING OF THE BBB

The cellular nature of the BBB at cerebral capillaries, first demonstrated by Reese and Karnovsky (1967), suggested to the author's group (Rapoport 1970; Rapoport et al. 1972) that the BBB might be made more permeable by applying hypertonic solutions on either side of the vascular wall and thereby osmotically shrinking vascular endothelial cells. Accordingly, this group investigated effects of hypertonic solutions, applied topically (extravascularly) for 10 minutes to the arachnoid surface of the rabbit brain, on the permeabilities of pial arterioles and venules to intravascular Evans blue-albumin. Minimal (threshold) concentrations were determined for various electrolytes and nonelectrolytes for increasing the permeability of the pial vessels to this tracer. When Evans blue was administered intravenously, 30 minutes after a threshold concentration of a particular test solution was applied to the brain surface for 10 minutes, the absence or presence of its extravasation demonstrated whether osmotic BBB opening was reversible.

An inverse relation between threshold concentration and octanol:water partition coefficient was demonstrated for reversibly acting agents, that is, those agents less lipid-soluble than ethylene glycol (octanol:water partition coefficient=0.012) (Rapoport et al. 1972; Rapoport 1976). This relation was interpreted to indicate that osmotic BBB opening was mediated by shrinkage of cerebrovascular endothelial cells, stressing and thereby widening interendothelial tight junctions. This suggested mechanism subsequently was confirmed, using electronmicroscopy and an electron dense tracer (horseradish peroxidase or ionic lanthanum) following intracarotid infusion of hypertonic urea or arabinose in animals (Brightman et al. 1973; Dorovini-Zis et al. 1983). Suggestions that osmotic BBB opening was mediated by increased transcellular vesicular transport later were shown to be unlikely (Rapoport and Robinson 1986; Robinson and Rapoport 1987). Indeed, tight junctional widening without stimulation of pinocytosis has been demonstrated at monolayers of cerebrovascular endothelia exposed to hypertonic arabinose solution (Dorovini-Zis et al. 1984).

In a series of quantitative studies in rabbits, rats, mice, and rhesus monkeys, the author's group and others showed that the BBB could be reversibly opened without damaging the brain by infusing any of several osmotic solutions into the carotid circulation, while maintaining appropriate oxygenation and blood flow to the brain. Two concentrated solutions proved most useful: 1.6 molal arabinose and 1.4 molar (1.6 molal) mannitol solution (Rapoport et al. 1980; Neuwelt 1989). At the author's laboratory, concentrated arabinose is used rather than mannitol solution in small animal experiments because of its lesser viscosity and lesser tendency to form crystals that produce embolic

125

neuropathology during the infusion procedure (Tomiwa et al. 1982; Rapoport and Robinson 1991). Postmortem studies demonstrated the absence of neurological abnormalities or neuropathology following the osmotic procedure (Rapoport and Thompson 1973; Tomiwa et al. 1982; Neuwelt et al. 1983; Cosolo et al. 1989), provided care was taken with regard to solution temperature, filtration, and animal maintenance. When this proscription was ignored, embolic brain damage occurred (Suzuki et al. 1988; Salahuddin et al. 1988). Brain edema follows osmotic treatment, as expected from the protective role of the intact BBB against edema (Rapoport 1985), but it is absent within 24 hours after the procedure (Rapoport et al. 1980).

Using a sensitive quantitative procedure to examine regional permeability of the BBB to [^{14}C]sucrose, Rapoport and colleagues (1980) showed that the BBB in pentobarbital-anesthetized rats was maximally opened at a threshold arabinose concentration of 1.6 molal for 30 seconds of intracarotid infusion. Higher concentrations had no incremental effect on BBB permeability, whereas 1.4 molal arabinose was minimally effective. However, the osmotic threshold is sensitive to the solute employed, to the animal species studied, as well as to the type of anesthetic used (Rapoport and Robinson 1991). Thus, 1.4 molar mannitol solution produces a maximal opening when infused into the carotid circulation of rats anesthetized with phenobarbital, ketamine-xylazine, or isoflurane but has a minimal BBB effect when methoxyflurane or fentanyl-doperidol is the anesthetic. The latter anesthetics make animals either more hypotensive or tachycardiac than does phenobarbital (Gumerlock and Neuwelt 1990).

The [^{14}C]sucrose method also was used to demonstrate that BBB opening is essentially reversed within 2 hours (Rapoport et al. 1980). Thus, the elevation of cerebrovascular permeability to [^{14}C]sucrose, following 1.6 molal arabinose infusion, has fallen dramatically by about 10 minutes after the procedure (suggesting that if drugs of similar size are to be employed they should be administered within this time). Furthermore, by using normally impermeant radiotracers of differing sizes, the author's group showed that the rate of decline of the permeability elevation following the osmotic procedure is greater for larger than for smaller tracer molecules. This observation is consistent with the interpretation that osmotic BBB modification is mediated by widening of tight junctions between endothelial cells but not by stimulation of transendothelial vesicular transport (see above) (Rapoport and Robinson 1986; Robinson and Rapoport 1987). It is likely that these open junctions (pores) are negatively charged, as permeability is increased more to positively charged than to neutral macromolecules (Armstrong et al. 1989). This suggests that entry of antibodies or other macromolecules into the brain following the osmotic procedure can be enhanced further by manipulating their charge.

In a series of animal studies, the author's group and collaborators also showed that the osmotic technique could be used to open the BBB to agents relevant to CNS disease: neutralizing antibodies to measles virus (Hicks et al. 1976); [^{3}H]norepinephrine and [^{125}I]albumin (Chiueh et al. 1978); lysosomal enzymes (Barranger et al. 1979); methotrexate (Ohata et al. 1985); bilirubin-albumin (Levine et al. 1985); and human interferon alpha (Greig et al. 1988). Clearances from brain, in relation to disease models, were determined for methotrexate and for bilirubin (Levine et al. 1985; Ohata et al. 1985) and illustrated the contribution of intracerebral binding or uptake on brain pharmacokinetics and pharmacodynamics. With regard to cancer chemotherapy, Neuwelt and colleagues (1983) evaluated the neurotoxicity of a number of antineoplastic agents that were allowed into the rat brain by the osmotic procedure; they concluded that doxorubicin, cis-platinum, bleomycin, 5-fluorouracil, and mitomycin are neurotoxic, whereas cyclophosphamide and methotrexate are not. Neuwelt (1989) summarizes additional studies on drug entry into the brain using the osmotic procedure.

Neuwelt and colleagues (1980) were the first to apply the osmotic procedure in the clinic for treating brain tumors (for a review, see Neuwelt 1989). They employed a combination of drugs—methotrexate, procarbazine, and cyclophosphamide—with the osmotic method. Their data provide an upper limit for morbidity and mortality associated with the osmotic procedure in humans as results were obtained on patients with brain tumors using anticancer drugs. When infusing a filtered, 1.4 molar mannitol solution at 37 °C into the carotid circulation, the incidence of permanent neurological damage equaled 0.8 percent (3 of 384 procedures) and that of seizures equaled 14 percent (55 of 384 procedures). No death could be related directly to the osmotic procedure (Rapoport 1988; Rapoport and Robinson 1990). Furthermore, in the absence of radiotherapy, there was no evidence that the procedure accelerated cognitive deterioration (Crossen et al., in press). Retinal pigment epithelial damage occurred in the eye unilateral to perfusion, as predicted from animal experiments, but visual loss was insignificant (Okisaka et al. 1976; Millay et al. 1986). Neuwelt and coworkers (1986, 1991) also reported, from Phase II studies, that the osmotic procedure with the aforementioned drugs significantly prolonged mean survival duration of patients with primary CNS lymphoma.

CHEMICAL MODIFICATION OF DRUGS

Lipophilicity and Passive Diffusion

Although a certain degree of lipid solubility is essential for a drug to cross the BBB, an agent that distributes excessively in octanol compared with water has some pharmacokinetic limitations. Uptake by brain as well as pharmacodynamic action may become limited if the octanol:water partition coefficient of the drug exceeds 100 ($log_{10}Partition>2$) (Hansch 1972; Rapoport 1976; Greig et al. 1990a). An excessively lipid-soluble agent may be difficult to solubilize and, when soluble, be heavily bound to plasma proteins. Indeed, studies by Sholtan (1968) demonstrate a linear relation between the binding of various drugs to human serum albumin and their lipophilicity. Furthermore, a very lipid-soluble drug may be rapidly cleared from plasma, as it is taken up into lipid compartments in body organs.

Modification studies by the author's group on the anticancer agent chlorambucil illustrate how the principle of lipid solubility can be employed with regard to drug pharmacokinetics and pharmacodynamics. As shown in figure 2, chlorambucil is a bifunctional, nitrogen mustard alkylating agent; it has proved useful in treating chronic lymphocytic leukemia and Hodgkin's disease (Greig et al. 1990a). However, it is largely ionized at physiological blood pH. As a charged anion, it minimally enters the brain, so that it is ineffective against potentially sensitive brain-sequestered tumors.

Chlorambucil

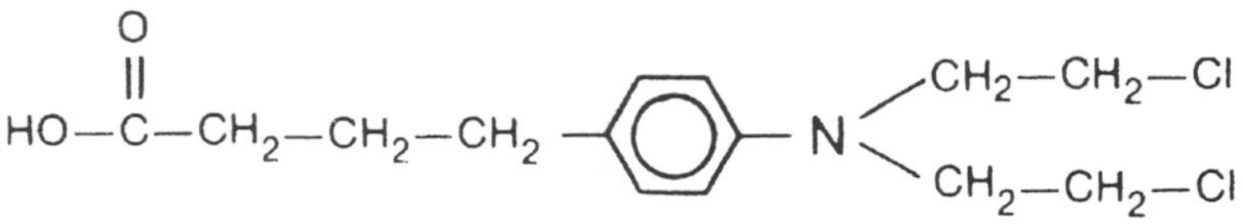

Chlorambucil-Tertiary Butyl Ester

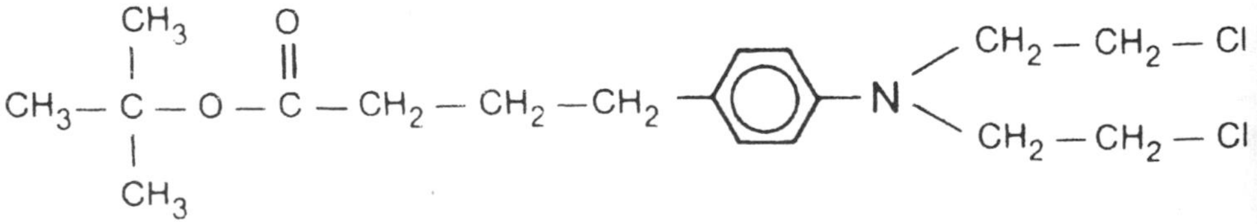

FIGURE 2.   *Chemical formulas of chlorambucil and of chlorambucil-tertiary butyl ester*

Postulating that masking the ionizable carboxylic acid moiety of chlorambucil by a lipophilic ester would increase its access to the brain but would not necessarily destroy its antitumor alkylating activity, Greig and colleagues (1990c, 1990d) reacted chlorambucil with many alcohols to form corresponding ester derivatives, without modifying its alkylating moieties. Each ester synthesized possessed significant intrinsic alkylating activity, although less than that of chlorambucil. However, none achieved or maintained greater concentrations in the rat brain after equimolar administration than did chlorambucil, with one exception, chlorambucil-tertiary butyl ester (figure 2). All but this latter ester were rapidly cleaved in plasma by esterases or were so lipophilic that they became tightly bound to plasma proteins (Sholtan 1968), thereby restricting their access into brain (equation 1). However, the steric hindrance of the branched chain chlorambucil-tertiary butyl ester reduced its rate of hydrolysis in plasma. Furthermore, despite its high lipophilicity ($\log_{10}$Partition=3.2), it can be readily formulated for IV administration, and a significant unbound fraction f exists in plasma. As illustrated in figure 3, administration of this ester to rats, compared with an equimolar amount of chlorambucil, resulted in significant uptake within brain.

With regard to pharmacodynamics, furthermore, the maximum tolerated dose of chlorambucil-tertiary butyl ester in rats was found to be sixfold higher than that of chlorambucil. Unlike chlorambucil, high doses of the ester did not cause seizures. Finally, chlorambucil-tertiary butyl ester, unlike chlorambucil,

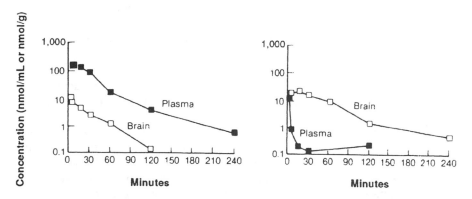

FIGURE 3. *Concentrations of chlorambucil (left) and of chlorambucil-tertiary butyl ester (right) in plasma and brain following equimolar IV administration in rats (10 mg/kg and 13 mg/kg, respectively)*

SOURCE: Greig et al. 1990a

significantly prolonged survival of rats with brain-implanted tumors and was found to be effective against human brain tumors in vitro that are insensitive to BCNU, the mainstay of brain tumor chemotherapy (Greig et al. 1990a; N.H. Greig, S. Genka, S.I. Rapoport, and F. Ali-Osman, unpublished observations).

Drug Modification for Carrier-Mediated Transport

An alternative goal of drug modification might be to synthesize an active compound that structurally resembles an endogenous agent that shares a facilitated transport system at the BBB. This principle has been demonstrated with regard to melphalan, the anticancer drug that is a nitrogen mustard derivative of L-phenylalanine (figure 4). Greig and colleagues (1987) showed that melphalan is transported into the CNS via the capillary carrier system for large neutral amino acids; its transport can be inhibited by L-phenylalanine, and it is concentration-dependent and saturable, with an affinity, however, that is less than those of the natural large neutral L-amino acids.

To more rationally identify which properties of large neutral L-amino acids determine affinity for the common carrier at the cerebrovasculature, Smith and coworkers (1987) examined affinities ($1/K_m$, where K_m equals half saturation concentration) of each of 14 neutral L-amino acids at cerebral capillaries of pentobarbital-anesthetized rats, using an in situ brain perfusion technique (Takasato et al. 1984). As illustrated by figure 5, the affinity of each L-amino acid was found to be proportional to the octanol:water partition coefficient, a measure of side-chain hydrophobicity (Yunger and Cramer 1981). Thus, although preferring the L-form of the amino acid, the carrier has weak requirements with regard to side-chain structure and size, other than how they influence hydrophobicity.

Under normal in vivo conditions, circulating large neutral L-amino acids compete with each other for the common carrier, which is saturated and has a high transport capacity. The very high affinity amino acids L-leucine and L-phenylalanine together occupy more than 50 percent of vascular carrier sites. Smith and coworkers (1989) later used the relation of figure 5 to design and study more than 100 synthetic amino acids of varying lipid solubilities to determine if some would have sufficiently high affinities to displace even L-phenylalanine and L-leucine from the carrier. They measured the ability of each amino acid to inhibit transport into rat brain of [1-^{14}C]L-phenylalanine, using their in situ perfusion technique. Even for the synthetic L-amino acids, affinity depended over a 10,000-fold range on side-chain hydrophobicity. Amino acid analogs with large hydrophobic side chains (e.g., L-napthylalanine) had much higher affinities than even L-phenylalanine (296 mM^{-1} compared with 95 mM^{-1} for phenylalanine) for the large neutral L-amino acid carrier.

	Saline Perfusion	
Compound	$PA \times 10^4$, s^{-1}	K_m
Tryptophan	966.7	0.009
Phenylalanine	790.0	0.010
Leucine	411.5	0.026
Tyrosine	356.0	0.050
Isoleucine	209.8	0.051
Methionine	77.3	0.075
Melphalan	10.8	0.150

$K_m = \mu moles/mL$

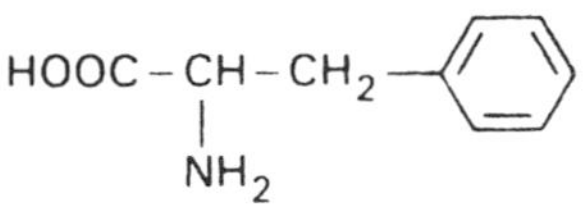

Phenylalanine

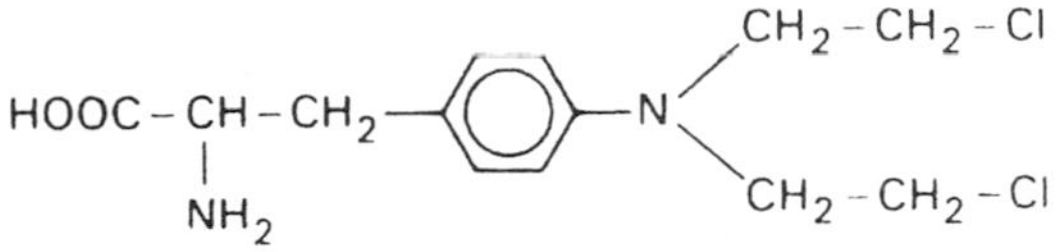

Melphalan

FIGURE 4. *Permeability-surface area products and half-saturation concentrations of large neutral L-amino acids and of melphalan at the BBB, as measured by the in situ brain perfusion technique of Takasato and colleagues (1984). Structures of phenylalanine and of melphalan are illustrated.*

SOURCE: Greig et al. 1987

On the basis of these studies, it should be possible to design drugs in the form of large neutral L-amino acids with hydrophobic side chains to take advantage of the high-capacity, large neutral L-amino acid carrier at the BBB. Similar approaches might be made with regard to other carrier systems, such as those subserving peptide transport at the BBB (Banks and Kastin 1990), although these usually have a lower transport capacity than does the large neutral L-amino acid carrier (Bradbury 1989).

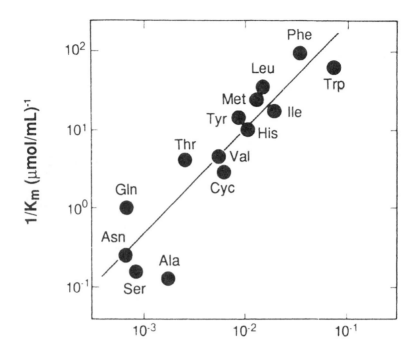

Octanol:Water Partition Coefficient

FIGURE 5.   *Relation between 1/K_m (K_m=half-saturation concentration) and octanol:water partition coefficient for 14 large neutral L-amino acids. Asn=asparagine; Ala=alanine; Cyc=cycloleucine; Glu=glutamine; His=histidine; Ile=isoleucine; Leu=leucine; Met=methionine; Phe=phenylalamine; Ser=serine; Thr=threonine; Trp=tryptophan; Tyr=tyrosine; Val=valine*

SOURCE: Smith et al. 1987

In conclusion, understanding the structure and function of the BBB can allow ways to be devised to increase BBB permeability to drugs or other agents or to design synthetic approaches to modify drugs so as to enhance their penetration into the brain passively or by means of existing carrier mechanisms.

REFERENCES

Armstrong, B.K.; Smith, Q.R.; Rapoport, S.I.; Strohalm, J.; Kopacek, J.; and Duncan, R. Osmotic opening of the blood-brain barrier permeability to N-(2-hydroxypropyl) methacrylamide copolymers. Effect of polymer MW, charge and hydrophobicity. *J Controlled Release* 10:27-35, 1989.

Banks, W.A., and Kastin, A.J. Peptide transport systems for opiates across the blood-brain barrier. *Am J Physiol* 259:E1-E10, 1990.

Barranger, J.A.; Rapoport, S.I.; Fredericks, W.R.; Pentchev, P.G.; MacDermot, K.D.; Steusing, J.K.; and Brady, R.O. Modification of the blood-brain barrier: Increased concentration and fate of enzymes entering the brain. *Proc Natl Acad Sci U S A* 76:481-485, 1979.

Bradbury, M.W. Transport across the blood-brain barrier. In: Neuwelt, E.A., ed. *Implications of the Blood-Brain Barrier and Its Manipulation. Basic Science Aspects*. Vol. 1. New York: Plenum, 1989. pp. 119-136.

Brightman, M.W.; Hori, M.; Rapoport, S.I.; Reese, T.S.; and Westergaard, E. Osmotic opening of tight junctions in cerebral endothelium. *J Comp Neurol* 152:317-325, 1973.

Chiueh, C.C.; Sun, C.L.; Kopin, I.J.; Fredericks, W.R.; and Rapoport, S.I. Entry of [^{3}H]norepinephrine, [^{125}I]albumin and Evans blue from blood into brain following unilateral osmotic opening of the blood-brain barrier. *Brain Res* 145:292-301, 1978.

Cornford, E.M. Blood-brain barrier permeability to anticonvulsant drugs. In: Levy, R.H.; Pittick, W.H.; Echlelbaum, M.; and Meyer, J., eds. *Metabolism of Antiepileptic Drugs*. New York: Raven Press, 1984. pp. 129-142.

Cosolo, W.C.; Martinello, P.; Louis, W.J.; and Christophidis, N. Blood-brain barrier disruption using mannitol: Time course and electron microscopy studies. *Am J Physiol* 256:R443-R447, 1989.

Crossen, J.R.; Goldman, D.L.; Kahlborg, S.A.; and Neuwelt, E.A. Neuropyschological assessment outcomes of non-AIDS primary central nervous system lymphoma patients before and after blood-brain barrier disruption chemotherapy. *Neurosurgery*, in press.

Dorovini-Zis, K.; Bowman, P.D.; Betz, A.L.; and Goldstein, G.W. Hyperosmotic arabinose solutions open the tight junctions between brain capillary endothelial cells in tissue culture. *Brain Res* 302:383-386, 1984.

Dorovini-Zis, K.; Santo, M.; Goping, G.; Rapoport, S.I.; and Brightman, M. Ionic lanthanum passage across cerebral endothelium exposed to hyperosmotic arabinose. *Acta Neuropathol (Berl)* 60:49-60, 1983.

Felgenhauer, K. Protein size and cerebrospinal fluid composition. *Klin Wochenschr* 52:1158-1164, 1974.

Fishman, J.B.; Rubin, J.B.; Handrahan, J.V.; Connor, J.R.; and Fine, R.E. Receptor-mediated transcytosis of transferrin across the blood-brain barrier. *J Neurosci Res* 18:299-304, 1987.

Greig, N.H.; Daly, E.M.; Sweeney, D.J.; and Rapoport, S.I. Pharmacokinetics of chlorambucil-tertiary butyl ester, a lipophilic chlorambucil derivative that achieves and maintains high concentrations in brain. *Cancer Chemother Pharmacol* 25:320-325, 1990c.

Greig, N.H.; Fredericks, W.R.; Holloway, H.W.; Soncrant, T.T.; and Rapoport, S.I. Delivery of human interferon-alpha to brain by transient osmotic blood-brain barrier modification in the rat. *J Pharmacol Exp Ther* 245:8-13, 1988.

Greig, N.H.; Genka, S.; Daly, E.M.; and Rapoport, S.I. Physico-chemical and pharmacokinetic parameters of 7 lipophilic chlorambucil esters designed for brain penetration. *Cancer Chemother Pharmacol* 25:311-319, 1990d.

Greig, N.H.; Genka, S.; and Rapoport, S.I. Delivery of vital drugs to the brain for the treatment of brain tumors. *J Controlled Release* 11:61-78, 1990a.

Greig, N.H.; Momma, S.; Sweeney, D.J.; Smith, Q.R.; and Rapoport, S.I. Facilitated transport of melphalan at the rat blood-brain barrier by the large neutral amino acid carrier system. *Cancer Res* 47:1571-1576, 1987.

Greig, N.H.; Soncrant, T.T.; Shetty, H.U.; Momma, S.; Smith, Q.R.; and Rapoport, S.I. Brain uptake and anticancer activities of vincristine and vinblastine are restricted by their low cerebrovascular permeability and binding to plasma contituents in rat. *Cancer Chemother Pharmacol* 26:263-268, 1990b.

Griffin, D.E., and Giffels, J. Study of protein characteristics that influence entry into the cerebrospinal fluid of normal mice and mice with encephalitis. *J Clin Invest* 70:289-295, 1982.

Gumerlock, M.K., and Neuwelt, E.A. The effects of anesthesia on osmotic blood-brain barrier disruption. *Neurosurgery* 26:268-277, 1990.

Hansch, C. Strategy in drug design. *Cancer Chemother Rep* 56:433-441, 1972.

Hicks, J.T.; Albrecht, P.; and Rapoport, S.I. Entry of neutralizing antibody to measles into brain and cerebrospinal fluid of immunized monkeys after osmotic opening of the blood-brain barrier. *Exp Neurol* 53:768-779, 1976.

Jones, D.R.; Hall, S.D.; Jackson, E.K.; Branch, R.A.; and Wilkinson, G.R. Brain uptake of benzodiazepines: Effects of lipophilicity and plasma protein binding. *J Pharmacol Exp Ther* 245:816-822, 1988.

Levine, R.L.; Fredericks, W.R.; and Rapoport, S.I. Clearance of bilirubin from the rat brain after reversible osmotic opening of the blood-brain barrier. *Pediatr Res* 19:1040-1043, 1985.

Levitan, H.; Zilyan, Z.; Smith, Q.R.; Takasato, Y.; and Rapoport, S.I. Brain uptake of a food dye, erythrocin B, prevented by plasma protein binding. *Brain Res* 323:131-134, 1984.

Millay, R.H.; Klein, M.L.; Shults, W.T.; Dahlborg, S.A.; and Neuwalt, E.A. Maculopathy associated with combination chemotherapy and osmotic opening of the blood-brain barrier. *Am J Ophthalmol* 102:626-632, 1986.

Neuwelt, E.A., ed. *Implications of the Blood-Brain Barrier and its Manipulation. Basic Science Aspects* and *Clinical Aspects.* Vols. 1 and 2. New York: Plenum, 1989.

Neuwelt, E.A.; Goldman, D.L.; Dahlborg, S.A.; Crossen, J.; Ramsey, F.; Roman-Goldstein, S.; Braziel, R.; and Dana, B. Primary CNS lymphoma treated with osmotic blood-brain barrier disruption: Prolonged survival and preservation of cognitive function. *J Clin Oncol* 9:1580-1590, 1991.

Neuwelt, E.A.; Frenkel, E.P.; Diehl, J.; Vu, L.H.; Rapoport, S.I.; and Hill, S.A. Reversible osmotic blood-brain barrier disruption in humans: Implications for the chemotherapy of brain tumors. *Neurosurgery* 7:44-52, 1980.

Neuwelt, E.A.; Frenkel, E.P.; Gumerlock, M.K.; Braziel, R.; Dana, B.; and Hill, S.A. Developments in the diagnosis and treatment of primary CNS lymphoma. A prospective series. *Cancer* 58:1609-1620, 1986.

Neuwelt, E.A.; Glasberg, M.; Frenkel, E.; and Barnett, P. Neurotoxicity of chemotherapeutic agents after blood-brain barrier modification: Neuropathological studies. *Ann Neurol* 14:316-324, 1983.

Ohata, M.; Fredericks, W.R.; Neuwelt, E.A.; Sandaram, U.; and Rapoport, S.I. [^{3}H]Methotrexate loss from the rat brain following enhanced uptake by osmotic opening of the blood-brain barrier. *Cancer Res* 45:1092-1096, 1985.

Ohno, K.; Pettigrew, K.D.; and Rapoport, S.I. Lower limits of cerebrovascular permeability to nonelectrolytes in the conscious rat. *Am J Physiol* 235:H299-H307, 1978.

Okisaka, S.; Kuwabara, T.; and Rapoport, S.I. Effect of hyperosmotic agents on the ciliary epithelium and trabecular meshwork. *Invest Ophthalmol* 15:617-625, 1976.

Pardridge, W.M.; Triguero, D.; and Buciak, J.L. β-Endorphin chimeric peptides: Transport through the blood-brain barrier in vivo and cleavage of disulfide linkage by brain. *Endrocrinology* 126:977-984, 1990.

Pomponi, M.; Giacobini, E.; and Brufani, M. Present state and future development of the therapy of Alzheimer's disease. *Aging* 2:125-153, 1990.

Rapoport, S.I. Effect of concentrated solutions on blood-brain barrier. *Am J Physiol* 219:270-274, 1970.

Rapoport, S.I. *Blood-Brain Barrier in Physiology and Medicine.* New York: Raven Press, 1976.

Rapoport, S.I. Reversible osmotic opening of the blood-brain barrier for experimental and therapeutic purposes. In: Levine, R.L., and Maisels, M.J., eds. *Hyperbilirubinemia in the Newborn.* Ross Conference on Pediatric Research. Columbus, OH: Ross Laboratories, 1983a. pp. 116-124.

Rapoport, S.I. Passage of proteins from blood to cerebrospinal fluid. Model for transfer by pores and vesicles. In: Wood, J.H., ed. *Neurobiology of Cerebrospinal Fluid.* New York: Plenum, 1983b. pp. 233-245.

Rapoport, S.I. A model for brain edema. In: Inaba, Y.; Klatzo, I.; and Spatz, M., eds. *Brain Edema. Proceedings of the Sixth International Symposium.* Berlin: Springer-Verlag, 1985. pp. 59-71.

Rapoport, S.I. Osmotic opening of the blood-brain barrier. *Ann Neurol* 24:677-680, 1988.

Rapoport, S.I.; Fitzhugh, R.; Pettigrew, K.D.; Sundaram, U.; and Ohno, K. Drug entry and distribution within brain and cerebrospinal fluid: [^{14}C]Urea pharmacokinetics. *Am J Physiol* 242:R339-R348, 1982.

Rapoport, S.I.; Fredericks, W.K.; Ohno, K.; and Pettigrew, K.D. Quantitative aspects of reversible osmotic opening of the blood-brain barrier. *Am J Physiol* 238:R421-R431, 1980.

Rapoport, S.I.; Hori, M.; and Klatzo, I. Testing of a hypothesis for osmotic opening of the blood-brain barrier. *Am J Physiol* 223:323-331, 1972.

Rapoport, S.I., and Robinson, P.J. Tight-junctional modification as the basis of osmotic opening of the blood-brain barrier. *Ann N Y Acad Sci* 481:250-267, 1986.

Rapoport, S.I., and Robinson, P.J. A therapeutic role for osmotic opening of the blood-brain barrier. Re-evaluation of literature and of importance of source-sink relations between brain and tumor. In: Johanson, B.B.; Owman, C.; and Widner, H., eds. *Pathophysiology of the Blood-Brain Barrier, Long Term Consequences of Barrier Dysfunction for the Brain.* Fernstrom Foundation Series. Vol. 14. Amsterdam: Elsevier, 1990. pp. 167-171.

Rapoport, S.I., and Robinson, P.J. Blood-tumor barrier controversies erupt. [Response to Letter to the Editor.] *J Cereb Blood Flow Metab* 11:165-168, 1991.

Rapoport, S.I., and Thompson, H.K. Osmotic opening of the blood-brain barrier in the monkey without associated neurological deficits. *Science* 180:971, 1973.

Reese, T.S., and Karnovsky, M.J. Fine structural localization of a blood-brain barrier to exogenous peroxidase. *J Cell Biol* 34:207-217, 1967.

Robinson, P.J., and Rapoport, S.I. Kinetics of protein binding determine rates of uptake of drugs by brain. *Am J Physiol* 251:R1212-R1220, 1986.

Robinson, P.J., and Rapoport, S.I. Size selectivity of blood-brain barrier permeability at various times after osmotic opening. *Am J Physiol* 253:R459-R466, 1987.

Salahuddin, T.S.; Johansson, B.B.; Kalimo, H.; and Olsson, Y. Structural changes in the rat brain after carotid infusions of hyperosmolar solutions. An electron mirocoscopic study. *Acta Neuropathol (Berl)* 77:5-13, 1988.

Sholtan, W. Die hydrophobe Bindung der Pharmaka an Humanalbumin und Ribonucleinsaure. *Arzneimittelforschung* 18:505-517, 1968.

Shulman, D.S.; Kaufman, J.J.; Eisenstein, M.M.; and Rapoport, S.I. Blood pH and brain uptake of ^{14}C-morphine. *Anesthesiology* 61:540-543, 1984.

Smith, Q.R.; Aoyagi, M.; and Rapoport, S.I. Structural specificity of the brain capillary neutral amino acid transporter. *Abstr Soc Neurosci* 15(2):1025, 1989.

Smith, Q.R.; Momma, S.; Aoyagi, M.; and Rapoport, S.I. Kinetics of neutral amino acid transport across the blood-brain barrier. *J Neurochem* 49:1651-1658, 1987.

Sourkes, T.L. Parkinson's disease and other disorders of the basal ganglia. In: Siegal, G.J.; Albers, R.W.; Agranoff, B.W.; and Katzman, R., eds. *Basic Neurochemistry*. 3d ed. Boston: Little, Brown, 1981. pp. 719-736.

Suzuki, M.; Yamamoto, T.; Konno, H.; and Kudo, H. Sequelae of the osmotic blood-brain barrier opening in rats. *J Neurosurg* 69:421-428, 1988.

Takasato, Y.; Rapoport, S.I.; and Smith, Q.R. An in situ brain perfusion technique to study cerebrovascular transport in the rat. *Am J Physiol* 247:H484-H493, 1984.

Tomiwa, K.; Hazama, F.; and Mikawa, H. Reversible osmotic opening of the blood-brain barrier: Prevention of tissue damage with filtration of perfusate. *Acta Pathol Jpn* 32:427-435, 1982.

Yunger, L.M., and Cramer, R.D. Measurement and correlation of partition coefficients of polar amino acids. *Mol Pharmacol* 20:602-608, 1981.

AUTHOR

Stanley I. Rapoport, M.D.
Chief
Laboratory of Neurosciences
National Institute on Aging
National Institutes of Health
Building 10, Room 6C-103
Bethesda, MD 20892

Cultured Brain Microvessel Endothelial Cells as In Vitro Models of the Blood-Brain Barrier

Yoshinobu Takakura, Kenneth L. Audus, and Ronald T. Borchardt

INTRODUCTION

A central nervous system (CNS) site of action generally requires that, following entry into the systemic circulation, substances must interact with the blood-brain barrier (BBB) en route to brain tissue targets. Many substances with CNS activity, including drugs of abuse, cross the BBB by simple passive diffusion (Oldendorf 1974; Levin 1980; Cornford et al. 1982). Accordingly, the BBB plays an important role in regulating access of drugs of abuse to the brain.

Recent evidence suggests that some drugs of abuse may alter BBB permeability characteristics. The permeability-altering activity of drugs of abuse at the BBB has been reported in chronic amphetamine intoxication (Rakic et al. 1989), acute ethanol exposure (Gulati et al. 1985), and opiate treatment (Baba et al. 1988). Ethanol addiction also has been reported to alter opiate interactions with the transport systems of the BBB (Banks and Kastin 1989). On the basis of these reports, one might infer that interactions of drugs of abuse with the BBB may have implications for the observed pharmacological and toxicological manifestations of exposure to these substances. These implications remain to be explored and confirmed. Consequently, the development of a fundamental understanding of the permeability and metabolic features of the BBB may contribute to a broader knowledge of the activity of drugs of abuse in the CNS.

The complexity of the whole animal as an experimental model has certain limitations when specific events at the cellular or molecular level are examined. In vitro models (i.e., brain microvessel suspensions or cultured brain endothelial cells) offer a promising alternative for the investigation of cellular- or molecular-level characteristics of the BBB (Audus et al. 1990; Audus and Borchardt 1987). The purpose of this chapter is to describe studies of the transport and metabolism characteristics of the BBB that employ cultured brain microvessel endothelial cells as in vitro BBB models. This chapter does not describe isolated suspensions of brain microvessel endothelial cells as in vitro models, since this subject has been reviewed by Betz and Goldstein (1984) and more recently by Takakura and coworkers (1991a). In addition, this chapter does not describe how cultured brain microvessel endothelial cells have been used to study the development and regulation of the BBB and pathological changes in the BBB, since these topics are discussed in other chapters in this monograph and have been reviewed previously by Takakura and coworkers (1991a).

ESTABLISHMENT AND CHARACTERIZATION OF CULTURED BRAIN MICROVESSEL ENDOTHELIAL CELLS AS IN VITRO BBB MODELS

Since Panula and colleagues (1978) demonstrated that rat brain microvessel endothelial cells could be maintained in tissue culture, various kinds of both primary and passaged cultures of isolated brain microvessel endothelial cells have been established from mouse, rat, bovine, human, canine, and porcine brain (for a review, see Audus et al. 1990).

In general, either enzymatic or mechanical dispersal, or a combination of both techniques, followed by either filtration or centrifugation steps are employed to isolate a homogeneous population of brain microvessel endothelial cells from the extremely heterogeneous population of cells found in brain tissues. For example, isolation of a viable, homogeneous population of brain capillary endothelial cells for establishment of a tissue culture system is accomplished by a two-step enzymatic digestion with dispase and a dispase/collagenase mixture of cerebral gray matter and successive centrifugation over dextran and percoll gradients (Bowman et al. 1983; Audus and Borchardt 1986a, 1987). In the authors' laboratories, primary cultures of bovine brain microvessel endothelial cell monolayers have been shown to retain morphological and biochemical properties typical of the BBB in vivo. These include tight junctions, attenuated pinocytosis, lack of fenestra, and the presence of proteins (e.g., γ-glutamyl transpeptidase, alkaline phosphatase, angiotensin-converting enzyme, factor VIII antigen) enriched in the endothelium of the BBB (Audus and Borchardt 1986a, 1987).

Basically, two types of experimental systems have been employed for study of transport phenomena using cultured brain microvessel endothelial cells: The first is the uptake study, and the second involves a transcellular transport study. The former system uses microvessel endothelial cell monolayers grown in culture dishes (Scriba and Borchardt 1989a, 1989b). Uptake experiments can be performed also using cerebral microvessel endothelial cells cultured on microcarriers (e.g., dextran beads) (Bottaro et al. 1986; Kempski et al. 1987). These systems allow examination of the first step of the transport process, that is, the uptake of the solutes into the brain capillary cells from the luminal side. The most sophisticated in vitro system for transport studies consists of cultured brain microvessel endothelial cell monolayers grown on microporous membranes. Transport studies can then be conducted in side-by-side diffusion cells or the cell-insert system (Audus et al. 1990). These systems afford an opportunity to look at bidirectional transendothelial movement (transfer from brain to blood and that from blood to brain) of solutes across the BBB in vitro since, at least for primary cultures of bovine microvessel endothelial cells, the cells are shown to be morphologically and functionally polarized in terms of ricin recycling (Raub and Audus 1990), transferrin transport (Newton and Raub 1988), and angiotensin II (Ang II) responsiveness (Guillot and Audus 1990, 1991a). The purity of these monolayers is greater than 95 percent (Guillot et al. 1990), and the transelectrical resistance is 160 ± 18 ohm/cm^2 (T.J. Raub, unpublished results).

Although bovine brain microvessel endothelial monolayers retain tight junctions, the tight junctions are not identical to those observed in vivo with regard to extent and complexity. This leads to higher leakiness in vitro than in vivo, which is a disadvantage in the use of cultured endothelial cells alone to study transcellular transport.

More impermeable monolayers of cultured brain microvessel endothelial cells may be developed in the future by exploiting the regulatory role of astrocytes in endothelial cell growth and development. It is widely accepted that the brain microvessel endothelial cells in vivo form the structural and functional bases of the BBB; however, some of the BBB functions are known to be regulated by astrocytes, which encircle the microvessel endothelial cells with their foot processes in vivo. Similar regulatory effects of astrocytes on the permeability properties of cultured endothelial cells in vitro have been reported. For example, Cancilla and DeBault (1983) demonstrated that contact with glial cells (a rat line of neoplastic astrocytes designated as C6 glioma cells) or exposure to glial-conditioned media enhances neutral amino acid uptake by passaged mouse cerebral endothelial cells in culture. Conditioned media prepared from astrocytes and C6 glioma cells have been shown to stimulate glucose uptake in passaged mouse cerebral endothelial cells (Maxwell et al. 1989) and in primary cultures of bovine brain microvessel endothelial cells (Takakura et al. 1991b). Conditioned media from rat astrocytes or C6 glioma cells also have been shown to decrease the permeability of various solutes across monolayers of bovine brain microvessel endothelial cells grown on microporous membranes (Trammel and Borchardt 1989; Raub et al. 1989). Recently, Dehouck and colleagues (1990) observed decreases in permeability

140

and increases in electrical resistance using an in vitro model system consisting of passaged brain microvessel endothelial cells grown on one side of a filter and astrocytes on the other side of the filter.

UPTAKE AND TRANSPORT STUDIES

Nutrients

Since glucose is an important source of energy for the brain, the mechanism of glucose transport across the BBB has been particularly well studied in vivo (Pardridge 1983). These studies support the concept that glucose is transported through the cerebral microvessel endothelium mainly by the mechanism of carrier-mediated facilitated diffusion. Glucose transport characteristics also were studied in cultured brain microvessel endothelial cells. For example, Vinters and coworkers (1985) demonstrated that the properties of 3-O-methylglucose (3MG) and 2-deoxyglucose uptake in established lines of cultured mouse cerebral microvessel endothelium are similar to those observed in vivo. Recently, characteristics of both uptake and transendothelial transport of 3MG were studied in primary cultures of bovine brain microvessel endothelial cells (Takakura et al. 1991c). The uptake characteristics of 3MG were shown to be identical to those observed in vivo and in vitro using isolated capillaries. Transport rates from the luminal to abluminal side and from the abluminal to luminal side, measured across the brain microvessel endothelial cells grown onto polycarbonate membranes, were nearly identical, suggesting symmetrical glucose transport across the monolayer of endothelial cells.

The passage of amino acids across the BBB was found to be saturable and stereospecific in vivo (Oldendorf 1971). Cancilla and DeBault (1983) showed the presence of A- and L-systems for uptake of neutral amino acids in cultured mouse cerebral endothelial cells. Using primary cultures of bovine brain microvessel endothelial cell monolayers grown onto microporous membranes, transport of a large neutral amino acid, leucine, was shown to be saturable, bidirectional, competitive with other amino acids, and energy independent (Audus and Borchardt 1986b). The kinetic parameters for leucine transport appear to be in good agreement with true kinetic parameters of the in vivo BBB. The transport of several amino acid drugs—including baclofen (van Bree et al. 1988), α-methyldopa (Chastain and Borchardt 1989), and acivicin (Chastain and Borchardt 1990)—by the amino acid carrier also has been explored in this system.

Because of a limited capability for de novo synthesis of choline, an important precursor to acetylcholine and phospholipid, the brain must depend on the blood for its supply of choline. Cornford and colleagues (1978) demonstrated the saturability of brain uptake of choline after intracarotid injection in rats. Recently, Estrada and associates (1990) studied choline uptake by bovine cerebral capillary endothelial cells in culture, demonstrating that these cells were able to incorporate choline by a carrier-mediated mechanism. The choline uptake was temperature dependent and was inhibited by choline analogs but was not affected by ouabain or dinitrophenol. Transendothelial transport of choline in cultured bovine brain microvessel endothelial cells has been characterized (Trammel and Borchardt 1987); it has been shown that the transport is saturable and is insensitive to ouabain and sodium azide, suggesting a facilitated diffusion mechanism.

Since the brain is one of the most active tissues for carrying out nucleotide and nucleic acid synthesis, the transport of nucleosides and purine bases across the BBB has been of interest. By employing the intracarotid injection technique in rats, Cornford and Oldendorf (1975) demonstrated the presence of two independent carrier systems for nucleic precursors: a nucleoside carrier and a purine base carrier. Beck and coworkers (1983) have described a carrier-mediated uptake of adenosine into mouse cerebral capillary endothelial cells in tissue culture. Characterization of the nucleoside uptake (e.g., adenosine, thymidine) into monolayers of cultured bovine brain endothelial cells also was studied, and the results suggested the presence of a carrier-mediated uptake of adenosine and thymidine (Shah and Borchardt 1989). Adenosine uptake is primarily via the carrier-mediated pathway, whereas thymidine enters by both a carrier-mediated and a passive pathway. Both nucleosides are extensively metabolized (e.g., phosphorylated) in the cultured bovine endothelial cells.

Peptides and Proteins

Although the physiological role of insulin in the regulation of brain functions remains to be elucidated, van Houten and Posner (1979) revealed that blood vessels throughout the CNS of the rat bind plasma insulin rapidly and with considerable specificity in vivo. The binding and receptor-mediated endocytosis of insulin and insulin-like growth factor I (IGF-I) also were studied using cultured bovine brain microvessel endothelial cells (Keller and Borchardt 1987; Keller et al. 1988). Rosenfeld and colleagues (1987) showed the similarity between the characteristics of the specific receptors for IGF-I and insulin-like growth factor II in the cultured bovine brain microvessel endothelial cells and in isolated rat brain microvessels.

Using monoclonal antibodies to the transferrin receptors, Jefferies and coworkers (1984) first reported that rat and human brain capillary endothelia have receptors for transferrin, an iron-transport protein in the circulation. Newton and Raub (1988) characterized the transferrin receptor in primary cultures of brain capillary endothelial cells, indicating saturable binding and internalization. They also demonstrated the transcytosis and the polarized efflux of transferrin using brain microvessel endothelial cells grown onto polycarbonate filters; these findings are in good agreement with the in vivo observations of Fishman and coworkers (1987) and Banks and coworkers (1988).

Atrial natriuretic factor (ANF), which is a 28-amino acid peptide produced by cardiac myocytes and released in response to increases in atrial pressure, expresses its natriuretic, diuretic, and hypotensive effects by acting on renal and vascular tissues. A specific receptor for ANF also was identified using primary cultures of bovine brain capillary endothelial cells (Smith et al. 1988). The binding of ANF was specific, saturable, and reversible. ANF also was shown to be rapidly internalized by a temperature-dependent process. A specific receptor for brain natriuretic peptide (BNP), which was found in the brain and has similarity to ANF in its structure and biological activities (Sudoh et al. 1988), was identified recently in primary cultures of bovine brain microvessel endothelial cells (M. Fukuta, M. Nonomura, Y. Takakura, and R.T. Borchardt, unpublished results). These studies suggested that ANF and BNP share the same receptor in bovine brain microvessel endothelium.

Speth and Harik (1985) reported that Ang II binds to microvessels isolated from dog brain in a specific, saturable, and reversible manner and with high affinity. It was suggested that specific Ang II receptor-binding sites are present in brain microvessels and that these receptors may have an important role in regulating the microcirculation of the brain. Work in the authors' laboratories indicates that bovine brain microvessel endothelial cell monolayers retain a high-affinity Ang II binding site that can be competed for by Ang II peptides (Guillot and Audus 1991b).

Recently, the transport of leu-enkephalin across the BBB by a carrier-mediated mechanism has been demonstrated in vivo (Zlokovic et al. 1987). In addition, Thompson and Audus (1989) showed that leu-enkephalin transfer across monolayers of brain microvessel endothelial cells occurs at a relatively high rate, which is consistent with a facilitated diffusion mechanism.

Vasopressin transport across the BBB has been examined with primary cultures of brain microvessel endothelial monolayers (Reardon and Audus 1989). Results suggest the existence of facilitated transport of the peptide from the abluminal to the luminal side of the monolayers. This finding is consistent with the in vivo characterization of a vasopressin BBB transport system (Banks et al. 1987). Van Bree and colleagues (1989) also have studied transport of vasopressin using an in vitro system and suggested that no carrier mediation is involved over a higher concentration range. Confirmatory studies are required to clarify the transport mechanism in detail.

Raeissi and Audus (1989) characterized the BBB permeability to delta sleep-inducing peptide (DSIP) in cultured microvessel endothelial cells. The results support in vivo observations indicating that intact DSIP crosses the BBB by simple transmembrane diffusion (Banks and Kastin 1987). Recently, Zlokovic and coworkers (1989) presented evidence in support of a facilitative BBB carrier for DSIP in vivo. Further work is ongoing concerning the solution structure of DSIP, which may help to explain its ability to readily penetrate the BBB (Audus and Manning 1990).

Native albumin, which is an acidic protein in plasma, is considered to pass through the BBB very slowly (Pardridge et al. 1985). However, increased BBB uptake and transport recently has been reported when it is chemically modified. Kumagai and colleagues (1987) demonstrated the enhanced binding and adsorptive-mediated endocytosis of cationized albumin by isolated bovine brain capillaries. The binding was saturable and inhibited by other polycations (e.g., protamine, protamine sulfate, and polylysine). Similar results have been reported for other types of polycationic proteins, including cationized immunoglobulin G (Triguero et al. 1989) and histone (Pardridge et al. 1989). Smith and Borchardt (1989) studied the binding, uptake, and transcellular transport of bovine serum albumin (BSA), cationized BSA (cBSA), and glycosylated BSA (gBSA) in cultured bovine brain microvessel endothelial cells. This study demonstrated that cBSA and gBSA bind to the cells specifically and are transported by an adsorptive-phase endocytotic mechanism. The use of cationized albumin in directed delivery of peptides through the BBB was examined by coupling β-endorphin to cationized albumin via a disulfide linkage (Kumagai et al. 1987).

Drugs

In contrast to water-soluble nutrients and peptides, which are transported by specific carrier- or receptor-mediated systems as mentioned above, most water-soluble solutes, including drugs, pass through the BBB by a passive diffusion mechanism. From in vivo studies, it has been well established that the permeability of these molecules across the BBB depends directly on their lipophilicity and inversely on their molecular size (Oldendorf 1974; Levin 1980; Cornford et al. 1982). Rim and coworkers (1986) and Shah and coworkers (1989) established a positive correlation between lipid solubility of a drug and its permeability across bovine brain microvessel endothelial monolayers grown

144

onto microporous membranes. As mentioned earlier in this chapter, brain microvessel endothelial monolayers are leakier than the BBB in vivo. Therefore, this leakiness in the monolayers must be corrected for by using impermeant marker molecules (e.g., sucrose, fluorescein, inulin, and dextran) when drug transport studies are conducted (Shah et al. 1989).

IN VITRO STUDIES ON BBB METABOLISM

Several different enzyme systems have been established in primary cultures of bovine brain microvessel endothelial cell monolayers. Both biochemical and histochemical techniques have been used to follow the expression of marker and catecholamine-metabolizing enzymes associated with these monolayers. For instance, enzyme systems considered markers for the BBB, γ-glutamyl transpeptidase and alkaline phosphatase, and for the endothelium, angiotensin-converting enzyme, are retained in the monolayers (Baranczyk-Kuzma et al. 1986). In addition, the brain microvessel endothelial cell monolayers retain the ability to degrade catecholamines through expression of monoamine oxidases A and B, catechol O-methyltransferase, and phenol sulfotransferase (Baranczyk-Kuzma et al. 1986, 1989a; Scriba and Borchardt 1989a, 1989b). Using monolayers of bovine brain microvessel endothelial cells, the metabolism of catecholamine esters (Scriba and Borchardt 1989a) and of 1-methyl-4-phenyl-1,2,3,6-tetrahydropyridine (MPTP) has been studied (Scriba and Borchardt 1989b).

The lysosomal compartment of endothelia is an important component of the transcytosis of macromolecules (Simionescu 1979). Current interest by the pharmaceutical industry in the delivery of therapeutic biotechnology products to the CNS (Audus et al. 1990) suggests a need for considering the activity of the lysosomal compartment of the BBB. However, little work has focused on lysosomal or acid hydrolase compartments within the BBB in vivo. By both quantitative and qualitative measures, bovine brain microvessel endothelial cells possess a lysosomal compartment that expresses typical acid hydrolases, acid phosphatase, β-galactose, and sulfatases (Baranczyk-Kuzma et al. 1989b). Peptidase activity has not yet been examined in the lysosomal fraction; however, aminopeptidase activity is characteristic of membrane and cytosolic fractions of the cells (Baranczyk-Kuzma and Audus 1987). Corresponding quantitative studies in in vivo enzyme systems and compartments have not been performed and may not be feasible. Therefore, the in vitro model may be a reasonable system in which to initiate further studies on the contributions of the lysosomal compartment to the fate of endocytosed peptides and proteins at the BBB (Baranczyk-Kuzma et al. 1989b).

CONCLUSIONS

The development of in vitro BBB models consisting of cultured brain microvessel endothelial cells has made possible the study of BBB transport and metabolism phenomena at the cellular level. Basic characteristics of BBB transport and metabolism of endogenous and exogenous solutes and their biochemical, pharmacological, ontogenic, and pathological regulation mechanisms have been investigated. This information has led not only to a better understanding of BBB transport but also to the construction of strategies for improving drug delivery to the CNS for diagnosis and therapeutics. To elucidate the complexity of BBB transport, in vivo studies are always necessary at some point; however, in vitro systems can be useful complements to in vivo systems. The tissue culture systems seem to be especially important in the clarification of cellular, biochemical, and molecular features of BBB transport. Appropriate systems should be selected or combined, depending on the purpose of the investigation.

REFERENCES

Audus, K.L.; Bartel, R.L.; Hidalgo, I.J.; and Borchardt, R.T. The use of cultured epithelial and endothelial cells for drug transport and metabolism studies. *Pharm Res* 7:435-451, 1990.

Audus, K.L., and Borchardt, R.T. Characterization of an in vitro blood-brain barrier model system for studying drug transport and metabolism. *Pharm Res* 3:81-87, 1986a.

Audus, K.L., and Borchardt, R.T. Characteristics of the large neutral amino acid transport system of bovine brain microvessel endothelial cell monolayers. *J Neurochem* 47:484-488, 1986b.

Audus, K.L., and Borchardt, R.T. Bovine brain microvessel endothelial cell monolayers as a model system for the blood-brain barrier. *Ann N Y Acad Sci* 507:9-18, 1987.

Audus, K.L., and Manning, M.C. In vitro studies of peptide transport through a cell culture model of the blood-brain barrier. *Eur J Pharmacol* 183:1636-1637, 1990.

Baba, M.; Oishi, R.; and Saeki, K. Enhancement of blood-brain barrier permeability to sodium fluorescein by stimulation of μ opioid receptors in mice. *Naunyn Schmiedebergs Arch Pharmacol* 337:423-428, 1988.

Banks, W.M., and Kastin, A.J. Saturable transport of peptides across the blood-brain barrier. *Life Sci* 41:1319-1338, 1987.

Banks, W.M., and Kastin, A.J. Inhibition of the brain to blood transport system for enkephalins and Tyr-MIF-1 in mice addicted to or genetically predisposed to drinking ethanol. *Alcohol* 410:53-57, 1989.

Banks, W.M.; Kastin, A.J.; Fasold, M.B.; Barrera, C.M.; and Augereau, G. Studies of the slow bidirectional transport of iron and transferrin across the blood-brain barrier. *Brain Res Bull* 21:881-885, 1988.

Banks, W.M.; Kastin, A.J.; Horvath, A.; and Michals, E.A. Carrier-mediated transport of vasopressin across the blood-brain barrier of the mouse. *J Neurosci Res* 18:326-332, 1987.

Baranczyk-Kuzma, A., and Audus, K. Characteristics of aminopeptidase activity from bovine brain microvessel endothelium. *J Cereb Blood Flow Metab* 7:801-805, 1987.

Baranczyk-Kuzma, A.; Audus, K.; and Borchardt, R.T. Catecholamine-metabolizing enzymes of bovine brain microvessel endothelial cell monolayers. *J Neurochem* 46:1956-1960, 1986.

Baranczyk-Kuzma, A.; Audus, K.; and Borchardt, R.T. Substrate specificity of phenol sulfotransferase from primary cultures of bovine brain microvessel endothelium. *Neurochem Res* 14:689-691, 1989a.

Baranczyk-Kuzma, A.; Raub, T.J.; and Audus, K. Demonstration of acid hydrolase activity in primary cultures of bovine brain microvessel endothelium. *J Cereb Blood Flow Metab* 9:280-289, 1989b.

Beck, D.W.; Vinters, H.V.; Hart, M.N.; Henn, F.A.; and Cancilla, P.A. Uptake of adenosine into cultured cerebral endothelium. *Brain Res* 271:180-183, 1983.

Betz, A.L., and Goldstein, G.W. Brain capillaries: Structure and function. In: Lajtha, A., ed. *Handbook of Neurochemistry.* Vol. 7. New York: Plenum Press, 1984. pp. 465-484.

Bottaro, D.; Shepro, D.; and Hechtman, B. Heterogeneity of intimal and microvessel endothelial barriers in vitro. *Microvasc Res* 32:389-398, 1986.

Bowman, P.D.; Ennis, S.R.; Rarey, K.E.; Betz, A.L.; and Goldstein, G.W. Brain microvessel endothelial cells in tissue culture: A model for study of blood-brain barrier permeability. *Ann Neurol* 14:396-402, 1983.

Cancilla, P.A., and DeBault, L.E. Neutral amino acid transport properties of cerebral endothelial cells in vitro. *J Neuropathol Exp Neurol* 42:191-199, 1983.

Chastain, J.E., Jr., and Borchardt, R.T. L-α-methyldopa transport across bovine brain microvessel endothelial cell monolayers, a model of the blood-brain barrier. *Neurosci Res Commun* 4:147-152, 1989.

Chastain, J.E., Jr., and Borchardt, R.T. Acivicin transport across bovine brain microvessel endothelial cell monolayers. A model of the blood-brain barrier. *Neurosci Res Commun* 6:51-55, 1990.

Cornford, E.M.; Baun, L.D.; and Oldendorf, W.H. Carrier mediated blood-brain barrier transport of choline analogs. *J Neurochem* 30:299-308, 1978.

Cornford, E.M.; Baun, L.D.; Oldendorf, W.H.; and Hill, M.N. Comparison of lipid-mediated blood-brain barrier penetrability in neonates and adults. *Am J Physiol* 243:C161-C168, 1982.

Cornford, E.M., and Oldendorf, W.H. Independent blood-brain barrier transport systems for nucleic acid precursors. *Biochim Biophys Acta* 394:211-219, 1975.

Dehouck, M.-P.; Meresse, S.; Delorme, P.; Fruchart, J.-C.; and Cecchelli, R. An easier, reproducible, and mass-production method to study the blood-brain barrier in vitro. *J Neurochem* 54:1798-1801, 1990.

Estrada, C.; Bready, J.; Berliner, J.; and Cancilla, P.A. Choline uptake by cerebral capillary endothelial cells in culture. *J Neurochem* 54:1467-1473, 1990.

Fishman, J.B.; Rubin, J.B.; Handrahan, J.V.; Connor, J.R.; and Fine, R.E. Receptor-mediated transcytosis of transferrin across the blood-brain barrier. *J Neurosci Res* 18:299-304, 1987.

Guillot, F.L., and Audus, K.L. Biochemistry of angiotensin peptide-mediated effects on fluid-phase endocytosis in brain microvessel endothelial cell monolayers. *J Cereb Blood Flow Metab* 10:827-834, 1990.

Guillot, F.L., and Audus, K.L. Angiotensin peptide regulation of bovine brain microvessel endothelial cell monolayers. *J Cardiovasc Pharmacol* 18:212-218, 1991a.

Guillot, F.L., and Audus, K.L. Some characteristics of specific angiotensin II binding sites on bovine brain microvessel endothelial cell monolayers. *Peptides* 12:535-549, 1991b.

Guillot, F.L.; Audus, K.L.; and Raub, T.J. Fluid-phase endocytosis by primary cultures of bovine brain microvessel endothelial cell monolayers. *Microvasc Res* 39:1-14, 1990.

Gulati, A.; Nath, C.; Shanker, K.; Srimal, R.C.; Dhawan, K.N.; and Bhargava, K.P. Effect of alcohols on the permeability of blood-brain barrier. *Pharmacol Res Commun* 17:85-93, 1985.

Jefferies, W.A.; Brandon, M.R.; Hunt, S.V.; Williams, A.F.; Gatter, K.C.; and Mason, D.Y. Transferrin receptor on endothelium of brain capillaries. *Nature* 312:162-163, 1984.

Keller, B.T., and Borchardt, R.T. Cultured bovine brain capillary endothelial cells (BBCEC)—a blood-brain barrier model for studying the binding and internalization of insulin and insulin-like growth factor 1. (Abstract 416.) *Federations Proc* 46:1997, 1987.

Keller, B.T.; Smith, K.R.; and Borchardt, R.T. Transport barriers to absorption of peptides. *Pharm Weekbl [Sci]* 10:38-39, 1988.

Kempski, O.; Villacara, A.; Spatz, M.; Dodson, R.F.; Corn, C.; Merkel, N.; and Bembry, J. Cerebromicrovascular endothelial permeability: In vitro studies. *Acta Neuropathol (Berl)* 74:329-334, 1987.

Kumagai, A.K.; Eisenberg, J.B.; and Pardridge, W.M. Absorptive-mediated endocytosis of cationized albumin and a β-endorphin-cationized albumin chimeric peptide by isolated brain capillaries. *J Biol Chem* 262:15214-15219, 1987.

Levin, V.A. Relationship of octanol/water partition coefficient and molecular weight to rat brain capillary permeability. *J Med Chem* 23:682-684, 1980.

Maxwell, K.; Berliner, J.A.; Bready, J.; and Cancilla, P.A. Stimulation of glucose analogue uptake by cerebral microvessel endothelial cells by a product released by astrocytes. *J Neuropathol Exp Neurol* 48:69-80, 1989.

Newton, C.R., and Raub, T.J. Characterization of the transferrin receptor in primary culture of bovine brain capillary endothelial cells. *J Cell Biol* 107:770a, 1988.

Oldendorf, W.H. Brain uptake of radiolabeled amino acids, amines, and hexoses after arterial injection. *Am J Physiol* 221:1629-1639, 1971.

Oldendorf, W.H. Lipid solubility and drug penetration of the blood brain barrier. *Proc Soc Exp Biol Med* 147:813-816, 1974.

Panula, P.; Joo, F.; and Rechardt, L. Evidence for the presence of viable endothelial cells in cultures derived from dissociated rat brain. *Experientia* 34:95-97, 1978.

Pardridge, W.M. Brain metabolism: A perspective from the blood-brain barrier. *Physiol Rev* 63:1481-1535, 1983.

Pardridge, W.M.; Eisenberg, J.; and Cefalu, W.T. Absence of albumin receptor on brain capillaries in vivo and in vitro. *Am J Physiol* 249:E264-E267, 1985.

Pardridge, W.M.; Triguero, D.; and Buciak, J. Transport of histone through the blood-brain barrier. *J Pharmacol Exp Ther* 251:821-826, 1989.

Raeissi, S., and Audus, K.L. In-vitro characterization of blood-brain barrier permeability to delta sleep-inducing peptide. *J Pharmacol Pharm* 41:848-852, 1989.

Rakic, L.M.; Zlokovic, B.V.; Davson, H.; Segal, M.B.; Begley, D.J.; Lipovac, M.N.; and Mitrovic, D.M. Chronic amphetamine intoxication and the blood-brain barrier permeability to polar molecules studies in the vascularly perfused guinea pig brain. *J Neurol Sci* 94:41-50, 1989.

Raub, T.J., and Audus, K.L. Adsorptive endocytosis and membrane recycling by cultivated primary bovine brain microvessel endothelial cell monolayers *J Cell Sci* 97:127-135, 1990.

Raub, T.J.; Kuentzel, S.L.; and Sawada, G.A. Characteristics of primary bovine cerebral microvessel endothelial cell monolayers on filters: Permeability and glial induced changes. *J Cell Biol* 109:315A, 1989.

Reardon, P.M., and Audus, K.L. Arginine-vasopressin distribution across the in vitro blood-brain barrier. *Pharm Res* 6:S-88, 1989.

Rim, S.; Audus, K.L.; and Borchardt, R.T. Relationship of octanol/buffer and octanol/water partition coefficients to transcellular diffusion across brain microvessel endothelial cell monolayers. *Int J Pharm* 32:79-84, 1986.

Rosenfeld, R.G.; Pham, H.; Keller, B.T.; Borchardt, R.T.; and Pardridge, W.M. Demonstration and structural comparison of receptors for insulin-like growth factor-I and -II (IGF-I and -II) in brain and blood-brain barrier. *Biochem Biophys Res Commun* 149:159-166, 1987.

Scriba, G.K.E., and Borchardt, R.T. Metabolism of catecholamine esters by cultured bovine brain microvessel endothelial cells. *J Neurochem* 53:610-615, 1989a.

Scriba, G.K.E., and Borchardt, R.T. Metabolism of 1-methyl-4-phenyl-1,2,3,6-tetrahydropyridine (MPTP) by bovine brain capillary endothelial cell monolayers. *Brain Res* 501:175-178, 1989b.

Shah, M.V.; Audus, K.L.; and Borchardt, R.T. The application of bovine brain microvessel endothelial-cell monolayers grown onto polycarbonate membranes in vitro to estimate the potential permeability of solutes through the blood-brain barrier. *Pharm Res* 6:624-627, 1989.

Shah, M.V., and Borchardt, R.T. Characterization of the nucleoside transport system in bovine brain microvessel endothelial cell (BBMEC) monolayers. *Pharm Res* 6:S-77, 1989.

Simionescu, N. The microvascular endothelium segmental differentiations; transcytosis; selective distribution of anionic sites. *Adv Inflamm Res* 1:61-70, 1979.

Smith, K.R., and Borchardt, R.T. Permeability and mechanism of albumin, cationized albumin, and glycosilated albumin transcellular transport across monolayers of cultured bovine brain capillary endothelial cells. *Pharm Res* 6:466-473, 1989.

Smith, K.R.; Kato, A.; and Borchardt, R.T. Characterization of specific receptors for atrial natriuretic factor on cultured bovine brain capillary endothelial cells. *Biochem Biophys Res Commun* 157:308-314, 1988.

Speth, R.C., and Harik, S.I. Angiotensin II receptor binding sites in brain microvessels. *Proc Natl Acad Sci U S A* 82:6340-6343, 1985.

Sudoh, T.; Kanagawa, K.; Minamiwa, N.; and Matsuo, H. A new natriuretic peptide in porcine brain. *Nature* 332:78-81, 1988.

Takakura, Y.; Audus, K.L.; and Borchardt, R.T. Blood-brain barrier: Transport studies in isolated brain capillaries and in cultured brain endothelial cells. In: August, J.T.; Anders, M.W.; and Murad, F., eds. *Advances in Pharmacology.* Vol. 22. Orlando, FL: Academic Press, 1991a. pp. 137-165.

Takakura, Y.; Kuentzel, S.L.; Raub, T.J.; Davies, A.; Baldwin, S.A.; and Borchardt, R.T. Hexose uptake in primary cultures of bovine brain microvessel endothelial cells. I. Basic characteristics and effects of D-glucose and insulin. *Biochim Biophys Acta* 1070:1-10, 1991c.

Takakura, Y.; Trammel, A.M.; Kuentzel, S.L.; Raub, T.J.; Davies, A.; Baldwin, S.A.; and Borchardt, R.T. Hexose uptake in primary cultures of bovine brain microvessel endothelial cells. II. Effects of conditioned media from astroglial and glioma cells. *Biochim Biophys Acta* 1070:11-19, 1991b.

Thompson, S.E., and Audus, K.L. Aspects of leu-enkephalin transport and metabolism at the blood-brain barrier. *Pharm Res* 6:S-175, 1989.

Trammel, A.M., and Borchardt, R.T. Choline transport in cultured brain microvessel endothelial cells. *Pharm Res* 4:S-41, 1987.

Trammel, A.M., and Borchardt, R.T. The effects of astrocytes and glioma cells on the permeability of cultured brain microvessel endothelial cells. *Pharm Res* 6:S-88, 1989.

Triguero, D.; Buciak, J.B.; Yang, J.; and Pardridge, W.M. Blood-brain barrier transport of cationized immunoglobulin G: Enhanced delivery compared to native protein. *Proc Natl Acad Sci U S A* 86:4761-4765, 1989.

van Bree, J.B.M.M.; Audus, K.L.; and Borchardt, R.T. Carrier-mediated transport of baclofen across monolayers of bovine brain endothelial cells in primary culture. *Pharm Res* 5:369-371, 1988.

van Bree, J.B.M.M.; de Bore, A.G.; Verhoef, J.C.; Danhof, M.; and Breimer, D.D. Transport of vasopressin fragments across the blood-brain barrier: In vitro studies using monolayer cultures of bovine brain endothelial cells. *J Pharmacol Exp Ther* 249:901-905, 1989.

van Houten, M., and Posner, B.I. Insulin binds to brain blood vessels in vivo. *Nature* 282:623-625, 1979.

Vinters, H.V.; Beck, D.W.; Bready, J.V.; Maxwell, K.; Berliner, J.A.; Hart, M.N.; and Cancilla, P.A. Uptake of glucose analogues into cultured cerebral microvessel endothelium. *J Neuropathol Exp Neurol* 44:445-458, 1985.

Zlokovic, B.V.; Lipovac, M.N.; Begley, D.J.; Davson, H.; and Rakic, L. Transport of leucine-enkephalin across the blood-brain barrier in the perfused guinea pig brain. *J Neurochem* 49:310-315, 1987.

Zlokovic, B.V.; Susic, V.T.; Davson, H.; Begley, D.J.; Jankov, R.M.; Mitrovic, D.M.; and Lipovac, M.N. Saturable mechanism for delta sleep-inducing peptide (DSIP) at the blood-brain barrier of the vascularly perfused guinea pig brain. *Peptides* 10:249-254, 1989.

ACKNOWLEDGMENTS

The authors' research on bovine brain microvessel endothelial cells as a model of the BBB was supported by grants from the Upjohn Company, Merck Sharp & Dohme-INTER$_x$ Corp., the American Heart Association, and the American Heart Association-Kansas Affiliate.

AUTHORS

Yoshinobu Takakura, Ph.D.
Assistant Professor

Kenneth L. Audus, Ph.D.
Associate Professor

Address all correspondence to:

Ronald T. Borchardt, Ph.D.
Summerfield Professor and Chairman
Department of Pharmaceutical Chemistry
University of Kansas School of Pharmacy
Malott Hall, Room 3006
Lawrence, KS 66045

Opioid Peptide Drug Development: Transport of Opioid Chimeric Peptides Through the Blood-Brain Barrier

William M. Pardridge

INTRODUCTION

There currently is a need for developing new drugs for the treatment of heroin addiction. Ideally, newer agents will lack the side effects of physical dependence or respiratory depression that are typical of μ-related opioid peptides but will still block heroin withdrawal symptoms. Among the three classes of opioid peptides (dynorphins, β-endorphin, and enkephalins), dynorphin analogs have shown some promise. These compounds have a high degree of κ-opioid receptor specificity (Goldstein et al. 1988). Moreover, studies over the past several years have shown that dynorphin 1-13 acts at spinal cord sites to suppress withdrawal symptoms in morphine-dependent rats and to play a role in tolerance and dependence mechanisms (Wen and Ho 1982; Wen et al. 1985; Green and Lee 1988; Stevens and Yaksh 1989). In addition, the termination of dynorphin treatment is not associated with withdrawal symptoms (Smith and Lee 1988). However, the use of opioid peptides in drug design is complicated by three principal problems: (1) rapid degradation of the native analogs by tissue peptidases, principally aminopeptidase; (2) lack of transport of peptide pharmaceuticals across the gut intestinal barrier; and (3) lack of transport of water-soluble peptides through the brain capillary endothelial wall, which makes up the blood-brain barrier (BBB) in vivo (Pardridge 1988).

With regard to the rapid inactivation of opioid peptides by tissue aminopeptidase, analogs have been synthesized that render the peptide much less resistant to aminopeptidase inactivation. For example, the substitution of the second amino acid with a D-Ala^2 results in significant resistance to aminopeptidase activity (Pert et al. 1979). With respect to circumventing the gut barrier, peptides may be administered by an intranasal insufflation route. For more than 10 years, this approach has been used successfully for the treatment of diabetes insipidus with a metabolically stable analog of arginine vasopressin (Cool et al. 1990). The vasopressin analog is only nine amino acids in length. However, peptides as large as insulin, which is approximately 50 amino acids in length, also have been successfully administered by intranasal insufflation (Salzman et al. 1985). Indeed, a series of peptides and even larger proteins have been shown to gain access to the bloodstream following nasal administration (Chien and Chang 1987). The availability of the transnasal route obviates the difficult problem of designing analogs that survive the acidity of the stomach and are transported through the gut intestinal barrier.

Since the problems of preparing peptidase-resistant analogs and of circumventing the gut barrier have existing solutions (Veber and Freidlinger 1985; Chien and Chang 1987), the major difficulty in opioid peptide drug design is the BBB transport problem. If BBB could be solved, there would be advantages to using opioid peptides in drug design, such as (1) no kidney or liver damage as in the case of nonpeptide benzomorphan or other nonpeptide drugs (Rapaka 1986), (2) easy synthesis of analogs in high yield that are peptidase resistant (Rapaka 1986), and (3) minimization of side effects by design of receptor-specific analogs with conformational restriction (Hruby and Mosberg 1982).

OVERVIEW OF STRATEGIES AVAILABLE FOR BBB DRUG DELIVERY

There are three principal approaches to delivery of drugs through the BBB: (1) invasive or neurosurgical-based, (2) pharmacologic-based, and (3) physiologic-based. Neurosurgical-based strategies include (1) the opening of the BBB following the intracarotid injection of hypertonic media and (2) the placement of intraventricular delivery catheters and continuous intraventricular drug infusion. Repetitive opening of the BBB with the injection of intracarotid hypertonic media has been associated with a high incidence of seizures as well as chronic neuropathologic changes in the brain (Neuwelt and Rapoport 1984; Salahuddin et al. 1988). The delivery of drugs by intraventricular infusion is complicated by the steep gradients of drug concentrations that are established in the brain with this procedure (Blasberg et al. 1975). These gradients arise from the rapid bulk flow of cerebrospinal fluid (CSF) through the ventricular spaces and absorption into the peripheral circulation at the superior sagittal sinus, relative to the slow rates of peptide diffusion down into brain parenchyma from the surface of the brain. For example, the CSF compartment in the human brain contains approximately 140 mL and is turned over every 4 hours by absorption at the arachnoid granulations into the superior sagittal sinus and peripheral bloodstream. Conversely, diffusion rates are relatively slow. For example, given a peptide with a molecular weight of 10,000 and a diffusion coefficient (D) of 1×10^{-6} cm^2/sec, it may be calculated that it takes this peptide 2.9 days to diffuse 5 mm (Pardridge 1991). Thus, the peptide is more likely to leave the brain into the peripheral circulation following release into the ventricular compartment than it is to diffuse down into the brain parenchyma. Moreover, as soon as the peptide enters brain parenchyma, it is subject to sequestration by the cells in brain, thus impeding its further diffusion into brain parenchyma. Conversely, the intraventricular drug delivery approach has proven successful in treating disorders that involve the surface of the brain. For example, there are high concentrations of opioid receptors on the surface of the spinal cord, and intraspinal morphine has proven effective in treatment of chronic pain syndromes (Coombs et al. 1983). Indeed, the intraventricular injection of β-endorphin in rodents produces analgesia, probably via the release of spinal methionine enkephalin and the interaction of this analog with δ-opioid receptors (Suh and Tseng 1990). However, the treatment of drug dependency syndromes likely involves significant peptidergic pathways in the cerebral cortex, and intraventricular drug administration would not allow for adequate drug delivery to these structures within the brain.

Pharmacologic-based approaches for BBB drug delivery include lipidization of peptides or the use of liposomes. Peptide lipidization involves the blocking of polar functional moieties on the peptide backbone with groups that greatly enhance the lipid solubility of the peptide. For example, carboxyl groups or hydroxyl groups on peptides may be blocked by esterification. Indeed, the high addictive properties of heroin (diacetyl morphine) depend on the extremely rapid rate of transport of heroin through the BBB owing to the acetylation of the two hydroxyl groups on the morphine nucleus (Oldendorf et al. 1972). The permeability of the BBB is enhanced a log order by the blockade of a single hydroxyl group on the drug nucleus (Pardridge 1988), and the rapid transport of heroin across the BBB relative to morphine contributes to the addictive properties of heroin relative to the parent morphine compound. The problem with peptide lipidization is that there is a size exclusion property of BBB lipid-mediated transport. For example, cyclosporin is a highly lipid-soluble, 11-amino acid peptide compound. The octanol/Ringer's partition coefficient of cyclosporin is approximately 1,000 and is equal to that of highly lipid-soluble steroid hormones that penetrate the BBB as fast as heroin or ethyl alcohol (Cefalu and Pardridge 1985). However, the BBB transport of cyclosporin is paradoxically low and, in the presence of plasma lipoproteins, is essentially negligible. Another lipid-soluble peptide, minisomatostatin, is composed of eight amino acids; and this peptide also has a relatively high degree of lipid solubility owing to the formation of internal hydrogen bonding within the cyclic peptide structure. However, the BBB transport of minisomatostatin is essentially nil, owing to the high molecular weight (approximately 1,000) of this compound (Pardridge et al. 1990a). Therefore, it seems unlikely that the lipidization of peptides that are composed of more than five to six amino acids is a feasible strategy for enhancing BBB drug transport, owing to the size exclusion property of lipid-mediated transport through the BBB (Pardridge 1988). This size exclusion property is also the principal reason why liposomes have not proven to be an efficacious mechanism for drug delivery across the BBB. Initial liposomes were large and found to be rapidly destabilized by plasma proteins and to be rapidly taken up by cells comprising the reticuloendothelial system (Gregoriadis 1976). Subsequently, small unilamellar vesicles were developed on the order of 50 nm in size. It may not be possible to synthesize liposomes that are much smaller than 20 to 50 nm in size (Freeman and Mayhew 1986). Nevertheless, this is still a relatively large size. For example, lipoproteins are some of the larger molecules in the bloodstream, and these proteins are on the order of 20 nm, or approximately 10 times the diameter of a peptide such as cyclosporin, which itself is subject to significant size exclusion with regard to BBB transport.

The prototypic physiologic-based strategy for BBB drug delivery is the use of L-dopa in the treatment of Parkinson's disease (Nutt et al. 1984). Dopamine, a catecholamine, is not transported through the BBB. Therefore, brain dopamine levels, which are greatly depressed in the caudate putamen nucleus in individuals with Parkinson's disease, cannot be repleted by dopamine administration. However, the precursor to dopamine, L-dopa, is transported through the BBB by virtue of its affinity for the neutral amino acid transporter within the BBB (Oldendorf 1971). That is, a knowledge of the underlying transport physiology of the BBB leads to the development of new strategies for drug delivery through this barrier. This principle has been extended further with regard to peptide transport into brain. Evidence accumulated over the past 5 years has demonstrated that the BBB is endowed with receptors for certain circulating peptides or plasma proteins, and these receptors act as transport mechanisms in a process called receptor-mediated transcytosis (Pardridge 1986). Subsequently, it was demonstrated that certain ligands that enjoy receptor-mediated or absorptive-mediated transcytosis through the BBB could function as drug transport vectors and ferry across peptide pharmaceuticals that by themselves are not capable of transport through the BBB. This approach, called the chimeric peptide strategy, is discussed in the next section of this chapter.

CHIMERIC PEPTIDE STRATEGY FOR BBB TRANSPORT OF PEPTIDE NEUROPHARMACEUTICALS

BBB Drug Transport Vectors

Chimeric peptides are composed of a nontransportable peptide pharmaceutical that is covalently coupled to a transportable peptide that is capable of receptor-mediated or absorptive-mediated transcytosis through the BBB. Receptor-mediated drug transport vectors include insulin, transferrin, and, possibly, insulin-like growth factor (IGF-2) (table 1). The discovery of a receptor-mediated BBB drug transport vector requires, first, the demonstration of a saturable receptor for the peptide on the brain capillary and, second, the demonstration that the receptor acts as a transport system allowing the net transcytosis of the peptide from blood into brain interstitial fluid. The simplest approach for identifying receptors on the BBB for a variety of peptide compounds is the use of the isolated brain capillary preparation. Capillaries may be isolated from either the brains of laboratory animals or the autopsied human brain using a relatively simple 3-hour procedure. As shown in figure 1, human brain capillaries can be isolated in high yield, free of contiguous brain tissues. These capillaries may then be used along with a radiolabeled peptide and standard radioreceptor methodology to quantify the binding characteristics of the BBB peptide receptor. As shown in table 1, the dissociation constant (K_D) and maximal binding capacity (B_{max}) have been measured for human brain capillary insulin, transferrin, and IGF-1 and IGF-2 receptors. The demonstration that these receptors may act as transport systems was first reported for insulin using morphologic techniques, including thaw-mount autoradiography (Pardridge 1986; Duffy and Pardridge 1987), and, subsequently, for transferrin using cell isolation techniques (Fishman et al. 1987). The transcytosis of peptides or plasma proteins through the BBB may be quantified using an internal carotid artery perfusion/capillary depletion method recently developed (Triguero et al. 1990).

TABLE 1.   *BBB peptide receptors*

Origin of Brain Capillary	Peptide or Protein	K_D (nM)	B_{max} (p_{mol} mg_p^{-1})
Human	Insulin	1.2 ± 0.5	0.17 ± 0.08
	IGF-1	2.1 ± 0.4	0.17 ± 0.02
	IGF-2	1.1 ± 0.1	0.21 ± 0.01
	Transferrin	5.6 ± 1.4	0.10 ± 0.02
Bovine	Histone	$15,200 \pm 2,800$	$7,700 \pm 1,000$
	Cationized IgG	900 ± 370	$1,400 \pm 400$
	Cationized albumin	$2,300 \pm 1,100$	$6,200 \pm 2,600$

SOURCE: Pardridge et al. 1985, 1989, 1990b; Kumagai et al. 1987; Duffy et al. 1988; Triguero et al. 1989

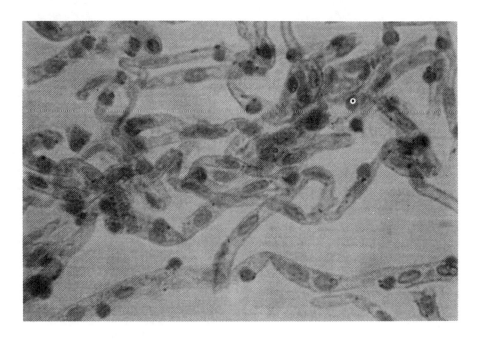

FIGURE 1. *Isolated human brain capillaries*

SOURCE: Pardridge et al. 1985, copyright 1985, Raven Press

There are two principal concerns in using natural peptides as drug transport vectors. First, the vector itself will have biologic activity. For example, the side effects of using insulin as a drug transport vector could include hypoglycemia. The use of transferrin may alter iron homeostasis, and the use of IGF-2 as a drug transport vector is complicated by the avid binding of this peptide by specific binding proteins in plasma (Duffy et al. 1988). Second, the interaction of peptide ligands with receptor binding sites is generally highly specific, and the addition of a nontransportable pharmaceutical onto an insulin or transferrin vector may result in markedly reduced rates of affinity of the modified insulin or transferrin for its native receptor. However, these two concerns are addressed with the use of polycationic proteins as BBB drug transport vectors. It has been known for many years that the cationization of proteins, in general, enhances the cellular uptake of these macromolecules (Basu et al. 1976; Shen and Ryser 1978). This property was demonstrated for BBB transport processes when it was shown that cationized albumin is transported across the BBB in vivo (Kumagai et al. 1987). Cationized albumin is prepared by converting surface carboxyl groups on the albumin molecule to extended primary amino groups using such derivatives as hexamethylenediamine. This raises the isoelectric point of the protein from approximately four to nine and causes the modified albumin to undergo rapid absorptive-mediated transcytosis through the BBB (Triguero et al. 1990). Native cationic proteins, such as histone, have been shown to undergo absorptive-mediated transcytosis through the BBB and to have saturable binding sites on brain capillaries (Pardridge et al. 1989), similar to cationized albumin or native peptides (table 1). However, histone has been shown to be toxic to the BBB and to cause changes in BBB permeability at relatively low doses. This property has not been observed following the infusion of cationized albumin (Triguero et al. 1990). Nevertheless, two concerns with regard to using cationized albumin as a drug transport vector are the potential toxicity of this polycationic protein and the immunogenicity of the cationized form of the native protein. These issues have been addressed recently in a study wherein 1 mg/kg of cationized rat albumin was administered daily to rats for periods of up to 8 weeks (Pardridge et al. 1990b). During the course of these studies, organs were analyzed by tissue histology, and serum chemistries were monitored. After 8 weeks, no discernible toxicity was found in 10 organs examined in the rat, and approximately 20 different metabolic, kidney, and hepatic function tests were found to be normal in the treated animals as compared with those animals receiving equal doses of native rat albumin. Moreover, the antibody response to the cationized rat albumin in rats was minimal owing to the use of a homologous system (i.e., the administration of cationized rat albumin to rats) (Pardridge et al. 1990b). The use of heterologous cationic proteins has been shown in previous studies to result in marked immunogenicity (Muckerheide et al. 1987). Nevertheless, the use of cationized homologous proteins has not been found to generate a significant immune response. On the basis of these other studies, cationized rat albumin is believed to be a suitable vector for the delivery of peptides across the BBB in a physiologic setting and to provide a model for pharmacologic paradigms involving repetitive drug administration (Pardridge et al. 1990b).

β-Endorphin Chimeric Peptides

A β-endorphin-cationized albumin chimeric peptide was prepared using the disulfide-based cross-linking reagent N-succinimidyl-3-(2-pyridyldithio)propionate (SPDP) (Carlsson et al. 1978). Disulfide-based cross-linkers were chosen because previous studies have shown that disulfide bonds are relatively stable in plasma but are labile in cells (Letvin et al. 1986), which is the necessary criterion that must be established for a drug delivery vehicle. The β-endorphin was coupled via N-terminal and lysine ε-amino groups on the opioid peptide to extended primary amino groups on the cationized albumin as follows (Kumagai et al. 1987):

| Cationized albumin | -CONH(CH$_2$)$_6$NHCO(CH$_2$)$_2$-S-S-(CH$_2$)$_2$CONH- | β-endorphin |

The cationized albumin-β-endorphin chimeric peptide was radiolabeled by first labeling the β-endorphin moiety with [^{125}I]-iodine or [^{3}H] prior to synthesis of the chimeric peptide. This allowed for the study of the transport and metabolism of the β-endorphin chimeric peptide by following the fate of the radiolabel.

The transport of chimeric peptides through the BBB is viewed within the context of four individual steps that are depicted in figure 2. The first step is absorptive-mediated endocytosis at the blood side of the BBB. The absorptive-mediated endocytosis of the cationized albumin-β-endorphin chimeric peptide was demonstrated with isolated brain capillaries using a mild acid wash technique (Kumagai et al. 1987).

The second step in the overall process is absorptive-mediated exocytosis at the brain side of the BBB, which completes the transcytosis of the chimeric peptide through the BBB, allowing for distribution of the chimeric peptide into brain interstitial fluid. This process was demonstrated using an internal carotid artery infusion/capillary depletion method (Pardridge et al. 1990c) recently developed in the author's laboratory (Triguero et al. 1990). Moreover, these studies showed that the rate of transcytosis of the β-endorphin-cationized albumin chimeric peptide through the BBB was essentially identical to the rate of transcytosis of the unmodified cationized albumin. These data supported the initial hypothesis that vectors that traverse the BBB via absorptive-mediated mechanisms (as opposed to receptor-mediated mechanisms) would be better able to tolerate the addition of bulky pharmaceuticals to the transport vector without significant impairment of BBB transport rates. This property is likely due to the fact that absorptive-mediated transport is triggered by the electrostatic interaction between cationic groups on the drug transport vector and anionic groups on the surface of the microvascular endothelium.

The third step in the overall chimeric peptide strategy is the cleavage of the disulfide bond joining the drug transport vector and the peptide pharmaceutical (figure 2). Moreover, it is necessary that the rate of cleavage of this disulfide bond is substantially faster than the rate of degradation of the pharmaceutical peptide while it is still attached to the drug transport vector. In the setting of slow cleavage of the disulfide bond by brain, there would be little free pharmacologically active peptide generated to interact with the respective peptide receptor on brain nerve endings. However, recent studies have shown that brain is endowed with high activities of the disulfide reductase enzymatic activity that cleaves the β-endorphin-cationized albumin chimeric peptide

160

Delivery of Chimeric Peptides
Through the Blood-Brain Barrier

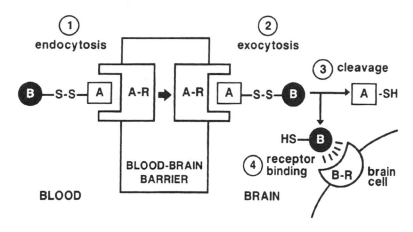

FIGURE 2. *Chimeric peptide drug delivery strategy. Scheme for delivery
of chimeric peptides through the BBB shows four steps in the
overall process: (1) receptor-mediated endocytosis of the
blood-borne chimeric peptide, (2) receptor-mediated exocytosis
of the chimeric peptide into the brain interstitium, (3) cleavage
of the disulfide bond liberating the unconjugated transport vector
and the pharmacologically active peptide, and (4) binding of
pharmacologically active peptide with its respective receptor on
brain cells. A=BBB transport vector (e.g., cationized albumin);
B=nontransportable (pharmacologically active) peptide (e.g.,
β-endorphin); A-R=peptide A receptor; B-R=peptide B receptor.*

SOURCE: Pardridge 1991, copyright 1991, Raven Press

(Pardridge et al. 1990c). As shown in figure 3, the conversion of the β-
endorphin-cationized albumin chimeric peptide into the free β-endorphin occurs
at a rate that is approximately 50 percent complete within 1 minute at 37 °C.
Moreover, the formation of free endorphin in brain occurs at a rate substantially
faster than the subsequent degradation of the β-endorphin (figure 3).

The fourth and final step of the chimeric peptide strategy depicted in figure 2
is the interaction of free pharmacologically active peptide with its respective
receptor on brain nerve endings. However, significant care must be
taken in choosing coupling strategies that allow for the generation of a

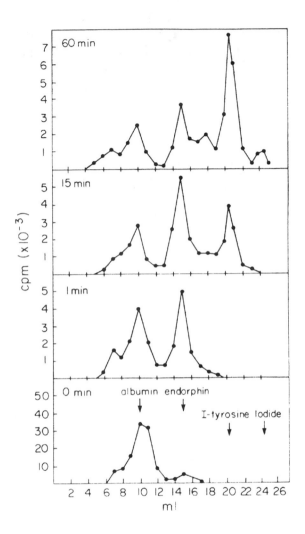

FIGURE 3. *Demonstration of cleavage of β-endorphin chimeric peptide by rat brain. Superose 12-HR fast protein liquid chromatography gel filtration of [^{125}I]-[D-Ala^2]-β-endorphin-cationized albumin chimeric peptide following incubation with rat brain homogenate for 0, 1, 15, or 60 minutes at 37 °C. The data show that monoiodotyrosine, which migrates at 20 mL, is formed subsequent to the formation of the unconjugated β-endorphin that is cleaved from the chimeric peptide by rat brain enzymes.*

SOURCE: Pardridge et al. 1990c, copyright 1990, The Endocrine Society

pharmacologically active peptide subsequent to the cleavage of the peptide from its drug transport vector. For example, the principal mode of attachment of a pharmaceutical peptide through the cationized albumin vector is via free amino groups on the pharmacologically active peptide. Subsequent to the cleavage of the chimeric peptide, there is a mercaptopropionate group remaining on the amino group that participated in the coupling reaction:

$$HS(CH_2)_2CONH-\boxed{\beta\text{-endorphin}}$$

Therefore, the construct for opioid peptide drug design must consider the structural requirements that are necessary for preservation of opioid peptide biologic activity following cleavage from the drug transport vector (see next section).

Chimeric Peptide Coupling Strategies

To prepare opioid chimeric peptides that are pharmacologically active following cleavage of the disulfide bond, there are several structural requirements that must be incorporated into the parent opioid peptide (Pardridge 1991).

1. The peptide must be relatively resistant to rapid aminopeptidase inactivation. This requires a substitution of glycine at the number two position with a D-alanine. The disadvantage of this substitution is that it causes the loss of κ-opioid peptide receptor selectivity (Goldstein et al. 1988). However, this substitution is essential for in vivo studies because the cerebral vasculature is endowed with high quantities of aminopeptidase (Pardridge and Mietus 1981).

2. The N-terminal α-amino group must be protected during the coupling procedure that converts free amino groups to pyridyl dithiopropionate (PDP) moieties. This procedure converts amino groups to active PDP groups that will then participate with free sulfhydryls on the transport vector to form the disulfide bond. In the case of opioid peptides that lack a cysteine sulfhydryl, PDP derivatives must be formed by reacting SPDP with free amino groups other than the N-terminal α-amino group, since this latter group must be free to maintain biologic activity of the opioid peptide (Bewley and Choh 1983). A blockade of the α-amino group with citraconic anhydride is a possibility; however, it is likely that this procedure will also block the internal (e.g., lysine ε-amino group) amino groups; and this, in turn, would prevent subsequent formation of the PDP derivative. This problem may be solved by preparing N-terminal t-butoxycarbonyl (boc)

derivatives of the opioid peptide by aminolytic cleavage of the peptide from the solid-phase resin using 1,5-diaminopentane, as described by Goldstein and coworkers (1988). This results in selective protection of the N-terminal α-amino group during the formation of the PDP derivative, and the boc group may then be cleaved with exposure to acid pH.

3. It is important to be able to radiolabel the opioid peptide so that following its conversion into a chimeric peptide, its transport through the BBB in vivo may be followed, and the pharmacokinetics of the clearance of the opioid chimeric peptide from blood in vivo may be determined. In addition, radiolabeled opioid chimeric peptide is needed to perform in vitro radioreceptor assays to assess biologic activity of the opioid peptide following its cleavage from the transport vector. The N-terminal tyrosine could be oxidatively iodinated directly. However, such [iodo-Tyr[1]] derivatives of opioid peptides exhibit reduced biologic activity (Li and Chung 1976). Therefore, an optimal approach for radiolabeling opioid peptides is to initially use boc derivatives of diiodotyrosine in the solid-state synthesis of opioid peptide. These iodo groups may then be removed by catalytic reduction, yielding high specific activity [^{3}H]-labeled opioid peptides (Miller et al. 1978).

4. The opioid peptide must be pharmacologically active following its release from the drug transport vector after cleavage of the disulfide bond. This requirement necessitates that the "molecular baggage" that is left on the opioid amino group following its cleavage from the chimeric peptide is placed in a portion of the molecule that is not involved in biologic activity and receptor binding. In the case of dynorphin derivatives, this problem may be solved by replacing lysine groups with arginines and preparing an analog with a C-terminal extended amino group that may participate in the coupling reaction, but that is not important for receptor binding site activity (Goldstein et al. 1988).

SUMMARY AND CONCLUSIONS

The use of chimeric peptides and physiologic-based strategies for drug delivery through the BBB may be applied to opioid peptides (dynorphins, endorphin analogs, and enkephalin analogs), and these agents have considerable advantages in drug development with respect to drug addiction. Recent research has allowed for the development of efficacious BBB drug transport vectors, as well as the demonstration that these vectors allow for shuttling of opioid peptides through the BBB in vivo. The major challenge to future research is the development of coupling strategies that allow for the release of biologically active opioid peptide from the drug transport vector following its cleavage by disulfide reductase enzymes, which are abundant in brain. These coupling strategies must be developed in advance since the amino groups necessary for coupling are incorporated into the opioid peptide at the level of solid-state synthesis.

REFERENCES

Basu, S.K.; Goldstein, J.L.; Anderson, R.G.W.; and Brown, M.S. Degradation of cationized low density lipoprotein and regulation of cholesterol metabolism in homozygous familial hypercholesterolemia fibroblasts. *Proc Natl Acad Sci U S A* 73:3178-3182, 1976.

Bewley, T.A., and Choh, H.L. Evidence for tertiary structure in aqueous solutions of human β-endorphin as shown by difference absorption spectroscopy. *Biochemistry* 22:2671-2675, 1983.

Blasberg, R.G.; Patlak, C.; and Fenstermacher, J.D. Intrathecal chemotherapy: Brain tissue profiles after ventriculo-cisternal perfusion. *J Pharmacol Exp Ther* 195:73-83, 1975.

Carlsson, J.; Drevin, H.; and Axen, R. Protein thiolation and reversible protein-protein conjugation. N-succinimidyl 3-(2-pyridyldithio)propionate, a new heterobifunctional reagent. *Biochem J* 173:723-733, 1978.

Cefalu, W.T., and Pardridge, W.M. Restrictive transport of a lipid-soluble peptide (cyclosporin) through the blood-brain barrier. *J Neurochem* 45:1954-1956, 1985.

Chien, Y.W., and Chang, S.-F. Intranasal drug delivery for systemic medications. *Crit Rev Ther Drug Carrier Syst* 4:67-194, 1987.

Cool, W.M.; Kurtz, N.M.; and Chu, G. Transnasal delivery of system drugs. In: Benedetti, C.; Chapman, C.R.; and Giron, G., eds. *Advances in Pain Research and Therapy*. Vol. 14. New York: Raven Press, 1990. pp. 241-258.

Coombs, D.W.; Saunders, R.L.; Gaylor, M.S.; Block, A.R.; Colton, T.; Harbaugh, R.; Pageau, M.G.; and Mroz, W. Relief of continuous chronic pain by intraspinal narcotics infusion via an implanted reservoir. *JAMA* 250(17):2336-2339, 1983.

Duffy, K.R., and Pardridge, W.M. Blood-brain barrier transcytosis of insulin in developing rabbits. *Brain Res* 420:32-38, 1987.

Duffy, K.R.; Pardridge, W.M.; and Rosenfeld, R.G. Human blood-brain barrier insulin-like growth factor receptor. *Metabolism* 37:136-140, 1988.

Fishman, J.B.; Rubin, J.B.; Handrahan, J.V.; Connor, J.R.; and Fine, R.E. Receptor-mediated transcytosis of transferrin across the blood-brain barrier. *J Neurosci Res* 18:299-306, 1987.

Freeman, A.I., and Mayhew, E. Targeted drug delivery. *Cancer* 58:573-583, 1986.

Goldstein, A.; Nestor, J.J., Jr.; Naidu, A.; and Newman, S.R. "DAKLI": A multipurpose ligand with high affinity and selectivity for dynorphin (κ-opioid) binding sites. *Proc Natl Acad Sci U S A* 85:7375-7379, 1988.

Green, P.G., and Lee, N.M. Dynorphin A-(1-13) attenuates withdrawal in morphine-dependent rats: Effect of route of administration. *Eur J Pharmacol* 145:267-272, 1988.

Gregoriadis, G. The carrier potential of liposomes in biology and medicine. *N Engl J Med* 295:704-710, 1976.

Hruby, V.K., and Mosberg, H.I. Conformational and dynamic considerations in peptide structure-function studies. *Peptides* 3:329-336, 1982.

Kumagai, A.K.; Eisenberg, J.; and Pardridge, W.M. Absorptive-mediated endocytosis of cationized albumin and a β-endorphin-cationized albumin chimeric peptide by isolated brain capillaries. Model system of blood-brain barrier transport. *J Biol Chem* 262:15214-15219, 1987.

Letvin, N.L.; Goldmacher, V.S.; Ritz, J.; Yetz, J.M.; Schlossman, S.F.; and Lambert, J.M. In vivo administration of lymphocyte-specific monoclonal antibodies in nonhuman primates. In vivo stability of disulfide-linked immunotoxin conjugates. *J Clin Invest* 77:977-983, 1986.

Li, C.H., and Chung, D. Isolation and structure of an untriakontapeptide with opiate activity from camel pituitary glands. *Proc Natl Acad Sci U S A* 73(4):1145-1148, 1976.

Miller, R.J.; Chang, K.-J.; Leighton, J.; and Cuatrecasas, P. Interaction of iodinated enkephalin analogues with opiate receptors. *Life Sci* 22:379-388, 1978.

Muckerheide, A.; Apple, R.J.; Pesce, A.J.; and Michael, J.G. Cationization of protein antigens. *J Immunol* 138:933-937, 1987.

Neuwelt, E.A., and Rapoport, S.I. Modification of the blood-brain barrier in the chemotherapy of malignant brain tumors. *Federations Proc* 43:214-219, 1984.

Nutt, J.G.; Woodward, W.R.; Hammerstad, J.P.; Carter, J.H.; and Anderson, J.L. The "on-off" phenomenon in Parkinson's disease. *N Engl J Med* 310:483-488, 1984.

Oldendorf, W.H. Brain uptake of radiolabeled amino acids, amines, and hexoses after arterial injection. *Am J Physiol* 221:1629-1639, 1971.

Oldendorf, W.H.; Hyman, S.; Braun, L.; and Oldendorf, S.Z. Blood-brain barrier: Penetration of morphine, codeine, heroin, and methadone after carotid injection. *Science* 178:984-986, 1972.

Pardridge, W.M. Receptor-mediated peptide transport through the blood-brain barrier. *Endocr Rev* 7:314-330, 1986.

Pardridge, W.M. Recent advances in blood-brain barrier transport. *Annu Rev Pharmacol Toxicol* 28:25-39, 1988.

Pardridge, W.M. *Peptide Drug Delivery to the Brain.* New York: Raven Press, 1991.

Pardridge, W.M.; Eisenberg, J.; and Yang, J. Human blood-brain barrier insulin receptor. *J Neurochem* 44:1771-1778, 1985.

Pardridge, W.M., and Mietus, L.J. Enkephalin and blood-brain barrier: Studies of binding and degradation in isolated brain microvessels. *Endocrinology* 109:1138-1143, 1981.

Pardridge, W.M.; Triguero, D.; and Buciak, J.B. Transport of histone through the blood-brain barrier. *J Pharmacol Exp Ther* 251:821-826, 1989.

Pardridge, W.M.; Triguero, D.; and Buciak, J.L. β-Endorphin chimeric peptides: Transport through the blood-brain barrier in vivo and cleavage of disulfide linkage by brain. *Endocrinology* 126:977-984, 1990c.

Pardridge, W.M.; Triguero, D.; Buciak, J.L.; and Yang, J. Evaluation of cationized rat albumin as a potential blood-brain barrier drug transport vector. *J Pharmacol Exp Ther* 255:893-899, 1990b.

Pardridge, W.M.; Triguero, D.; Yang, J.; and Cancilla, P.A. Comparison of in vitro and in vivo models of drug transcytosis through the blood-brain barrier. *J Pharmacol Exp Ther* 253:884-891, 1990a.

Pert, C.B.; Klee, W.; Costa, E.; Pert, A.; and Davis, G.C. Basic and clinical studies of endorphins. *Ann Intern Med* 91:239-251, 1979.

Rapaka, R.S. Research topics in the medicinal chemistry and molecular pharmacology of opioid peptides—Present and future. *Life Sci* 39:1825-1843, 1986.

Salahuddin, T.S.; Johansson, B.B.; Kalimo, H.; and Olsson, Y. Structural changes in the rat brain after carotid infusions of hyperosmolar solutions. An electron microscopic study. *Acta Neuropathol (Berl)* 77:5-13, 1988.

Salzman, R.; Manson, J.E.; Griffing, G.T.; Kimmerle, R.; Ruderman, N.; McCall, A.; Stoltz, E.I.; Mullin, C.; Small, D.; Armstrong, J.; and Melby, J.C. Intranasal aerosolized insulin: Mixed-meal studies and long-term use in type I diabetes. *N Engl J Med* 312:1078-1084, 1985.

Shen, W.-C., and Ryser, H.J.-P. Conjugation of poly-L-lysine to albumin and horseradish peroxidase: A novel method of enhancing the cellular uptake of proteins. *Proc Natl Acad Sci U S A* 74(4):1872-1876, 1978.

Smith, A.P., and Lee, N.M. Pharmacology of dynorphin. *Annu Rev Pharmacol Toxicol* 28:123-140, 1988.

Stevens, C.W., and Yaksh, T.L. Time course characteristics of tolerance development to continuously infused antinociceptive agents in rat spinal cord. *J Pharmacol Exp Ther* 251(1):216-223, 1989.

Suh, H.H., and Tseng, L.F. Delta but not mu-opioid receptors in the spinal cord are involved in antinociception induced by β-endorphin given intracerebroventricularly in mice. *J Pharmacol Exp Ther* 253(3):981-986, 1990.

Triguero, D.; Buciak, J.B.; and Pardridge, W.M. Capillary depletion method for quantifying blood-brain barrier transcytosis of circulating peptides and plasma proteins. *J Neurochem* 54:1882-1888, 1990.

Triguero, D.; Buciak, J.B.; Yang, J.; and Pardridge, W.M. Blood-brain barrier transport of cationized immunoglobulin G. Enhanced delivery compared to native protein. *Proc Natl Acad Sci U S A* 86:4761-4765, 1989.

Veber, D.F., and Freidlinger, R.M. The design of metabolically-stable peptide analogs. *Trends Neurosci* 6:392-396, 1985.

Wen, H.L., and Ho, W.K.K. Suppression of withdrawal symptoms by dynorphin in heroin addicts. *Eur J Pharmacol* 82:183-186, 1982.

Wen, H.L.; Mehal, Z.D.; Ong, B.H.; Ho, W.K.K.; and Wen, K.Y.K. Intrathecal administration of β-endorphin and dynorphin (1-13) for the treatment of intractable pain. *Life Sci* 37:1213-1220, 1985.

AUTHOR

William M. Pardridge, M.D.
Professor
Department of Medicine
Brain Research Institute
University of California, Los Angeles School of Medicine
Los Angeles, CA 90024-1682

Redox Approaches to Drug Delivery to the Central Nervous System

Marcus E. Brewster and Nicholas Bodor

INTRODUCTION

Targeted drug delivery is a highly desirable goal in the practice of medicinal chemistry. The preparation of molecular systems that act to concentrate a pharmacologically active agent at its pathophysiologically relevant site would provide a variety of advantages over agents lacking this specificity. For example, since a greater portion of the administered dose of a drug is sequestered at a particular locus, the delivery system should be highly efficacious and the drug dose could be reduced. In addition, nontarget site toxicities would be attenuated since lower concentrations of the drug are present. The lowering of the effective dose and the increasing of the dose of drug required to initiate toxicity results in a significant improvement in the therapeutic index. This ratio is arguably the most important parameter that must be optimized during the drug design and testing process.

One organ system for which drug targeting would be beneficial is the central nervous system (CNS). The reason for this importance, aside from the vital role that the CNS plays in body functioning and homeostasis, is that a variety of drugs are barred from entering the brain, making the treatment of cerebral disease difficult. The basis of this impermeability is the blood-brain barrier (BBB) (Neuwelt 1989; Rapoport 1976; Suckling et al. 1986), which acts as a functional barricade to separate the brain from the systemic circulation. Structurally, the component endothelial cells of the CNS capillaries are joined tightly together, precluding intercellular bulk transport (Reese and Karnovsky 1967). This architecture forces compounds to diffuse directly through the cell membranes if they are to gain access to the brain parenchyma; and as the cell membranes are phospholipoidal in nature, only lipophilic agents may breach the BBB, meaning that many water-soluble substances are excluded. In the periphery, capillaries are leaky, allowing nonspecific intercellular transport. Brain capillaries also are characterized by a high concentration of various enzymes that help to maintain the delicate cerebral milieu by preventing the uptake of blood-borne neurotransmitters and other substances. Enzymes found in high concentration in the cerebral vascular system include monoamine oxidase, catechol-O-methyltransferase, γ-glutamyl transpeptidase, γ-aminobutyric acid transaminase, aromatic amino acid decarboxylase, various enkephalinases, and others (Pardridge et al. 1975; Levin 1977).

These anatomical and enzymatic differences explain the barrier properties of the BBB but incompletely describe the system. Many essential nutrients such as glucose and metabolic wastes such as acetate must be taken up or expelled. These compounds, because of their high polarity, would not be expected to rapidly diffuse through cell membranes, and thus, an apparent problem arises. This paradox is explained by the presence of specialized carrier systems that are located in the BBB (Neuwelt 1989; Pardridge 1981). These protein macromolecular systems are characterized by saturability and high molecular selectivity. Carriers are facilitative in nature and have been identified for hexoses; neutral, acidic, and basic amino acids; monocarboxylic acids; nucleosides and nucleoside bases; choline; and various other biologically important molecules. This avenue, therefore, provides for the bidirectional movement of selective molecules; but with few exceptions (Greig et al. 1987), these systems are not relevant to drug delivery. Thus, the CNS has evolved to exclude polar metabolites and other compounds that may prove harmful. Unfortunately, this barrier system also may exclude many potentially useful therapeutic agents.

Therefore, general methods for improving drug flux into the brain would be useful. Brain uptake of compounds can be improved by derivatization of the drug molecules via prodrug formation (Stella 1975; Bodor 1981; Bodor and Kaminski 1987; Bundgaard 1985). A prodrug is a pharmacologically inactive compound that results from transient chemical modification of a biologically active species. The chemical change is designed to improve some deficient physicochemical property of the drug, such as membrane permeability or water solubility. After administration, the prodrug by virtue of its improved characteristics is brought closer to the receptor site for longer periods where it can convert to the active species. Prodrugs usually require a single activating step. When the BBB is considered, increased drug penetration is usually well correlated with the lipophilicity or the octanol:water partition coefficient of a drug (Levin 1980; Fenstermacher 1985). To improve the entry of a hydroxy-, amino-, or carboxylic-acid-containing drug, esterification or amidation may be performed. This greatly enhances the lipid solubility of the drug, and as a result, the drug can better enter the brain parenchyma. Once the drug is in the CNS, hydrolysis of the lipophilicity-modifying group will release the active compound.

170

Unfortunately, simple prodrugs suffer from several important limitations. Whereas increasing the lipophilicity of a molecule may improve its movement through the BBB, the uptake of the compound into other tissues is likewise augmented, leading to a generally greater tissue burden (Stella and Himmelstein 1980). This nonselectivity of delivery is especially detrimental when potent drugs such as steroids or cytotoxic agents are considered because nontarget site toxicities are exacerbated. In addition, although drug uptake into the CNS may be facilitated by increasing the lipophilicity of a drug, its efflux also is enhanced. This results in poor tissue retention of the drug and short biological action. Finally, whereas the only metabolism associated with prodrugs should be by conversion to the parent drug, other routes can occur and may contribute to the toxicity of the compounds (Gorrod 1980). These effects (i.e., poor selectivity, poor retention, and the possibility for reactive catabolism) often conspire to decrease, not increase, the therapeutic index of drugs when masked as a prodrug.

CHEMICAL DELIVERY SYSTEMS

Some of the limitations associated with the prodrug approach are derived from the fact that only one chemical conversion occurs in the activation of the compound. In many circumstances, multiple, facile conversions may not only lead to selectivity in delivery but also may act to decrease the toxicity of a drug as well as sustain its action. A chemical delivery system (CDS) is defined as a biologically inert molecule that requires several steps in its conversion to the active drug and that enhances drug delivery to a particular organ or site (Bodor and Brewster 1983; Bodor et al. 1981; Bodor 1987). In designing a CDS for the CNS, the unique architecture of the BBB was exploited. As with a prodrug, a CDS should be sufficiently lipophilic to allow for brain uptake. Subsequent to this step, the molecule should undergo an enzymatic or other conversion to promote retention within the CNS but, at the same time, to accelerate peripheral elimination of the entity. Finally, the intermediate should degrade, releasing the active compound in a sustained manner.

One system that possesses these attributes is summarized in figure 1. In this CDS, a carrier molecule is used as a lipophilicity modifier. Although many moieties may serve such functions, 1,4-dihydrotrigonellinates have proved to be the most useful. In this approach, a hydroxy-, amino-, or carboxylic-acid-containing drug is esterified, aminated, or otherwise covalently linked to nicotinic acid or a nicotinic acid derivative. This compound is then quaternized to generate the 1-methylnicotinate salt or trigonellinate and chemically reduced to give the 1,4-dihydrotrigonellinate or CDS. This dihydro moiety greatly enhances the lipophilicity of the drug to which it is attached. Upon systemic administration, the CDS, due to its enhanced lipophilicity, can partition into

171

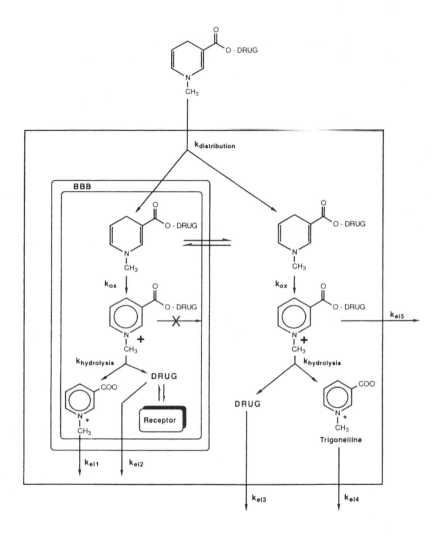

FIGURE 1. *The CDS is a reduced 1-methyl nicotinic acid conjugate of an active drug. Systemic administration of the dihydronicotinate or nicotinamide results in relatively extensive distribution due to the lipophilicity of the species. Subsequent to distribution, the labile dihydronicotinamide undergoes oxidation resulting in the formation of a nicotinate salt conjugate (k_{ox}). This more polar species is rapidly eliminated from the periphery but is retained in the CNS (k_{e15} is rapid). In the CNS, the locked-in salt can slowly hydrolyze, liberating the drug of interest as well as the spent carrier.*

several body compartments, some of which are inaccessible to the unmanipulated compound. At this point, the CDS is working as a lipoidal prodrug. The carrier molecule is specially designed, however, to undergo an enzymatically mediated oxidation that converts the membrane-permeable dihydrotrigonellinate to a hydrophilic, membrane-impermeable trigonellinate salt. This conversion occurs ubiquitously. The now polar, oxidized carrier-drug conjugate is trapped behind the lipoidal BBB and is, in essence, depoted in the CNS. Any of this oxidized salt that is present in the periphery will be rapidly lost as it is now polar and an excellent candidate for elimination by the kidney and liver. The conjugate that is trapped behind the BBB can then slowly hydrolyse to give the active species in a slow and sustained manner. By the system design, concentrations of the active drug are very low in the periphery, reducing systemic, dose-related toxicities. In addition, the drug in the CNS is present mostly in the form of an inactive conjugate, thus lowering any central toxicities. This approach should allow for a more potent compound in that a larger portion of the administered dose is shunted to its site of action. In addition, this system should allow for increased dosing interval.

Since it was first proposed in 1978, the brain-targeting CDS has been applied extensively to various pharmacologically active agents. Reviews of work conducted prior to 1983 and 1986 are available (Bodor and Brewster 1983; Bodor 1987).

BRAIN-ENHANCED DELIVERY OF ANTIVIRAL AGENTS

Viral encephalitic diseases are major health problems in the United States and throughout the world. These diseases have the reputation of being extraordinarily pernicious and difficult to treat. The basis of this refractoriness can be traced to several factors, not the least of which is the inability of many potentially useful drugs to penetrate into brain tissue. This section examines the application of the CDS to antiviral agents—specifically, drugs useful in the treatment of acquired immunodeficiency syndrome (AIDS), herpes encephalitis, cytomegaloviral encephalitis, and Japanese encephalitis.

Zidovudine or azidothymidine (AZT) is the first approved drug for the treatment of AIDS. In a few cases, this modified riboside has been shown to be useful in improving the neuropsychiatric course of AIDS encephalopathy, but the doses required to elicit this improvement precipitate severe anemia (Yarchoan et al. 1987). This usually leads to cessation of therapy. When the drug is withdrawn in response to this neutropenia, all the abated symptoms promptly return. Interestingly, AZT does enter the cerebrospinal fluid (CSF) after oral or intravenous (IV) dosing, and it achieves significant concentrations (Balis et al. 1989; Klecker et al. 1987; Blum et al. 1988). Unfortunately, these CSF levels appear to greatly overestimate brain parenchymal and neuronal levels as AZT poorly penetrates the BBB (Terasaki and Pardridge 1988). In an effort to ameliorate the prognosis of AIDS encephalopathy, the CDS approach was applied to AZT (Little et al. 1990; Brewster et al. 1988a; Gallo et al. 1989; Gogu et al. 1989; Torrence et al. 1988; Chu et al. 1990; Aggarwal et al. 1990). This antiviral agent has a primary alcohol functionality in the 5'-position, which was considered for carrier attachment. As shown in figure 2, AZT was treated with nicotinoyl chloride hydrochloride in pyridine to yield the 5'-nicotinate. This ester was subsequently quaternized with methyl iodide to yield the 5'-trigonellinate (1-methylnicotinate) and reduced in basic aqueous sodium dithionite to give the 5'-(1,4-dihydrotrigonellinate) derivative of AZT (AZT-CDS).

The AZT-CDS is a crystalline solid that is stable at room temperature for several months when protected from light and moisture. The lipophilicity of the AZT-CDS and its metabolites (AZT and the AZT-5'-trigonellinate salt [AZT-Q^+]) is important in determining the efficiency of the CDS. The n-octanol:water partition coefficient (log P) was determined to be 0.06, -2.00, and 1.5 for AZT, AZT-Q^+, and AZT-CDS, respectively, as shown in figure 2. This indicates that

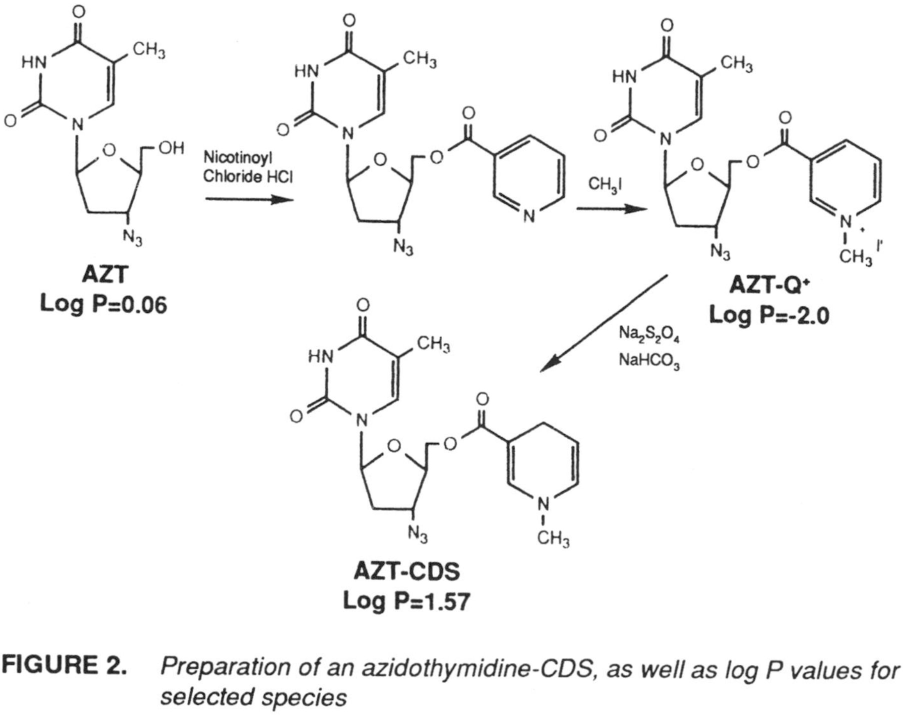

FIGURE 2. *Preparation of an azidothymidine-CDS, as well as log P values for selected species*

the CDS is 34-fold more lipophilic than the parent riboside and more than 3,900-fold more lipophilic than the AZT-Q$^+$. These parameters should correlate with rapid brain uptake of the CDS (log P>1.0) and rapid systemic elimination of the AZT-Q$^+$ (Greig 1987).

The in vitro stability of the AZT-CDS and its metabolite/precursor, AZT-Q$^+$, was determined in pH 7.4 phosphate buffer, 20 percent rat brain homogenate, and whole rat blood. The CDS is relatively stable in buffer but rapidly oxidizes in enzymatic media. In addition, the depot form AZT (i.e., the AZT-Q$^+$) was shown to gradually release the parent compound.

The CDS form of AZT was subsequently examined in a rat model. This study compared the CNS delivery of AZT after dosing animals with either the parent drug or the AZT-CDS. Figure 3 gives the brain and blood concentration of AZT after an IV dose of 0.136 mmol/kg AZT. As shown, blood levels were initially high but disappeared rapidly, with a half-life of approximately 20 minutes. By 2 hours, no AZT was detected. In the brain, AZT levels never surpassed blood concentrations and were at their peak at the first sampling point. AZT was not found in the brain at 60 minutes. The profile of drug distribution after CDS administration was significantly different. In blood, high levels of the AZT-CDS occurred initially but disappeared rapidly, with a $t_{1/2}$ of 5 minutes (figure 4). The AZT-Q$^+$ also was present in high levels at early time points, but the concentration of this also fell rapidly ($t_{1/2}=7$ minutes). Finally, low levels of AZT could be detected in blood, but the drug was completely cleared from the body by 2 hours. The amount of AZT present in the blood after AZT-CDS administration was much lower than that generated after AZT dosing. In brain (figure 5), no CDS was detected consistent with its in vitro lability. AZT-Q$^+$ concentrations were characterized by an appearance phase reaching a C_{max} at 15 minutes and then by a slow decline. The appearance phase is typical for CDS derivatives and is a consequence of the in vivo conversion of the CDS to its corresponding pyridinium salt. AZT-Q$^+$ was detectable in the brain at the last time point examined (4 hours). These sustained levels of AZT-Q$^+$ were associated with release of AZT in the CNS, which reached peak levels at 30 minutes post-drug administration and were detectable up to 120 minutes. When the parent drug was considered, the areas under the brain AZT concentration curve were threefold higher after AZT-CDS dosing compared with AZT administration (figure 6). This was a consequence not only of a higher C_{max} value but also of a longer CNS mean residence time. This is important in that the estimated virustatic concentration of AZT (1.0 µmol/L) is maintained twice as long after AZT-CDS administration compared with AZT dosing. This, in combination with the lower blood levels of AZT, results in a favorable increase in the brain:blood ratio for the parent compound when administered as its CDS.

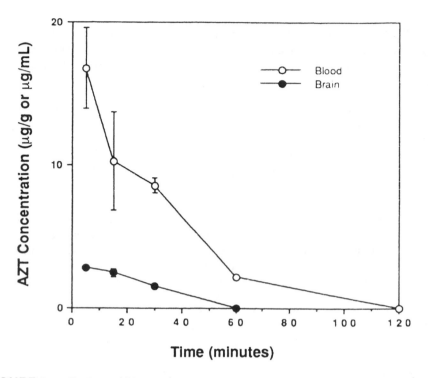

FIGURE 3. *Brain and blood concentrations of AZT (mean±SEM) after an IV dose of 0.136 mmol/kg AZT using dimethyl sulfoxide (DMSO) (0.5 mL/kg) as a vehicle*

Similar distribution studies have been completed by Chu at the University of Georgia using a mouse model (Chu et al. 1990). In the evaluation, National Institutes of Health-Swiss mice were dosed with either AZT (50 mg/kg) or equimolar AZT-CDS (72.7 mg/kg) via the tail vein. Animals were sacrificed at various times post-drug administration; and brain and serum were analyzed for AZT in the case of AZT dosing and for AZT, AZT-Q+, and AZT-CDS in the case of the AZT-CDS experiments. Whereas similar areas under the serum concentration-time curves (AUC) were observed for AZT when administered either as such or as its CDS, the brain AUC for AZT was almost tenfold higher after systemic use of the AZT-CDS. This dramatic increase was related with a long $t_{1/2}$ for AZT in the CNS subsequent to AZT-CDS dosing compared with AZT administration (15.8 hours and 0.54 hours, respectively).

The behavior of the CDS for AZT also has been examined in the rabbit. This model is useful in that simultaneous brain, CSF, and blood data can be obtained in terminal samples. AZT administration generated a distributional

176

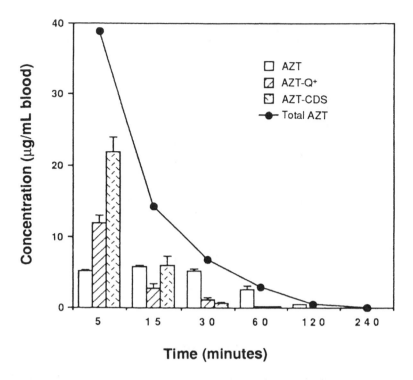

FIGURE 4. *Blood concentrations of AZT-CDS and its metabolites, AZT-Q⁺ and AZT, after an IV dose of 0.136 mmol/kg of AZT-CDS*

profile similar to that observed in rats (figure 7). Administration of the AZT-CDS generated a somewhat different profile. In rabbits, AZT-CDS was not detectable at the first sampling point (15 minutes). This is slightly different from previously obtained data in rats, which showed that, at least in blood, AZT-CDS was present through 30 minutes. The quaternary metabolite was found in brain and blood, although in much lower concentrations than reported in other animals models. In brain, AZT-Q⁺ salt levels peaked at 30 minutes and then decreased to undetectable levels at 3 hours. In blood, significant levels occurred only at the first time point (15 minutes). When AZT was considered, relatively high and sustained levels of the nucleoside were generated in brain tissue. Blood levels, while high initially, fell below brain levels by 30 minutes. CSF levels were significantly lower than brain or blood levels throughout the study (figure 8). When AZT levels were compared subsequent to either AZT or AZT-CDS treatment, a clear increase in the area under the brain concentration curves was evident. The inversion in the magnitude of brain:blood ratio for AZT after AZT-CDS administration resulted in a more favorable value compared with

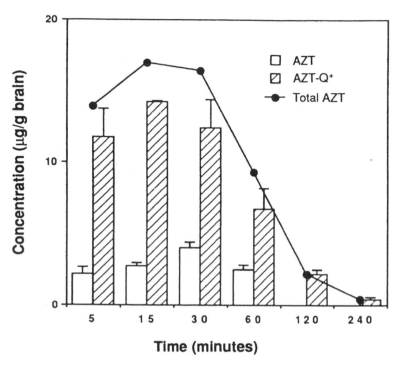

FIGURE 5. *Brain concentrations of AZT and AZT-Q⁺ after an IV dose of 0.136 mmol/kg of AZT-CDS*

AZT dosing. As illustrated in figure 9, AZT brain:blood ratios reached three by 60 minutes after AZT-CDS treatment but were consistently less than one after AZT treatment.

Subsequent to the investigations in rodents, AZT-CDS was studied in a canine model. In a preliminary study, a mongrel dog (BW=20 kg) was given 11 µmol/kg AZT in a vehicle containing 2.5-percent DMSO in polyethylene glycol (400) followed 1 week later with a dose of 11 µmol/kg AZT-CDS. In both administrations, samples of CSF and blood were obtained. Blood levels of AZT after IV administration of either the AZT or the AZT-CDS are given in figure 10. After administration of the parent compound, blood levels of AZT disappeared in an apparent biphasic manner, as previously reported. Blood levels of AZT after the CDS were much lower initially than those obtained after the parent drug. By 100 minutes, the blood concentration curves were superimposed after the two treatments. In the CSF (figure 11), AZT administration produced significant

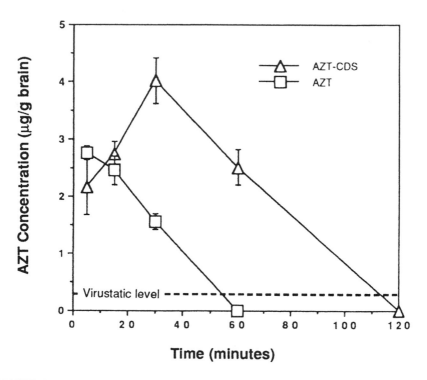

FIGURE 6. *Brain levels of AZT in rat after a 0.136 mmol/kg dose of either AZT or AZT-CDS*

levels of AZT at early times. However, these levels were below the 1.0 μmol/L therapeutic threshold for virustatic activity. In addition, these levels fell quickly, with an estimated half-life of 30 minutes. Equimolar AZT-CDS generated therapeutically significant concentrations of AZT in the CSF for up to 3 hours postdosing. These data indicate that the area under the AZT concentration curve in CSF was doubled after AZT-CDS dosing compared with AZT administration.

A variety of in vitro studies also have suggested that AZT-CDS may be a useful compound in the treatment of AIDS encephalopathy. Aggarwal and colleagues (1990), for example, found that the delivery system was more active in inhibiting human immunodeficiency virus replication than AZT and similarly was less cytotoxic. In addition, the uptake of the AZT-CDS into H9 cell was significantly greater than that of the AZT.

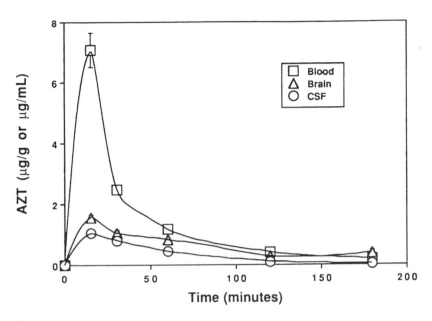

FIGURE 7. *Brain, blood, and CSF concentrations of AZT in rabbits (μg/mL) after an 17.2 mg/kg dose of AZT*

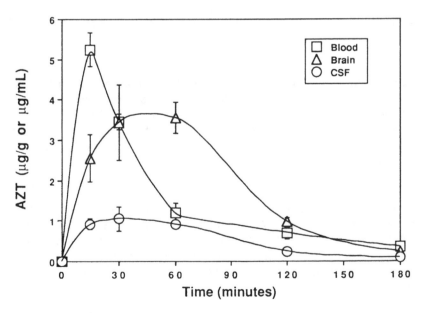

FIGURE 8. *Brain, blood, and CSF concentrations of AZT in rabbits (μg/mL) after a dose of AZT-CDS equimolar to 17.2 mg/kg AZT*

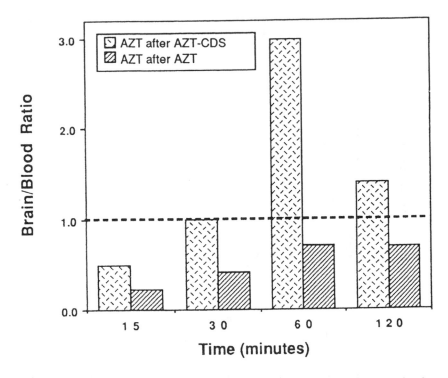

FIGURE 9. *Brain to blood ratio of AZT after an IV dose of AZT or equimolar AZT-CDS*

Ribavirin (RV) was first synthesized in 1972 and, since that time, has been shown to be a useful, broad spectrum antiviral agent (Conner 1984; Huggins et al. 1984; Sidwell et al. 1979; Canonico et al. 1988). This riboside has been demonstrated to inhibit the cytopathicity of various RNA viruses and has been found clinically useful in the treatment of respiratory syncytial virus (Rodriguez and Parrott 1987) and Lassa fever (McCormick et al. 1988). However, RV is highly water soluble and poorly lipophilic (log P=-2.06) (Sidwell et al. 1979). This property renders this potentially useful drug useless in the treatment of RNA viral encephalitic diseases, such as Japanese B encephalitis, Rift Valley fever, and Dengue fever. Application of the CDS to RV may, therefore, improve its spectrum of activity. RV has three hydroxy groups (2'-, 3'-, and 5'-positions) that are amenable to derivatization. The brain-targeting 1,4-dihydrotrigonellinate moiety can be placed at any or all of these loci. In addition, the underivatized hydroxy groups can be masked with lipophilicity modifying ester to optimize delivery. The simple 5'-1,4-dihydrotrigonellinate derivative of RV was prepared according to figure 12. RV was protected as the

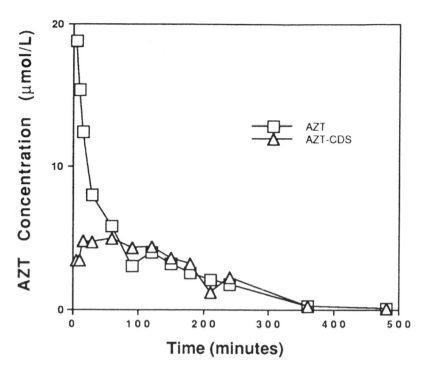

FIGURE 10. *Blood levels of AZT in dog after an 11 µmol/kg dose of either AZT-CDS or AZT*

2',3'-acetonide. This compound then was nicotinoylated with nicotinic anhydride and deprotected using formic acid. The 5'-nicotinate then was methylated to give the 5'-trigonellinate of RV (RV-Q+) and reduced in aqueous dithionite to give the RV-5'-CDS. This compound, independently prepared, was tested in C57BL/6 mice that had been infected intraperitoneally (i.p.) with 10 LD_{50}s of the Peking strain of Japanese encephalitic virus. The CDS was administered i.p. at doses of 45 mg/kg/day for 9 days. A survival rate of 40 to 50 percent was described even though vehicle or RV itself were totally ineffective (100 percent mortality) (Canonico et al. 1988).

A variety of other systems were generated. Acylation of the 2'- and 3'-hydroxy groups of RV-CDS produces a family of triacylated derivatives, including the 2',3'-bis-O-acetate, 2',3'-bis-O-isobutyrate, 2',3'-bis-O-pivaloate, and 2',3'-bis-O-benzoate adducts of 5'-(1,4-dihydrotrigonellinate) RV. In addition, placement of the dihydrotrigonellinate targeting group at the 2'- or 3'-locus was considered. The most efficient way to produce these compounds appeared to be

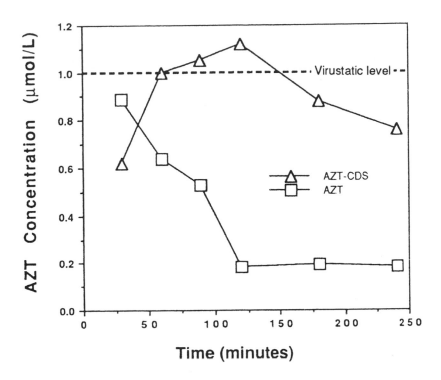

FIGURE 11. *CSF levels of AZT in dog after an 11 μmol/kg dose of either AZT-CDS or AZT*

nonselective benzoylation followed by nicotinoylation. In this way, the 2'-O-(1,4-dihydrotrigonellinate)-3'-benzoate and 2'-O-benzoate-3'-O-(1,4-dihydrotrigonellinate) derivatives of RV were obtained. Several of these compounds were found to exert antiviral activity in a murine model in which *Punta Toro* virus (Balliet strain) was inoculated intracranially into Swiss Webster mice (figure 13). The 2'-O-(1,4-dihydrotrigonellinate)-3'-O-benzoate derivative of RV caused a significant increase in animals surviving the viral challenge compared with vehicle controls as well as a decrease in brain viral titres. A variety of other compounds, including the bis-O-pivaloate and bis-O-isobutyrate derivatives of RV-CDS, acted to significantly increase the mean survival time of animals inoculated with *Punta Toro* virus.

BRAIN-SUSTAINED DELIVERY OF ESTROGENS

Estrogens are lipophilic steroids that are not impeded in their entry to the CNS. These compounds readily penetrate the BBB and achieve high central levels after peripheral administration. Unfortunately, estrogens are poorly retained by

183

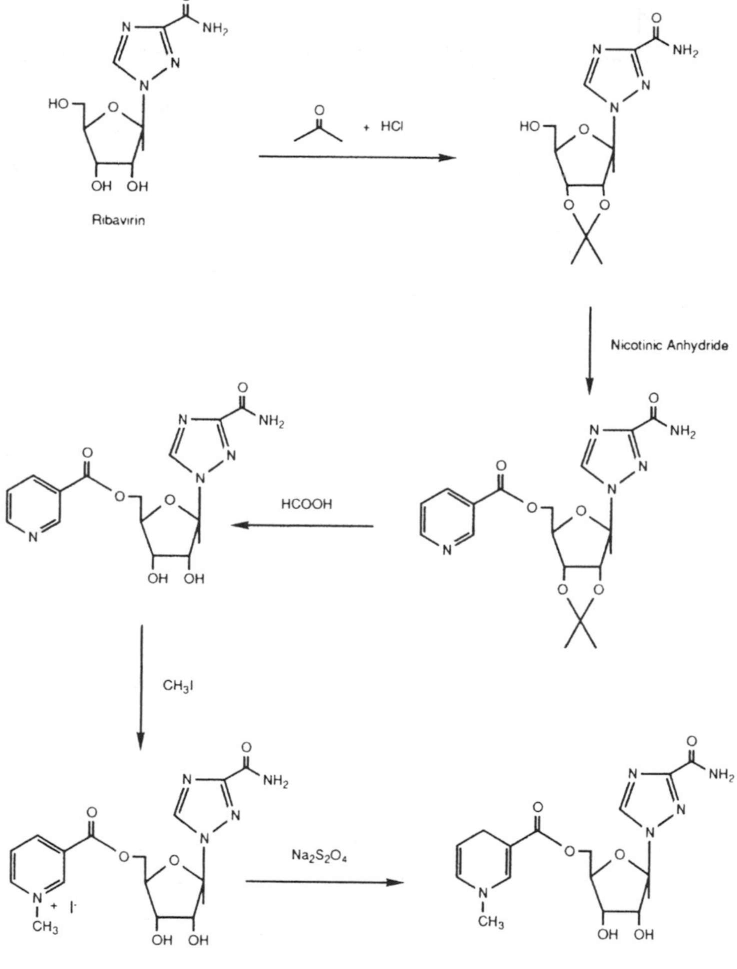

FIGURE 12. *Synthesis of an RV-CDS. RV was protected as a 2',3'-0-acetonide, reacted with nicotinic anhydride, the acetonide group removed, and the resulting nicotinate quaternized with methyl iodide and reduced using sodium dithionite.*

Increased Survival

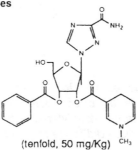

(43%, 75 mg/Kg)   (50%, 175 mg/Kg)

Increased Mean Survival Time

(17%, 3.5 mg/Kg)   (15%, 34.4 mg/Kg)

(14%, 50 mg/Kg)   (12%, 43.8 mg/Kg)

Decreased Brain Viral Titres

(tenfold, 50 mg/Kg)

FIGURE 13. *Antiviral efficacy of selected RV-CDS using a murine Punta Toro viral model*

185

the brain. This circumstance requires that frequent doses of these steroids be administered to maintain therapeutically significant concentrations. Constant peripheral exposure of estrogen has been related, however, to several pathological conditions, including cancer, hypertension, and altered metabolism (Fotherby 1985; Kaplan 1978). As the CNS is the target site for many of the actions of estrogens, a brain-targeted delivery form of these compounds may provide for safer and more effective estrogens. A CDS for 17β estradiol was generated by treatment of estradiol with nicotinoyl chloride hydrochloride to give the 3,17-bis nicotinate (figure 14). Treatment of this ester with methanol potassium bicarbonate resulted in selective cleavage of the phenolic nicotinate. The obtained secondary nicotinate was then quaternized and reduced to provide the 17-(1,4-dihydrotrigonellinate) ester of β-estradiol or E_2CDS (Bodor et al. 1987; Brewster et al. 1987).

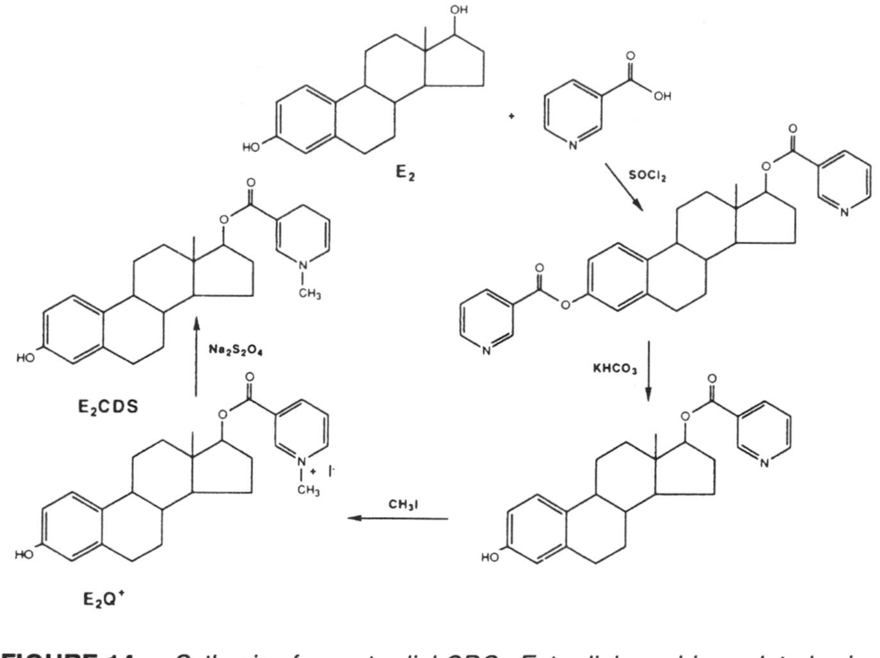

FIGURE 14.   *Sythesis of an estradiol-CDS. Estradiol was bis-acylated using nicotinoyl chloride, the phenol ester cleaved in base, and the resulting 17-nicotinide methylated with methyl iodide and reduced with sodium dithionite to give the CDS.*

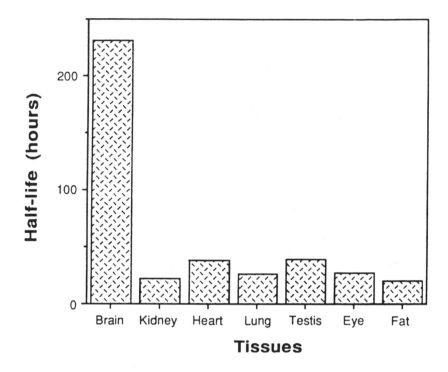

FIGURE 15. *Half-life of elimination of E_2-Q^+ formed after E_2CDS administration in brain, kidney, heart, lung, testis, eye, and fat*

The E_2CDS was shown to be readily converted to its corresponding quaternary salt (E_2-Q^+) subsequent to systemic administration in rats, dogs, and monkeys. The rate of loss of the E_2-Q^+ was found to be relatively slow from the CNS compared to peripheral tissues (figure 15) (Mullersman et al. 1988). The high, sustained E_2-Q^+ levels in the CNS were associated with a prolonged but significant release of the parent compound (Sarkar et al. 1989). This release was sufficient to reduce luteinizing hormone (LH) secretion in ovariectomized rats for periods over 1 month subsequent to a single 1 mg/kg dose (Simpkins et al. 1986). The LH suppression occurred even though serum levels of estradiol were low and, in fact, identical with those obtained after estradiol treatment. Estradiol resulted only in a transient effect (24 days) on LH levels (Estes et al. 1987). The E_2CDS was also shown to be efficient in stimulating male sexual activity in castrate rats (Anderson et al. 1987), in decreasing weight gain in rodents (Estes et al. 1988), and in reducing food intake in rats (Simpkins et al. 1989). All of the parameters are thought to be CNS-mediated effects.

Given the highly successful animal pharmacology of this compound, toxicity studies and human clinical trials were planned and carried out. Prior to clinical evaluation, extensive safety studies were performed on E_2CDS to ensure, as much as possible, that the drug would not provoke untoward reactions in humans. The E_2CDS formulated in a water-soluble vehicle (2-hydroxypropyl-β-cyclodextrin, E_2CDS-CD) was shown to lack mutagenic potential in bacteria as measured in a standard Ames test. This excipient was chosen as it is not parenterally toxic and gives adequate aqueous solubility for the E_2CDS (Brewster et al. 1988b, 1990a). The E_2CDS-CD system was then tested in Sprague-Dawley rats and cynomolgus monkeys over a period of either 14 (subacute) or 90 (subchronic) days. In the subacute studies, groups of 10 rats (5 males and 5 females) or 2 monkeys (1 male and 1 female) were injected IV with normal saline, 2-hydroxypropyl-β-cyclodextrin in sterile water, or E_2CDS in the cyclodextrin vehicle at doses of 0.025, 0.25, 1.5, and 5.0 mg/kg. The treatments were administered every second day, resulting in cumulative doses of 0.2, 2, 12, and 40 mg/kg. Twenty-four hours after the eighth dose, animals were sacrificed and necropsied. Histopathological samples were prepared from various organs, and blood was drawn for hematologic and clinical chemistry evaluation. No effects of the vehicle were apparent. The estrogen caused expected changes in hematology (increased neutrophils) in both species. In rats, various expected estrogenic reactions were observed, including weight loss and pituitary hypertrophy. In the subchronic paradigm, 20 rats (10 males and 10 females) and 8 monkeys (4 males and 4 females) were used. Again, one group received normal saline and another the cyclodextrin vehicle at a dose of 200 mg/kg. E_2CDS was administered to monkeys at doses of 1.0 and 5.0 mg/kg and to rats at a dose of 2.5 mg/kg. Drug treatment was performed every other day, resulting in cumulative doses of 46 and 230 mg/kg in monkeys and 115 mg/kg in rats. Twenty-four hours after the 46th dose, animals were necropsied and biological samples obtained for evaluation. There were no mortalities in this study as in the subacute trials, and no abnormal cageside behaviors were observed. Again, various estrogen-sensitive parameters were significantly altered as a result of E_2CDS dosing, including decreased body weight and white blood cell count and increased pituitary weight in rats and decreased protein and glucose concentrations with increased triglycerides in monkeys. The toxicological evaluation of the data obtained from the subchronic studies indicated that the no-observable *adverse effect* dose was the maximum dose used in the protocol (i.e., 5 mg/kg in monkeys and 2.5 mg/kg in rats).

Since the CDS, by its design, targets drugs to the CNS, the neurotoxicological potency of these compounds should be examined. This was done for E_2CDS by evaluating the effect of the CDS on central neurochemical function (Brewster et al. 1988c). In the experiment, E_2CDS, saline, or the cyclodextrin vehicle was administered to conscious, restrained cynomolgus monkeys IV every other day for 2 weeks. The cumulative dose of E_2CDS ranged from 0.2 to 40 mg/kg, and two monkeys (one male and one female) were included in each group. Twenty-four hours after the eighth dose, animals were euthanized and samples of striatum removed and frozen. During the study, animals were observed twice a day for such locomotor impairments as rigidity, akinesia, and hypoactivity. No altered motor activity was observed. Neurochemical analysis of brain samples was performed by high-performance liquid chromatography with electrochemical detection, as earlier described. The results demonstrate that E_2CDS did not affect striatal dopaminergic concentration. The unaffected dopamine levels and the lack of behavioral changes suggest neurotoxicological safety of these materials.

The first human examination of E_2CDS was designed as a rising dose safety study (Howes et al. 1988; Brewster et al. 1990b). In this evaluation, menopausal women served as the test population in that plasma LH and follicle-stimulating hormone (FSH) could be readily assayed as indicators of pharmacological action. The initial report evaluated 10 subjects. In the protocol, all subjects were healthy, postmenopausal females as defined by age and time of last menstrual period, which was confirmed by plasma FSH and LH levels. Each subject received a single dose of E_2CDS as an IV injection of the drug dissolved in 20 percent (w/v) 2-HPCD. Subjects remained for 48 hours in the clinic, and subjective side effects and vital signs were recorded. Blood samples were obtained for analysis of LH, FSH, and 17-β-estradiol at 15 minutes, at 30 minutes, and at 1, 2, 4, 8, 24, and 48 hours after drug administration. Subjects then were released from the clinic but were asked to return on the mornings of days 4 and 7 for additional blood sampling. In addition, prestudy and poststudy blood samples were taken for clinical evaluation.

In the study, all subjects met the entry criteria for inclusion. There were no dropouts, and all subjects completed the protocol. No adverse effects were reported that could be attributed to the E_2, and all hematological and clinical chemistry values were unaffected by drug administration. In examining the data, the results appeared to cluster into three groups: 10 to 40 µg dose (n=3), which showed minimal changes; 80 to 640 µg (n=5), which showed threshold effects; and 1,280 µg (n=2), which showed substantial and sustained decreases in plasma LH levels. Grouping the data for interpretation also had the benefit of reducing the effects of interindividual variation as only one subject was given a particular dose of drug in most cases.

Figure 16 illustrates the relationship between these three dose groups and the percent maximum fall in LH value. Mean peak decreases of 11, 34, and 50 percent were noted for the 10 to 40 µg, 80 to 640 µg, and 1,280 µg dosing

189

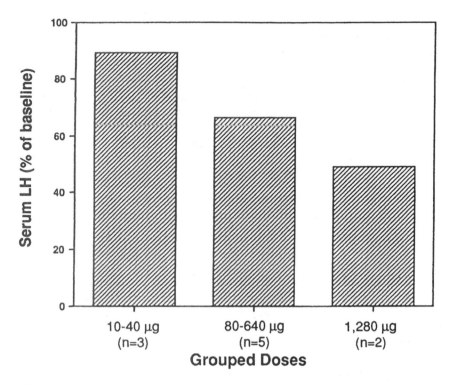

FIGURE 16. *Effect of various grouped doses of E₂CDS on mean LH suppression relative to baseline values in postmenopausal women*

groups, respectively. This fall in LH favorably compares with mean peak decreases of 28 to 36 percent seen after 1 month of dosing with estradiol transdermal patches (Judd 1987; Steingold et al. 1985).

Figure 17 illustrates the duration of LH changes as a function of the magnitude of the LH decrease (i.e., at least 10-, 20-, or 40-percent decreases from baseline values). The duration of the effect also shows a substantial dose-dependent relationship (e.g., a >20-percent decrease lasted for up to 48 hours after 1,280 µg, 18 hours at 80 to 640 µg, and 0 hour at 10 to 40 µg). In these studies, it was difficult to quantitate the magnitude of improved action obtained using the CDS relative to the natural hormone estradiol, in that no studies had been published that specifically examined the effect of moderate IV dose of E_2 on serum LH and E_2. This lack of experimental data was not totally unexpected in that estradiol is poorly water soluble. This makes parenteral dosing especially difficult when moderate to high E_2 doses are considered. The

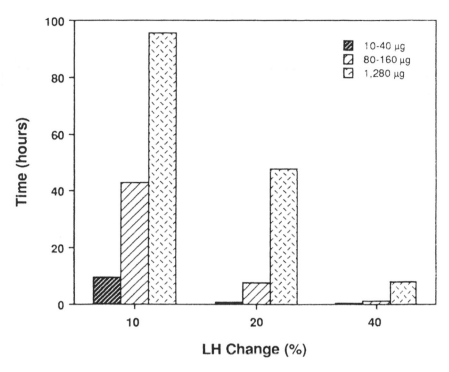

FIGURE 17. *Effect of various grouped doses of E_2CDS on the duration of action of LH suppression. Duration is measured by return to baseline values in at least two consecutive measurements. Suppression of 10, 20, and 40 percent of LH values is presented.*

recent development of nontoxic, highly water-soluble modified β-cyclodextrins has allowed for the IV administration of highly water-insoluble compounds such as sex steroids. The paucity of historic controls and the timely development of safe, useful, and water-soluble inclusion complexes of estradiol led to an IV study using this technology to examine E_2 and LH levels with time after moderate doses of estradiol.

Figure 18 illustrates the effect of E_2 and E_2CDS, both administered in an aqueous-modified β-cyclodextrin vehicle, on LH levels at various times posttreatment in postmenopausal human volunteers. In this study, the dose of E_2 was 900 µg and the equimolar dose of E_2CDS was 1,280 µg. The data were reported as percent of control where control values were obtained by averaging the LH levels obtained at time 0 and on the day prior to treatment. As illustrated, LH is dampened in a clinically meaningful way through 96 hours

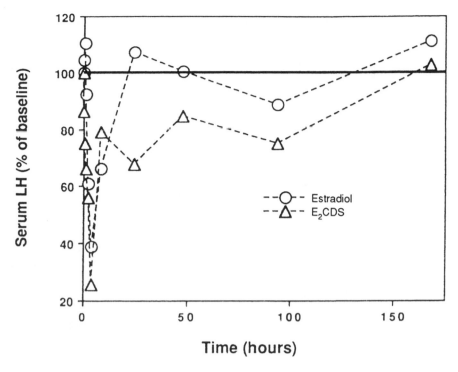

FIGURE 18.   *Effect of E$_2$CDS (1,280 µg) and E$_2$ (900 µg) on LH values in a human postmenopausal volunteer. Data are reported as percent of control.*

after E$_2$CDS treatment, whereas LH values have already returned to control by 24 hours after E$_2$ dosing. The LH suppression induced by E$_2$CDS returns to control values by 168 hours. As would be expected for a long-acting drug such as E$_2$CDS, the ratio of the areas under the LH suppression curve obtained after either E$_2$CDS or E$_2$ dosing increases as a function of time. In addition, if the initial LH drop that is common to both treatments is discounted, the apparent E$_2$CDS/E$_2$ enhancement is even greater. Thus, the suppression of LH elicited by E$_2$CDS was 12.6-fold greater than that produced by E$_2$ between 24 and 168 hours.

The effect of E$_2$ and E$_2$CDS on serum E$_2$ is given in figure 19. Administration of estradiol in an HPCD vehicle rapidly generates high serum E$_2$ levels as expected, and these levels fall rapidly. In contrast, E$_2$CDS produces relatively low initial levels of estradiol. These concentrations also are cleared rapidly. Past 8 hours, the profiles of E$_2$ elimination are superimposed after either E$_2$

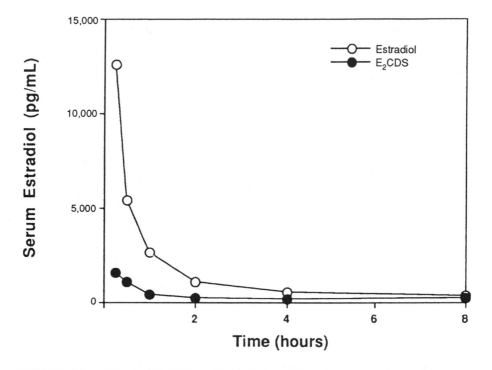

FIGURE 19. *Effect of E_2CDS or E_2 on E_2 levels in a human postmenopausal volunteer. The data point at 15 minutes obtained after E_2 treatment represented E_2 levels, which were too high to be calculated with the standard curve used in the assay (>6000 pg/mL). This point was estimated using a curve-fitting procedure. The model used was $y=a+b/x+c/x2$, which gave an $r^2>0.999$.*

or E_2CDS administration. The relative E_2CDS areas under the estradiol concentration curve increase with time starting at 0.2 at 4 hours and approach 1.0 at 168 hours.

Two important pieces of information are derived from this study. One, the initial levels of plasma E_2 generated by E_2CDS are fivefold to tenfold less than those generated after estradiol. This dampened surge should improve the therapeutic index of E_2CDS relative to estradiol, especially in circumstances where estrogens are counterindicated, such as in breast cancer. The levels of E_2 following E_2CDS treatment, however, do seem to be sufficient to support bond development in postmenopausal women. Two, LH is clearly suppressed at 24, 48, and 96 hours in a clinically relevant manner after E_2CDS treatment, whereas *no* LH suppression is evident at 24 hours and beyond after E_2 treatment. This occurs in spite of the fact that the serum levels of immunoreactive estradiol are similar for the two groups. This strongly suggests that E_2CDS is indeed working via brain-mediated mechanism in that serum differences in E_2 *cannot* account for the LH suppression.

BRAIN-ENHANCED DELIVERY OF AMINO ACIDS AND PEPTIDES

L-tryptophan is an essential amino acid that is used pharmacologically as a nutrient and, more recently, as an antidepressant. Several reports have indicated that acute administration of tryptophan can lower blood pressure in spontaneously hypertensive and other rat models (Wolf and Kuhn 1984a, 1984b; Sved et al. 1982; Fuller et al. 1979). In addition, administration of this amino acid to humans has shown a hypotensive effect (Feltkamp et al. 1984). Many mechanisms have been proposed for the antihypertensive effect of tryptophan, including changes in NaCl ingestion, increased serotonin turnover, and alteration of angiotensin II binding (Ito and Schanberg 1974; Fuller et al. 1979; Wurtman 1981). In any case, the brain figures highly in most of these hypotheses. Tryptophan is transported into the CNS by a stereospecific large neutral amino acid carrier (Pardridge 1985). In addition, tryptophan is the only amino acid that significantly binds to serum albumin. These mechanisms attenuate transport of the amino acid to the CNS and require high systemic doses to significantly alter brain levels. Unfortunately, there is evidence that tryptophan can cause bladder cancer and blood dyscrasias, especially eosinophilia, after large oral doses (Caterall 1988).

Synthesis of a nicotinamide CDS for tryptophan therefore was considered (Pop et al. 1990). Tryptophan esters were treated with nicotinoyl chloride to give the corresponding amide-esters (figure 20). Quaternization and reduction of these derivatives produced the Try-CDS. The compounds were found to be of sufficient lipophilicity to pass the BBB readily and also to convert to the corresponding quaternary salt. The Try-CDS containing an ethyl ester was tested in a deoxycorticosterone acetate (DOCA) model of hypertension (Fregly and Fater 1986; Fregly et al. 1987, 1988). Although vehicle or tryptophan was ineffective in changing blood pressure, an IV dose of the Try-CDS of 14.2 mg/kg significantly reduced blood pressure in rats, 14 percent by 3 hours and 25 percent by 4 hours. Lowering the dose by 63 percent generated an equivalent hypotensive effect at 3 hours that was not as prominent at 4 hours postdosing (figure 21).

The inability to deliver peptides to the CNS is due to two characteristics of the BBB: its exclusion of hydrophilic substances and its histochemistry. This latter point is important in that many peptides degrade in transit through the vascular

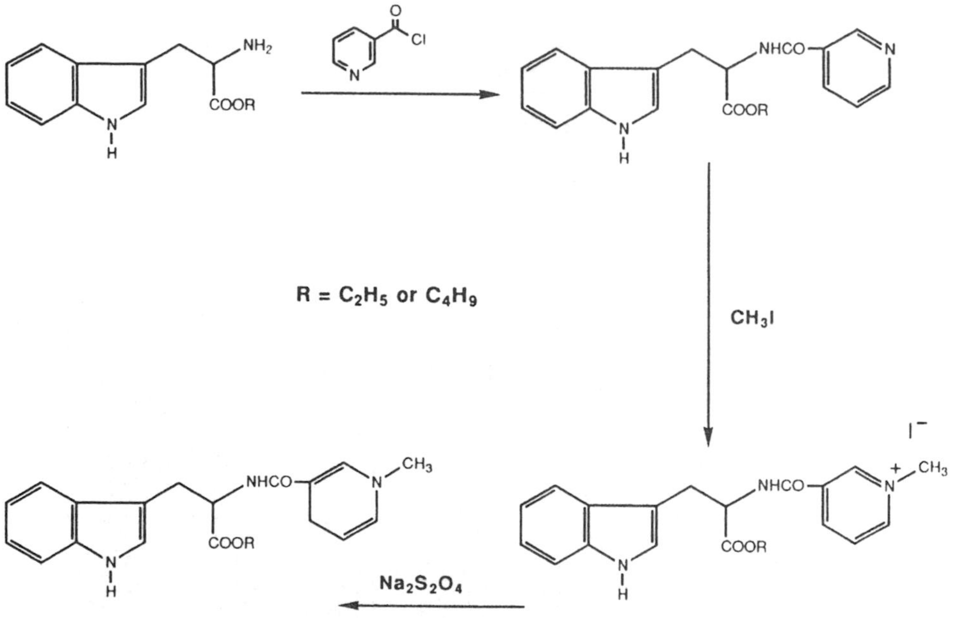

FIGURE 20. *Synthesis of tryptophan-CDS. Various alkyl esters of tryptophan were condensed with nicotinic acid giving the corresponding nicotinamides. Quaternization and reduction afforded the CDS.*

epithelium. Even lipophilic peptides such as cyclosporin may breach the luminal vascular membrane but then are degraded rapidly by amino and other peptidases. Direct introduction of peptides to the CSF does not seem feasible, as the low diffusion coefficient for peptides in brain tissue would restrict distribution to little more than 1.2 mm over a period of 1 hour. Given the active catabolic processes available in the CNS, it is unlikely any peptide would traverse the necessary distance intact to be of much use. Other approaches for increasing peptide delivery include osmotic opening of the BBB using hypertonic nonelectrolytes, cationic liposomes, or chemical manipulation.

Application of the CDS to peptides is possible and, in fact, has been completed in the case of a pentapeptide. Results indicate significant activity and high concentrations of the corresponding quaternary salt in the CNS.

195

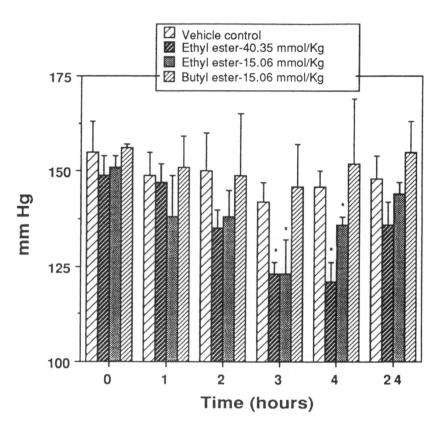

FIGURE 21.   *Effect of CDS for tryptophan on systolic blood pressure in a DOCA-induced hypertension rat model*

REFERENCES

Aggarwal, S.K.; Gogu, S.R.; Rangan, S.R.; and Aggarwal, K.C. Synthesis and biological evaluation of prodrugs of zidovudine. *J Med Chem* 33:1505-1510, 1990.

Anderson, W.R.; Simpkins, J.; Brewster, M.E.; and Bodor, N. Evidence for the reestablishment of copulatory behavior in castrated male rats with a brain-enhanced estradiol-chemical delivery system. *Pharmacol Biochem Behav* 27:265-271, 1987.

Balis, F.; Pizzo, P.; Murphy, R.; Eddy, J.; Jarosinski, P.; Fallon, J.; Broder, S.; and Poplock, D. The pharmacokinetics of zidovudine administered by continuous infusion in children. *Ann Intern Med* 110:279-285, 1989.

Blum, R.; Liao, S.; Good, S.; and deMiranda, P. Pharmacokinetics and bioavailability of zidovudine in humans. *Am J Med* 85(Suppl 2A):189-194, 1988.

Bodor, N. Novel approaches to prodrug design. *Drugs Future* 6:165-182, 1981.

Bodor, N. Redox drug delivery for targeting drugs to the brain. *Ann N Y Acad Sci* 507:289-306, 1987.

Bodor, N., and Brewster, M. Problems of delivery of drugs to the brain. *Pharmacol Ther* 19:337-386, 1983.

Bodor, N.; Farag, H.; and Brewster, M. Site-specific, sustained release of drugs to the brain. *Science* 214:1370-1372, 1981.

Bodor, N., and Kaminski, J. Prodrugs and site-specific chemical delivery systems. *Annu Rep Med Chem* 22:303-313, 1987.

Bodor, N.; McCornack, J.; and Brewster, M. Improved delivery through biological membranes 22. Synthesis and distribution of brain-selective estrogen delivery systems. *Int J Pharm* 35:47-59, 1987.

Brewster, M.E.; Estes, K.S.; and Bodor, N. Improved delivery through biological membranes 32. Synthesis and biological activity of brain-targeted delivery systems for various estradiol derivatives. *J Med Chem* 31:244-249, 1987.

Brewster, M.E.; Estes, K.S.; and Bodor, N.S. An intravenous toxicity study of 2-hydroxypropyl-β-cyclodextrin, a useful drug solubilizer, in rats and monkeys. *Int J Pharm* 59:231-243, 1990a.

Brewster, M.E.; Estes, K.; Loftsson, T.; Perchalski, R.; Derendorf, H.; Mullersman, G.; and Bodor, N. Improved delivery through biological membranes 31. Solubilization and stabilization of an estradiol chemical delivery system by modified β-cyclodextrins. *J Pharm Sci* 77:981-985, 1988b.

Brewster, M.E.; Estes, K.S.; Perchalski, R.; and Bodor, N. A dihydropyridine conjugate which generates high and sustained levels of the corresponding pyridinium salt in the brain does not exhibit neurotoxicity in cynomolgus monkeys. *Neurosci Lett* 87:277-282, 1988c.

Brewster, M.; Little, R.; Venkatraghavan, V.; and Bodor, N. Brain-enhanced delivery of antiviral agents. (Abstract.) *Antiviral Res* 9:127, 1988a.

Brewster, M.; Simpkins, J.; and Bodor, N. Brain delivery of estrogens. *Rev Neurosci* 2:241-285, 1990b.

Bundgaard, H., ed. *Design of Prodrugs*. Amsterdam: Elsevier Science Publishers, 1985.

Canonico, P.; Kende, M.; and Gabrielsen, B. Carrier-mediated delivery of antiviral agents. *Adv Virus Res* 35:271-312, 1988.

Caterall, W.C. Tryptophan and bladder cancer. *Biol Psychiatry* 24:733-734, 1988.

Chu, C.K.; Bhadti, V.S.; Doshi, K.J.; Etse, J.T.; Gallo, J.M.; Boudinot, F.D.; and Schinazi, R.F. Brain targeting of anti-HIV nucleosides: Synthesis and in vitro and in vivo studies of dihydropyridine derivatives of 3'-azido-2',3'-dideoxyuridine and 3'-azido-3'-deoxythymidine. *J Med Chem* 33:2188-2192, 1990.

Conner, C.S. Ribavirin. *Drug Intell Clin Pharm* 18:137-138, 1984.

Estes, K.S.; Brewster, M.E.; and Bodor, N. A redox system for brain targeted estrogen delivery causes chronic body weight decrease in rats. *Life Sci* 42:1077-1084, 1988.

Estes, K.S.; Brewster, M.E.; Simpkins, J.W.; and Bodor, N. A novel redox system for CNS-directed delivery of estradiol causes sustained LH suppression in the castrate rat. *Life Sci* 40:1327-1334, 1987.

Feltkamp, H.; Meurer, K.H.; and Godchardt, F. Tryptophan-induced lowering of blood pressure and changes of serotonin uptake by platelets in patients with essential hypertension. *Klin Wochenschr* 62:1115-1119, 1984.

Fenstermacher, J.D. Current models of blood-brain transfer. *Trends Neurol Sci* 8:449-452, 1985.

Fotherby, K. Oral contraceptives, lipids and cardiovascular disease. *Contraception* 31:367-394, 1985.

Fregly, M.J., and Fater, D.C. Prevention of DOCA-induced hypertension in rats by chronic treatment with tryptophan. *Clin Exp Pharmacol Physiol* 13:767-776, 1986.

Fregly, M.J.; Lockley, O.E.; and Cade, J.R. Effect of chronic dietary treatment with L-tryptophan on the development of renal hypertension in rats. *Pharmacology* 36:91-100, 1988.

Fregly, M.J.; Lockley, O.E.; vanderVoort, J.; Sumner, C.; and Henley, W. Chronic dietary administration of tryptophan prevents the development of deoxycorticosterone acetate salt induced hypertension in rats. *Can J Physiol Pharmacol* 65:753-764, 1987.

Fuller, R.W.; Holland, D.R.; Yen, T.T.; Bemis, K.G.; and Stamm, N. Antihypertensive effects of fluoxetine and L-5-hydroxytryptophan in rats. *Life Sci* 25:1237-1242, 1979.

Gallo, J.; Boubinot, F.; Doshi, D.; Etse, J.; Bhandti, V.; Schinazi, R.; and Chu, C.K. Evaluation of brain targeting of anti-HIV nucleosides delivered via dihydropyridine prodrugs. (Abstract.) *Res Pharm* 6:S161, 1989.

Gogu, S.R.; Aggarwal, S.K.; Rangan, S.R.; and Agrawal, K.C. A prodrug of zidovudine with enhanced efficacy against human immunodeficiency virus. *Biochem Biophys Res Commun* 160:656-661, 1989.

Gorrod, J. Potential hazards of the prodrug approach. *Chem Indust* 11:458-462, 1980.

Greig, N. Optimizing drug delivery to brain tumors. *Cancer Treat Rev* 14:1-28, 1987.

Greig, N.H.; Momma, S.; Sweeney, D.J.; Smith, Q.R.; and Rapoport, S.I. Facilitated transport of melphalan at the rat blood-brain barrier by the large neutral amino acid carrier system. *Cancer Res* 47:1571-1576, 1987.

Howes, J.; Bodor, N.; Brewster, M.E.; Estes, K.; and Eve, M. A pilot study with PR-63 in post-menopausal volunteers. (Abstract.) *J Clin Pharmacol* 28:951, 1988.

Huggins, J.W.; Robins, R.K.; and Canonico, P.G. Synergistic antiviral effects of ribavirin and the C-nucleoside analogs of tiazofurin and selenazofurin against togaviruses, bunyaviruses, and arenaviruses. *Antimicrob Agents Chemother* 26:476-480, 1984.

Ito, A., and Schanberg, S. Central nervous system mechanism responsible for blood pressure elevation induced by p-chlorophenylalanine. *J Pharmacol Exp Ther* 181:65-74, 1974.

Judd, H. Efficacy of transdermal estradiol. *Am J Obstet Gynecol* 156:1326-1331, 1987.

Kaplan, N.M. Cardiovascular complications of oral contraceptives. *Annu Rev Med* 29:31-40, 1978.

Klecker, R.; Collins, J.; Yarchoan, R.; Thomas, R.; Jenkins, J.; Broder, S.; and Myer, C. Plasma and cerebrospinal fluid pharmacokinetics of 3'-azido-3'-deoxythymidine: A novel pyrimidine analog with potential application for the treatment of patients with AIDS and related diseases. *Clin Pharmacol Ther* 41:407-412, 1987.

Levin, E. Are the terms blood-brain barrier and brain capillary permeability synonymous? *Exp Eye Res* 25:191-199, 1977.

Levin, V.A. Relationship of octanol/water partition coefficients and molecular weight to rat brain capillary permeability. *J Med Chem* 23:682-684, 1980.

Little, R.; Bailey, D.; Brewster, M.; Estes, K.; Clemmons, R.; Saab, A.; and Bodor, N. Improved delivery through biological membranes 33. Brain-enhanced delivery of azidothymidine. *J Biopharm Sci* 1:1-18, 1990.

McCormick, J.; King, I.; Webb, P.; Scribner, C.; Craven, R.; Johnson, K.; Elliott, L.; and Belmont-Williams, R. Lassa fever: Effective therapy with ribavirin. *N Engl J Med* 314:20-26, 1988.

Mullersman, G.; Derendorf, H.; Brewster, M.E.; Estes, K.S.; and Bodor, N. High-performance liquid chromatographic assay of a central nervous system (CNS)-directed estradiol chemical delivery system and its application after intravenous administration in rats. *Pharm Res* 5:172-177, 1988.

Neuwelt, E.A., ed. *Implications of the Blood-Brain Barrier and Its Manipulations.* New York: Plenum Medical Book Co., 1989.

Pardridge, W.M. Transport of nutrients and hormones through the blood-brain barrier. *Diabetologia* 20:246-254, 1981.

Pardridge, W.M. Strategies for drug delivery through the blood-brain barrier. In: Borchardt, R.; Repta, A.; and Stella, V.J., eds. *Directed Drug Delivery.* Clifton, NJ: Humana Press, 1985. pp. 83-96.

Pardridge, W.M.; Connor, J.D.; and Crawford, I.L. Permeability changes in the blood-brain barrier: Causes and consequences. *CRC Crit Rev Toxicol* 3:159-199, 1975.

Pop, E.; Anderson, W.; Prokai-Tatrai, K.; Brewster, M.; Fregly, M.; and Bodor, N. Antihypertensive activity of redox derivatives of tryptophan. *J Med Chem* 33:2216-2221, 1990.

Rapoport, S.I. *The Blood-Brain Barrier in Physiology and Medicine.* New York: Raven Press, 1976.

Reese, B., and Karnovsky, M.J. Fine structural localization of a blood-brain barrier to exogenous peroxides. *J Cell Biol* 34:207-217, 1967.

Rodriguez, W., and Parrott, R. Ribavirin aerosol treatment of serious respiratory syncytial virus infection in infants. *Infect Dis Clin North Am* 1:425-439, 1987.

Sarkar, D.K.; Friedman, S.J.; Yen, S.S.C.; and Frautschy, S.A. Chronic inhibition of hypothalamic-pituitary-ovarian axis and body weight gain by brain-directed delivery of estradiol-17β in female rats. *Neuroendocrinology* 50:204-210, 1989.

Sidwell, R.; Robins, R.; and Hillyard, I. Ribavirin: An antiviral agent. *Pharmacol Ther* 6:123-146, 1979.

Simpkins, J.W.; Anderson, W.R.; Dawson, R.; and Bodor, N. Effect of a brain-enhanced chemical delivery system for estradiol on body weight and food intake in intact and ovariectomized rats. *Pharm Res* 6:592-600, 1989.

Simpkins, J.W.; McCornack, J.; Estes, K.S.; Brewster, M.E.; Shek, E.; and Bodor, N. Sustained brain-specific delivery of estradiol causes long-term suppression of luteinizing hormone secretion. *J Med Chem* 29:1809-1812, 1986.

Steingold, K.A.; Lauter, L.; Chetkowski, R.J.; Defazio, J.; Matt, D.W.; and Meldrum, D.R. Treatment of hot flashes with transdermal estradiol administration. *J Clin Endocrinol Metab* 61:627-632, 1985.

Stella, V.J. Prodrugs: An overview and definition. In: Higuchi, T., and Stella, V.J., eds. *Prodrugs as Novel Drug Delivery Systems.* Washington, DC: American Chemical Society, 1975. pp. 1-115.

Stella, V.J., and Himmelstein, K.J. Prodrugs and site-specific drug delivery. *J Med Chem* 23:1275-1282, 1980.

Suckling, A.J.; Rumsby, M.G.; and Bradbury, M.W., eds. *The Blood-Brain Barrier in Health and Disease.* Chichester, England: VCH Publishers, 1986.

Sved, A.; Van Itallie, C.M.; and Fernstrom, J.D. Studies on the antihypertensive action of L-tryptophan. *J Pharmacol Exp Ther* 221:329-333, 1982.

Terasaki, T., and Pardridge, W. Restricted transport of 3'-azido-3'-deoxythymidine and dideoxynucleosides through the blood-brain barrier. *J Infect Dis* 158:630-632, 1988.

Torrence, P.; Kinjo, J.; Lesiak, K.; Balzarini, J.; and DeClercq, E. AIDS dementia: Synthesis and properties of a derivative of 3'-azido-3'-deoxythymidine (AZT) that may become "locked" in the central nervous system. *FEBS Lett* 234:134-140, 1988.

Wolf, W.A., and Kuhn, D.M. Antihypertensive effects of L-tryptophan are not mediated by brain serotonin. *Brain Res* 295:356-359, 1984a.

Wolf, W.A., and Kuhn, D.M. Effect of L-tryptophan on blood pressure in normotensive and hypertensive rats. *J Pharmacol Exp Ther* 230:324-329, 1984b.

Wurtman, R.J. "Process and Composition for Reducing Blood Pressure in Animals." U.S. Patent 4,296,119, 1981.

Yarchoan, R.; Brouwers, P.; Spitzer, A.; Grafman, J.; Safai, B.; Perno, C.; Larson, M.; Berg, G.; Fischl, M.; Wichman, A.; Thomas, R.; Brunetti, A.; Schmidt, P.; Myers, C.; and Broder, S. Response of human immunodeficiency-virus-associated neurological disease to 3'-azido-3'-deoxythymidine. *Lancet* 1:132-135, 1987.

AUTHORS

Marcus E. Brewster, Ph.D.
Director of Research
Pharmatec, Inc.
P.O. Box 730
Alachua, FL 32615

Nicholas Bodor, Ph.D., D.Sc.
Graduate Research Professor and Director
Center for Drug Discovery
University of Florida
  College of Pharmacy
P.O. Box J-497, JHMHC
Gainesville, FL 32610

Drug Delivery to the Brain Using an Anti-Transferrin Receptor Antibody

Phillip M. Friden, Lee Walus, Marjorie Taylor, Gary F. Musso, Susan A. Abelleira, Bernard Malfroy, Fariba Tehrani, Joseph B. Eckman III, Anne R. Morrow, and Ruth M. Starzyk

INTRODUCTION

The blood-brain barrier (BBB) poses a formidable obstacle to the effective treatment of neurological disorders. Access to the brain by nonlipophilic drugs is blocked by the endothelial cells that compose the vascular network within the brain (Goldstein and Betz 1986; Pardridge 1986). These cells, unlike those in other organs, are joined together by complex, tight intercellular junctions that form a continuous wall against the passive movement of substances from the blood to the brain (Brightman 1977; Reese and Karnovsky 1967). Brain capillary endothelial cells are also unusual in that they have few pinocytic vesicles that would allow somewhat nonselective transport across the capillary wall. Moreover, continuous gaps or channels connecting the luminal and abluminal membranes are lacking. Because the brain requires, in a controlled manner, many blood-borne compounds (such as glucose, amino acids, and hormones), brain capillary endothelial cells possess an array of transport systems that allow selective passage across the BBB (Pardridge 1986). Together, these features of brain capillary endothelial cells ensure that the homeostasis of the brain is maintained.

In shielding the brain from toxic substances as well as fluctuations in the levels of blood-borne compounds, such as ions and hormones, the BBB also restricts the entry of many drugs. Highly lipophilic drugs, such as chloramphenicol and heroin, readily pass through the membranes of brain capillary endothelial cells and enter the brain unaided (Goldstein and Betz 1986). However, the majority of drugs with potential for treating neurological disorders are water soluble and, therefore, require some assistance in reaching their site of action within the brain. Current methods for the delivery of nonlipophilic drugs to the brain include disruption of the tight junctions between endothelial cells through the intracarotid injection of hyperosmolar sugar solutions (Cosolo et al. 1989; Neuwelt et al. 1982) and more invasive means such as intracerebroventricular injection of drug into the cerebrospinal fluid or implantation of drug-releasing polymers during neurosurgery. All these procedures are quite hazardous and have many drawbacks. The development of a noninvasive method for the delivery of drugs to the brain would have a significant impact on the treatment of neurological disorders.

One potential solution to this problem involves the use of a redox delivery system (Bodor 1987). In this scheme, the drug to be delivered is modified by the attachment of a lipophilic group that enables the drug to pass freely through the membranes of the brain capillary endothelial cells. In addition, the chemical modification that allows the drug to enter the brain is designed to be rapidly converted to a charged, hydrophilic moiety, thus trapping the modified drug within the brain. The modifying group is subsequently released, leaving active drug within the brain. Some success has been reported in enhancing the delivery of certain drugs to the brain using this approach, but there are several limitations. Such a delivery system appears to be best suited for small drugs, and then only for those that can accommodate the required chemical modifications. Also, because there is no selectivity in this system, the enhanced lipophilicity of the modified drug allows it to more readily penetrate all cellular membranes.

Another approach to drug delivery to the brain utilizes cationic and cationized proteins as drug carriers (Pardridge et al. 1989; Triguero et al. 1989). Proteins with a net positive charge, such as cationized immunoglobulin G (IgG) or histone, can interact with the negatively charged surface of the capillary endothelial cells. Absorptive-mediated endocytosis at the luminal membrane and exocytosis at the abluminal membrane are thought to mediate the transcytosis of these compounds across the brain capillary endothelial cells and, thus, the BBB. In vitro and in vivo data suggest that positively charged proteins traverse the endothelial cell layer upon intracarotid injection and gain access to the brain parenchyma. However, the attachment of "passenger" drugs to cationic or cationized proteins will no doubt have some effect on the net charge as well as other physical/chemical properties of the carrier protein, possibly making it difficult to use this system for the delivery of small drugs, which would require a high drug-to-carrier ratio to achieve therapeutic doses in the brain. Cationization of an antibody for imaging, on the other hand, may be a more appropriate use for this system, provided that the cationization procedure does not alter functional properties of the protein and that sufficient quantities cross the BBB. Other potential problems with this approach are enhanced immunogenicity due to the cationization and renal toxicity (Lambert et al. 1984; Muckerheide et al. 1987).

Other types of carrier-based systems for the delivery of drugs across the BBB include antibodies or ligands that bind to receptors on brain capillary endothelial cells or, to achieve higher levels of targeting, antibodies that recognize brain-specific antigens. The authors have explored one of these possibilities by examining whether an antibody, which recognizes the transferrin receptor (a protein known to transport its ligand, transferrin, across brain capillary endothelial cells), can function as a carrier for drug delivery to the brain.

The transferrin receptor is an integral membrane glycoprotein consisting of two identical 95,000 dalton subunits that are linked by a disulfide bond (McClelland et al. 1984; Omary and Trowbridge 1981). It has been reported in the literature that brain capillary endothelial cells have a high density of transferrin receptor on their membrane surface, which is unusual for cells in a nonproliferative state (Jefferies et al. 1984). This observation may be due to the fact that the transcytosis of iron-loaded transferrin across the BBB is the primary, if not the only, method for the delivery of iron to the brain parenchyma (Fishman et al. 1987; Pardridge et al. 1987). Therefore, to ensure that the proper levels of iron are maintained within the brain, capillary endothelial cells must be capable of binding and transporting sufficient transferrin to satisfy their own needs as well as those of other cells within the brain such as neurons and astrocytes.

The uptake of iron by individual cells is a multistep process. Iron-loaded ferrotransferrin binds to the receptors on the cell surface and is internalized by endocytosis (Klausner et al. 1984). In most cells, the endocytic vesicles then are acidified to a pH of less than 5.5 (Dautry-Varsat et al. 1983). This process results in the release of free iron from transferrin. The iron then is separated from the apotransferrin-receptor complex, which recycles to the cell surface where the apotransferrin is released and the receptor is made available for another round of endocytosis. Brain capillary endothelial cells must possess an alternative pathway for iron uptake (Pardridge 1986). A substantial portion of the endocytic vesicles containing ferrotransferrin-receptor complexes must escape acidification so that the iron-loaded transferrin will be transported to and released at the abluminal surface instead of within the endothelial cells. Once inside the barrier, the ferrotransferrin can be taken up by cells within the brain following the pathway utilized by cells in other tissues. Thus, it may be possible to exploit this endogenous transport system for the delivery of drugs to the brain.

IMMUNOHISTOCHEMICAL STUDIES

The system chosen for testing the feasibility of using anti-transferrin receptor antibodies for the delivery of drugs to the brain was the rat, utilizing the anti-rat transferrin receptor antibody OX-26 (Jefferies et al. 1985). It has been reported in the literature that this murine monoclonal antibody preferentially binds to brain capillary endothelial cells following in vivo administration (Jefferies et al. 1984). Immunohistochemistry on fresh-frozen brain sections prepared from rats injected intravenously with OX-26 was used to confirm the selectivity of this antibody (Friden et al. 1991). The tail vein was chosen as the site of injection as it more closely mimics the route of administration that is envisioned for treatment in humans, as opposed to injection into the carotid artery, for example. The avidin:biotinylated horseradish peroxidase (HRP) complex technique was used with 3, 3'-diaminobenzidine as the chromogenic substrate for the detection of OX-26 in tissue sections.

As can be seen in figure 1, very intense staining of the brain vasculature, indicative of the presence of the OX-26 antibody, was observed 1 hour following the injection of 0.5 mg of OX-26 via the tail vein. A dose as low as 0.05 mg of OX-26 per rat gave rise to detectable staining in the brain vasculature. Increasing doses of antibody from 0.05 to 2.0 mg per rat resulted in increased staining, with saturation occurring at approximately 0.5 mg OX-26 per rat. Injection of comparable amounts of a control murine monoclonal antibody of the same subclass as OX-26 (IgG2a) did not lead to detectable immunostaining of the brain vasculature.

A time course experiment in which animals were sacrificed at various times postinjection of OX-26 was performed to determine how soon after injection the antibody could be found in the brain vasculature as well as how long after injection it persisted. Uniform staining of capillaries was observed throughout the brain as early as 5 minutes postinjection of OX-26 and became more intense over time. Between 2 and 4 hours postinjection, the staining pattern developed a punctate appearance that lasted until approximately 8 hours postinjection. By 24 hours postinjection, the staining pattern for OX-26 returned to a fainter, more uniform pattern.

The changes in the pattern of localization of OX-26 in the brain suggest a time-dependent sequestration of the antibody followed by eventual dispersal. The punctate staining observed with OX-26 is similar to the results obtained by Broadwell and colleagues (1988) following the injection of a wheat germ agglutinin (WGA)-HRP conjugate into the jugular vein of rats. Electron microscopy was used by these researchers to demonstrate that the punctate staining observed between 6 and 24 hours after the injection of WGA-HRP was due to the accumulation of the conjugate in pericytes. These cells, which are embedded in the basement membrane surrounding brain capillary endothelial cells, are thought to have some macrophage-like properties and may represent a second line of defense against unwanted compounds entering the brain (Farrell et al. 1987; Van Deurs 1976). If the punctate staining observed with

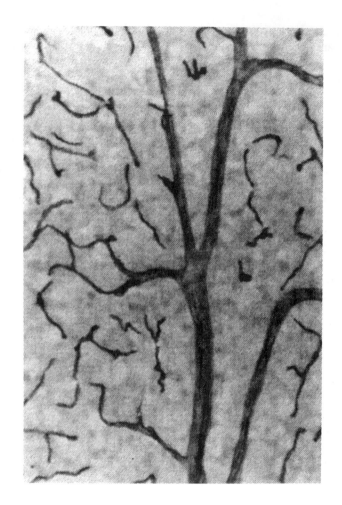

FIGURE 1. *Immunohistochemical detection of OX-26 in rat brain sections following intravenous (IV) administration via the tail vein. Fresh-frozen brain sections (~30 μm) were prepared from rats sacrificed 1 hour following the injection of 0.5 mg of OX-26. Biotinylated horse anti-mouse IgG antisera and an avidin/biotinylated HRP mixture with diaminobenzidine as the chromogenic substrate were used for immunodetection. Larger vessels as well as capillaries show the dark staining indicative of the presence of OX-26 (X 100).*

SOURCE: Friden et al. 1991

OX-26 indicates uptake into pericytes, it would suggest that the antibody has traversed the endothelial cell layer that composes the BBB. Electron microscopy experiments are under way to confirm this.

If an anti-transferrin receptor antibody is to function as a drug carrier, it must retain its ability to target to brain capillary endothelial cells in vivo when conjugated with passenger molecules. As a model for a small drug passenger, methotrexate (MTX) was conjugated to OX-26 via a hydrazone linkage (approximately six molecules of MTX per antibody) (G. Musso and S. Abelleira, unpublished manuscript). To prepare this conjugate, MTX γ-hydrazide was reacted with aldehydes that were formed by the oxidation of the carbohydrate groups located in the Fc portion of the antibody. By directing the attachment of the drug in this manner, the chance of interference with the antigen binding sites should be decreased. Following in vivo administration via the tail vein, anti-mouse IgG or anti-MTX antisera were used to localize the carrier or the passenger portions of the conjugate, respectively, in fresh-frozen brain sections as described above. Patterns of immunolocalization identical to that of unconjugated antibody were obtained using either antisera, suggesting that there is colocalization of the carrier and the drug in the brain vasculature and that the attachment of drug molecules to the antibody does not alter its targeting to the brain. Free MTX injected intravenously did not localize to the brain vasculature. Similar results were obtained with conjugates of OX-26 to other small drugs.

The ability of the anti-transferrin receptor antibody OX-26 to deliver large molecules, such as proteins, also was examined. HRP was chosen as a prototype protein passenger because it is easily detected using immunohistochemical methods and it is of average size (40 kD). Conjugates of HRP and OX-26 (approximately 2:1 molar ratio) were synthesized using a periodate linkage that crosslinks oxidized carbohydrate groups on HRP with free amino groups on the antibody. Targeting of the OX-26-HRP conjugate to brain capillary endothelial cells following IV administration was assessed immunohistochemically either directly for HRP or indirectly for the carrier using anti-mouse IgG antisera. Identical patterns of localization were obtained using either detection method; as for the drug conjugate, the patterns were the same as those obtained for unconjugated antibody. These results suggest that OX-26 can deliver proteins to brain capillary endothelial cells via IV administration.

Both the MTX and the HRP conjugates of OX-26 displayed the punctate staining observed with unconjugated antibody at similar times postinjection. This indicates that the process responsible for the punctate staining pattern— which the authors believe to be accumulation in pericytes—is unaffected by the presence of passenger molecules on OX-26. Another interesting observation in this regard is that neither $F(ab')_2$ nor Fab fragments of OX-26, which do bind to brain capillary endothelial cells following in vivo administration, display the punctate staining. These results suggest that the process responsible for this phenomenon is mediated by the Fc portion of the antibody, which the antibody fragments lack.

QUANTITATIVE STUDIES

The results of the immunohistochemistry experiments show qualitatively that the anti-rat transferrin receptor antibody OX-26 can bind to brain capillary endothelial cells following administration via the tail vein and that the binding is not affected by the attachment of either drugs or proteins to the antibody. However, these experiments do not provide any information as to the quantity of antibody or conjugate that reaches the brain or conclusive evidence that any of the material that binds to the capillaries ever crosses the BBB. Two types of experiments were utilized to address these questions.

In the first type of experiment, the amount of antibody that is specifically associated with the brain was measured in brain homogenates following the IV administration of radiolabeled OX-26. The antibody was labeled with either ^{3}H-succinimidyl propionate or ^{14}C-acetic anhydride (Kummer 1986; Montelaro and Rueckert 1975). In addition, a control antibody (^{3}H-labeled in the case of ^{14}C-labeled OX-26 or vice versa) was coinjected with the anti-transferrin receptor antibody so that nonspecific accumulation in the brain due to contaminating blood could be determined.

A peak level of OX-26 associated with the brain (approximately 0.9 percent of the injected dose [%ID]) was reached by 1 hour postinjection and remained relatively constant until 4 hours postinjection (figure 2). The amount of OX-26 associated with the brain then decreased until approximately 48 hours postinjection, at which time it leveled off at approximately 0.3 %ID. The association of radiolabeled OX-26 with the brain was significantly reduced by the coinjection of unlabeled OX-26.

In contrast to the brain level, the blood level of OX-26 dropped quite rapidly, such that by 1 hour postinjection, approximately 80 percent of the labeled antibody had been cleared from the circulation. Gel electrophoresis of serum IgG followed by autoradiography demonstrated that the radiolabeled OX-26 remaining in the blood at 48 hours following injection was intact.

The receptor-mediated transcytosis of blood-borne compounds across the BBB is proposed to consist of the following steps: (1) binding of the blood-borne molecule to its receptor on the luminal surface of the brain capillary endothelial

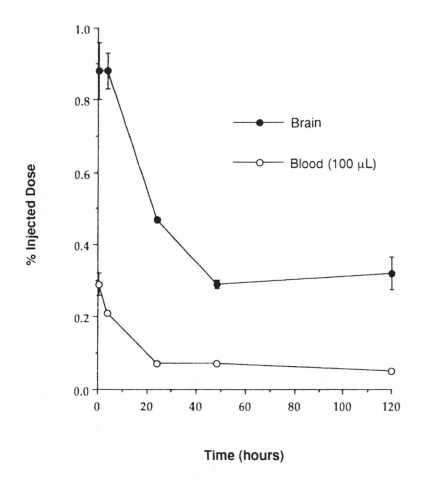

FIGURE 2.   *Brain uptake of ¹⁴C-labeled OX-26 in rats. The %ID of radiolabeled antibody per brain and per 100 μL of blood is plotted vs. time postinjection. All injections were made via the tail vein. The amount of antibody due to blood associated with the brain has been subtracted. The values shown are means±SEM (n=3 rats per time point). These results are representative of other studies that have been done.*

cell, (2) internalization of occupied receptors into endocytic vesicles that are directed to the abluminal membrane of the cell, and (3) fusion of the vesicle with the abluminal endothelial cell membrane and release of receptor-bound material (Broadwell et al. 1988; Pardridge 1986). The results of the immunohistochemistry experiments indicate that step 1—binding to receptors on brain capillary endothelial cells—does occur.

Capillary depletion experiments also were performed to address the question of whether the anti-transferrin receptor antibody or antibody conjugates are taken up by the endothelial cells and cross the BBB. This procedure was used by Triguero and colleagues (1990) to study the transcytosis of cationized proteins across the BBB. As for the experiments described above, homogenates were prepared from brains taken from animals injected with radiolabeled antibody. The homogenates then were depleted of vasculature by centrifugation through dextran to yield a vascular pellet and a supernatant that consisted of the brain parenchyma. This method removes greater than 90 percent of the microvasculature from the homogenate. Because there is no enzymatic digestion of the homogenate prior to centrifugation, the pericytes are included in the vascular pellet. Based on the results of the immunohistochemistry experiments, high levels of radiolabeled OX-26 should be associated with the capillary fraction of the brain at early times postinjection. If transcytosis of the antibody does take place, the amount of OX-26 associated with the brain parenchyma fraction should increase, whereas the amount associated with the capillary fraction should decrease over time. If the antibody that binds to the brain capillary endothelial cells is not transported across the BBB, the amount of radiolabeled OX-26 associated with the brain parenchyma fraction should not increase.

The results of these experiments were consistent with the transcytosis of OX-26 across the BBB (figure 3). At 30 minutes postinjection, more of the radiolabeled OX-26 was associated with the vascular fraction of the brain (0.47 %ID) than with the parenchyma fraction (0.29 %ID). By 24 hours postinjection, the distribution had changed such that the majority of the radiolabeled antibody was associated with the parenchyma fraction (0.43 %ID vs. 0.12 %ID for the capillary fraction).

Similar experiments were performed with radiolabeled conjugates of OX-26 with either MTX or HRP to determine if drugs or proteins can be delivered across the BBB using an anti-transferrin receptor antibody. Methotrexate labeled at the 3', 5', and 7 positions with ^3H was conjugated with OX-26 using the γ-hydrazone linkage as described above. At 30 minutes postinjection, there was approximately twofold more of the labeled conjugate in the capillary fraction of the brain as compared with the parenchyma fraction (figure 4). At 24 hours

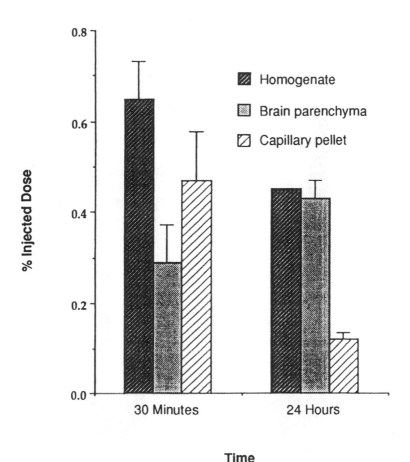

FIGURE 3. *Time-dependent changes in the disposition of ^{14}C-labeled OX-26 between brain parenchyma and vasculature. Capillary depletion was performed on homogenates prepared from brains taken from animals 30 minutes and 24 hours postinjection of radiolabeled OX-26. The %IDs of antibody for the whole homogenate, brain parenchyma fraction, and vascular pellet are shown. The amount of antibody due to blood associated with the brain has been subtracted. The values shown are means±SEM (n=3 rats per time point). These results are representative of other studies that have been done.*

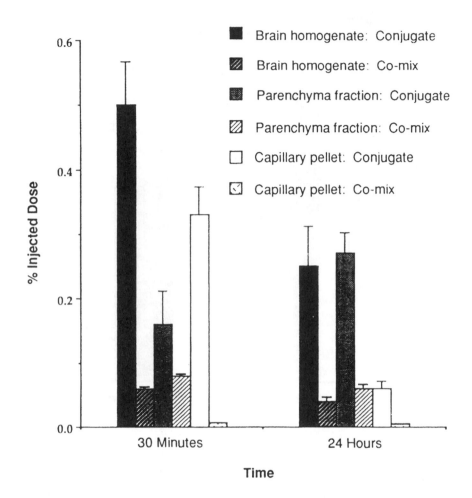

FIGURE 4. *Enhanced delivery of MTX across the BBB using OX-26 as a drug carrier. Capillary depletion experiments were used to compare the brain distribution of an OX-26-MTX conjugate to that of free drug. The data are expressed as in figure 3. The values shown are means±SEM (n=3 rats per time point). These results are representative of other studies that have been done.*

SOURCE: Friden et al. 1991

postinjection, the distribution was reversed, with approximately fivefold more of the radioactivity in the parenchyma fraction. These time-dependent changes in the distribution of the OX-26-MTX conjugate were similar to those observed for antibody alone and suggested that transcytosis of the conjugate across the BBB had occurred.

To ensure that the ^{3}H-MTX that accumulated in the brain parenchyma was derived from the OX-26-MTX conjugate and not from residual free ^{3}H-MTX associated with the conjugate or ^{3}H-MTX that had been cleaved from the conjugate in the blood, a co-mix of ^{3}H-MTX and OX-26 having the same molar composition as the conjugate was injected into rats for capillary depletion. The amount of ^{3}H-MTX in the different brain fractions was significantly lower for the co-mix as compared with the conjugate with OX-26 (figure 4). In addition, the ^{3}H-MTX in the co-mix did not show the same time-dependent changes in distribution within the brain as were seen with the conjugate or antibody alone. These results indicate that the delivery of MTX to the brain parenchyma was facilitated greatly when administered in the form of a covalent conjugate with an anti-transferrin receptor antibody.

Capillary depletion experiments also were performed using a conjugate of OX-26 with HRP coupled via a periodate linkage. In this case, the label (^{3}H) was on the antibody and the HRP. A peak of labeled material associated with the capillary fraction of the brain was seen early (approximately 1 hour) after injection. This was followed by a rise in the amount of material associated with the parenchyma fraction of the brain (figure 5). Similar results were obtained using a conjugate in which the radioactive label was only on the HRP portion of the conjugate. These results suggest that HRP can be delivered across the BBB using an anti-transferrin receptor antibody as a carrier.

CONCLUSION

Using both qualitative and quantitative in vivo assays, the authors have shown that the anti-rat transferrin receptor antibody OX-26 binds to brain capillary endothelial cells following in vivo administration and, over time, is transported across the BBB. The results obtained are consistent with the proposed mechanism of receptor-mediated transcytosis across the BBB. In addition, the anti-transferrin receptor antibody can function as a carrier for the delivery of both small drugs and larger molecules, such as proteins, to the brain parenchyma. Although the transferrin receptor is found on all cell types, this delivery system appears to be somewhat brain-selective due to a high density of receptors located on the luminal surface of brain capillary endothelial cells. It is envisioned that this carrier system will be somewhat generic in that it could be

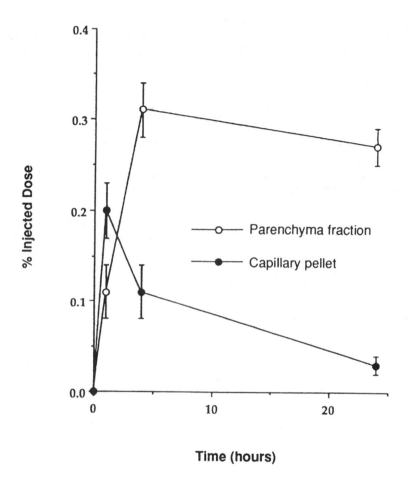

Time (hours)

FIGURE 5. *Enhanced delivery of HRP using OX-26 as a carrier. The results of capillary depletion experiments using a ^{3}H-labeled conjugate of OX-26 and HRP are shown as in figure 4. The values shown are the means of the %ID in the different brain fractions at the times shown±SEM (n=3 rats per time point). These results are representative of other studies that have been done.*

used for any drug for which a suitable linker can be developed. Also, antibody fragments or chimeric antibodies having specific physical and biological characteristics could be constructed at the DNA level using the tools of molecular biology. In this way, second-generation carriers could be designed to optimize the drug delivery aspects of the antibody. Thus, anti-transferrin receptor antibodies appear to have potential as a noninvasive means for circumventing the BBB for the treatment of neurological diseases. The crucial test for this drug delivery system will be to demonstrate that therapeutic levels of a drug can be delivered to the brain. Experiments to examine the efficacy of this carrier in an animal model of a neurological disorder are in the planning stages.

REFERENCES

Bodor, N. Redox drug delivery systems for targeting drugs to the brain. In: Juliano, R.L., ed. *Biological Approaches to the Controlled Delivery of Drugs.* New York: New York Academy of Sciences, 1987. pp. 289-306.

Brightman, M.W. Morphology of blood-brain interfaces. *Exp Eye Res* 25(Suppl):1-25, 1977.

Broadwell, R.D.; Balin, B.J.; and Salcman, M. Transcytotic pathway for blood-borne protein through the blood-brain barrier. *Proc Natl Acad Sci U S A* 85:632-636, 1988.

Cosolo, W.C.; Martinello, P.; Louis, C.L.; and Christophidis, N. Blood-brain barrier disruption using mannitol: Time course and electron microscopy studies. *Am J Physiol* 256:R443-R447, 1989.

Dautry-Varsat, A.; Ciechanover, A.; and Lodish, H.F. pH and recycling of transferrin during receptor-mediated endocytosis. *Proc Natl Acad Sci U S A* 80:2258-2262, 1983.

Farrell, C.R.; Stewart, C.L.; Farrell, C.L.; and Del Maestro, R.F. Pericytes in human cerebral microvasculature. *Anat Rec* 218:466-469, 1987.

Fishman, J.B.; Rubin, J.B.; Handrahan, J.V.; Connor, J.R.; and Fine, R.E. Receptor-mediated trancytosis of transferrin across the blood-brain barrier. *J Neurosci Res* 18:299-304, 1987.

Friden, P.M.; Walus, L.R.; Musso, G.F.; Taylor, M.A.; Malfroy, B.; and Starzyk, R.M. Anti-transferrin receptor antibody and antibody-drug conjugates cross the blood-brain barrier. *Proc Natl Acad Sci U S A* 88:4771-4775, 1991.

Goldstein, G.W., and Betz, A.L. The blood-brain barrier. *Sci Am* 255(3):74-83, 1986.

Jefferies, W.A.; Brandon, M.R.; Hunt, S.V.; Williams, A.F.; Gatter, K.C.; and Mason, D.Y. Transferrin receptor on endothelium of brain capillaries. *Nature* 312:162-163, 1984.

Jefferies, W.A.; Brandon, M.R.; Williams, A.F.; and Hunt, S.V. Analysis of lymphopoietic stem cells with a monoclonal antibody to the rat transferrin receptor. *Immunology* 54:333-341, 1985.

Klausner, R.D.; Harford, J.; and van Renswoude, J.V. Rapid internalization of the transferrin receptor in K562 cells is triggered by ligand binding or treatment with phorbol ester. *Proc Natl Acad Sci U S A* 81:3005-3009, 1984.

Kummer, U. Tritium radiolabeling of antibodies to high specific activities with N-succinimidyl [2,3-^{3}H]propionate: Use in detecting and analyzing monoclonal antibodies. *Methods Enzymol* 121:670-678, 1986.

Lambert, P.P.; Doriaux, J.; Sennesael, J.; Vanholder, R.; and Lammens-Verslijpe, M. Pathogenicity of cationized albumin in the dog: Renal and extrarenal effects. *Clin Sci* 67:19-33, 1984.

McClelland, A.; Kuhn, L.C.; and Ruddle, F.H. The human transferrin receptor gene: Genomic organization, and the complete primary structure of the receptor deduced from a cDNA sequence. *Cell* 39:267-274, 1984.

Montelaro, R.C., and Rueckert, R.R. Radiolabeling of proteins and viruses in vitro by acetylation with radioactive acetic anhydride. *J Biol Chem* 250(4):1413-1421, 1975.

Muckerheide, A.; Apple, R.J.; Pesce, A.J.; and Michael, J.G. Cationization of protein antigens. I. Alteration of immunogenic properties. *J Immunol* 138(3):833-837, 1987.

Neuwelt, E.; Barnett, P.A.; Bigner, D.D.; and Frenkel, E.P. Effects of adrenal cortical steroids and osmotic blood-brain barrier disruption in the delivery of methotrexate. *Proc Natl Acad Sci U S A* 79:4420-4423, 1982.

Omary, M.B., and Trowbridge, I.S. Covalent binding of fatty acid to the transferrin receptor in human cells in vitro. *J Biol Chem* 256:12888-12895, 1981.

Pardridge, W.M. Receptor-mediated peptide transport through the blood-brain barrier. *Endocr Rev* 7(3):314-330, 1986.

Pardridge, W.M.; Eisenberg, J.; and Yang, J. Human blood-brain barrier transferrin receptor. *Metabolism* 36(9):892-895, 1987.

Pardridge, W.M.; Triguero, D.; and Buciak, J. Transport of histone through the blood-brain barrier. *J Pharmacol Exp Ther* 251(3):821-826, 1989.

Reese, T.S., and Karnovsky, M.J. Fine structural localization of a blood-brain barrier to exogenous peroxidase. *J Cell Biol* 34:207-217, 1967.

Triguero, D.; Buciak, J.; and Pardridge, W.M. Capillary depletion method for quantification of blood-brain barrier transport of circulating peptides and plasma proteins. *J Neurochem* 54(6):1882-1888, 1990.

Triguero, D.; Buciak, J.B.; Yang, J.; and Pardridge, W.M. Blood-brain barrier transport of cationized immunoglobulin G: Enhanced delivery compared to native protein. *Proc Natl Acad Sci U S A* 86:4761-4765, 1989.

Van Deurs, B. Observations on the blood-brain barrier in hypertensive rats, with particular reference to phagocytic pericytes. *J Ultrastruct Res* 56:65-77, 1976.

AUTHORS

Phillip M. Friden, Ph.D.
Senior Research Scientist

Lee Walus, B.A.
Senior Research Associate

Marjorie Taylor, M.S.
Research Associate

Gary F. Musso, Ph.D.
Senior Research Scientist

Susan A. Abelleira, M.S.
Senior Research Associate

Bernard Malfroy, Ph.D.
Director of Development

Fariba Tehrani, B.A.
Research Associate

Joseph B. Eckman III, B.A.
Research Associate

Anne R. Morrow, B.A.
Research Associate

Ruth M. Starzyk, Ph.D.
Senior Research Scientist

Alkermes, Inc.
26 Landsdowne Street
Cambridge, MA 02139-4234

Permeation of the Blood-Brain Barrier for Drug Delivery to the Brain

Heidi C. Horner, Kari Barbu, Frederique Bard, Deborah Hall, Mary Janatpour, Katy Manning, Janine Morales, Seth Porter, Paulette E. Setler, Laura Tanner, and Lee R. Rubin

INTRODUCTION

Advances in molecular neurobiology are rapidly bringing researchers closer to understanding the etiology of acute and degenerative diseases of the brain. A natural consequence of this improved insight is the development of therapeutics to treat neurological disorders and dysfunctions such as stroke, brain tumor, Alzheimer's disease, and substance abuse. It is quite likely that many of these therapeutics will be drugs that do not penetrate the blood-brain barrier (BBB). The ability to manipulate the permeability properties of the BBB is a critical factor in treating diseases of the central nervous system (CNS). Hence, the safe and reversible enhancement of BBB permeability is essential for therapeutic efficacy. To that end, the authors have developed an in vitro model of the BBB and used it to begin preliminary screening of compounds that cause enhanced penetration of normally impermeant or weakly permeant substances. This chapter describes the authors' in vitro model of the BBB; the use of the model to identify second messengers that are involved with regulating permeability at the cellular level; and finally, a screening strategy to evaluate the in vivo efficacy of agents that are, from in vitro indications, most likely to enhance experimental drug delivery to the brain.

More than 100 years ago Paul Ehrlich (1885) noticed that systemic administration of basic dyes stained all tissues except the brain. However, the idea that brain capillaries constitute the BBB only began to be fully accepted in the late 1960s when Reese and Karnovsky (1967) and, later, Brightman and Reese (1969) showed by electron microscopy that horseradish peroxidase does not penetrate the endothelial tight junctions of brain capillaries. It is now generally believed that the BBB is made up of a single layer of specialized endothelial cells (ECs). These cells are morphologically and biochemically distinct from their peripheral counterparts. Unlike peripheral ECs, they form tight junctions (zonulae occludens) between apposing cells and have increased mitochondrial content (Oldendorf et al. 1977) and decreased pinocytotic activity. These hallmark features of brain capillary endothelium allow the cells to serve as a functional barrier between the blood and brain. Some biochemical differences, such as increased concentrations of the glucose transporter protein and increased gamma-glutamyl transpeptidase (GTase), most likely permit selective entry of substances to brain parenchyma. Thus, the brain is protected from unwanted blood-borne elements while still being furnished with essential nutrients, precursors, and cofactors.

These specialized properties are bestowed on ECs by the brain tissue. Stewart and Wiley (1981) have demonstrated that peripheral capillaries that vascularize brain tissue acquire the ability to exclude trypan blue, a dye that normally penetrates peripheral tissue. These cells develop tight junctions and have increased mitochondria. Conversely, brain capillaries that vascularize peripheral tissue lose features characteristic of the brain EC phenotype, including the ability to exclude trypan blue. In an extension of this work, Janzer and Raff (1987) transplanted rat astrocytes into rat eye and onto the chorioallantoic membrane of chick embryos. In both cases the astrocytes became vascularized by capillaries that excluded Evans blue. Meresse and coworkers (1989) and Meyer and coworkers (1990) have shown that ECs isolated from brain capillaries selectively lose GTase activity as they proliferate in culture. Several investigators (DeBault and Cancilla 1980; Beck et al. 1986; Maxwell et al. 1987; Bauer et al. 1990) have reported the induction of endothelial GTase by astrocytes or astrocyte-conditioned medium (ACM). Thus, there is good evidence that the functional and biochemical phenotype of brain ECs is dependent on a brain-derived factor(s).

These are important issues to consider when establishing a cell culture system that accurately reflects the BBB in vivo. Although several groups have reported on various features of ECs cocultured with astrocytes or ACM (DeBault et al. 1979; Bowman et al. 1983; Larson et al. 1987; van Bree et al. 1988; Shah et al. 1989), relatively few have described cell culture systems in which ECs were shown to maintain properties corresponding to those seen in vivo, including the presence of high-resistance tight junctions, exclusion of small hydrophilic molecules, and low rates of pinocytosis.

The authors' goal was to establish a cell culture system in which a monolayer of ECs with these properties could be grown on a permeable membrane separating two chambers, one representing the blood and the other the brain. Such a system serves as a relatively simple model, useful for discovering technologies that will enhance penetration of therapeutic agents into the CNS.

Data on compounds that increase permeability in vitro enabled the authors to compile a list of putative BBB permeators and to design a screening strategy to evaluate the capacity of these agents to increase permeability in vivo. Initially, the compounds are tested for their capacity to increase radiolabeled sucrose and bovine serum albumin (BSA) uptake into mouse brain. If the test agent causes increased brain uptake of these normally impermeant tracers, it is assayed for its capacity to decrease the doses of morphine required to elicit analgesia in mice. The compound is subsequently evaluated for effects on the cardiovascular system, including effects on heart rate, blood pressure, and blood gases. This approach allows the efficacy of an agent as a BBB permeator to be assessed by a variety of different in vitro and in vivo assays and to develop a drug to be used clinically for drug delivery to the CNS.

THE IN VITRO MODEL

As discussed above, ECs in the intact BBB possess many specialized features that distinguish them from peripheral ECs. It appears that those features that are responsible for their functional role as a barrier are the features necessary to reproduce in vitro. These include (1) a homogeneous monolayer of cells having the staining characteristics of ECs, (2) the presence of high electrical resistance as an indication of tight junction formation, (3) the exclusion of small hydrophilic molecules that typically distribute through peripheral ECs, and (4) low levels of pinocytosis. Bovine brain capillaries were chosen because they are a readily available, abundant, and inexpensive source of brain ECs. In a few experiments, ECs were isolated from human brain biopsy samples that were transported directly from the operating room to the laboratory. Briefly, brain ECs were isolated from capillaries by modifications of standard protocols (Bowman et al. 1983; Audus and Borchardt 1986) and plated on collagen/fibronectin-coated tissue culture flasks in ACM (see below). After about 7 days, the cells were trypsinized off the flasks and plated on Costar polycarbonate porous membranes, also coated with collagen and fibronectin. Cells were grown in Eagle's Minimal Essential Medium with either 5-percent fetal calf serum or plasma-derived horse serum. Two days after plating onto the membranes, the cells were fed growth medium supplemented with the chlorophenylthio derivative of cyclic 5'-adenosine monophosphate (cAMP) and a phosphodiesterase inhibitor, PDE1. To obtain ACM, rat brain Type I astrocytes were prepared from 1-day rat cortex, essentially as described by Lillien and colleagues (1987). ACM was collected by feeding confluent cultures with fresh medium and collecting after 48 hours. The ACM was mixed with an equal volume of fresh medium before use.

The resulting monolayers are brightly stained for Factor VIII and show robust uptake of acetylated low-density lipoprotein, consistent with their endothelial phenotype. There is occasional contamination by smooth muscle as revealed by staining with an anti-smooth muscle actin antibody. In the absence of ACM and cAMP/PDE1, contaminating cells proliferate and form a multilayered membrane. Furthermore, the cells show diffuse cytoplasmic staining with rhodamine-phalloidin, a reagent that detects the band of filamentous actin beneath the tight junctional complex. Cells treated with ACM and cAMP/PDE1 grow as a single monolayer and display dramatic changes in morphology. The cells become elongated, and the rhodamine-phalloidin staining is confined to the cell periphery. In addition, the ECs stain brightly with the ZO-1 antibody, a reagent that detects a tight junctional component in high resistance epithelial cells (Stevenson et al. 1986). Thus, treatment with ACM and cAMP/PDE1 promotes brain EC growth as a uniform monolayer with actin and a junctional protein circumferentially distributed in belt-like fashion, typical of that seen in high-resistance epithelial monolayers.

The electrical resistance of cells growing on a semipermeable filter is easily measured in vitro by passing current across the cells. Studies conducted by Crone and Olesen (1982) in amphibian brain microvessels suggest that resistance across the intact BBB is in the range of 1,900 ohms-cm^2. In the authors' research, brain ECs grown in the absence of ACM and cAMP/PDE1 displayed low electrical resistance, varying from 10 to 40 ohms-cm^2, which is comparable with that of peripheral ECs. The electrical resistance of brain ECs grown in ACM alone is typically in the 100 to 150 ohms-cm^2 range. The addition of cAMP/PDE1 and agents that increase intracellular cAMP dramatically improves electrical resistance (table 1). Resistance in brain ECs has reached almost 800 ohms-cm^2 and is, on average, greater than 500 ohms-cm^2. Isoproterenol and 5-hydroxytryptamine (5-HT), agents that bind to G-protein coupled receptors and secondarily increase cAMP, increase resistance to a similar magnitude as cAMP itself—that is, more than fourfold over control. Forskolin, which stimulates adenylate cyclase directly, causes an eightfold increase in resistance.

For the intact BBB, the penetration of a substance can be predicted by its octanol:water partition coefficient, the measure of the degree of lipophilicity of the compound. If the isolated brain ECs maintain their barrier characteristics in vitro, the movement of a substance across a monolayer should obey the principles of exclusion according to lipophilicity. That is, the more lipophilic a molecule, the greater penetration into brain parenchyma; the more hydrophilic, the less entry into the brain unless there is a specific transporter for the substance (e.g., D-glucose). Even quite small molecules such as sucrose (MW 340) cannot cross the BBB due to its hydrophilic nature. Traditionally, cultures of brain ECs have been leaky to hydrophilic molecules. Presumably, these low-resistance monolayers lack tight junctions that are responsible for

TABLE 1. *Effect of increasing brain EC levels on resistance. Bovine brain ECs were grown to confluence on collagen/fibronectin-coated filters. Cells were left untreated (control) or treated for 24 hours with 250 μM cAMP, 10 μM isoproterenol, 10 μM 5-HT, or 10 μM forskolin. All treated cultures had 35 μM PDE1, in addition. Each value represents the average of three experiments. The resistance of untreated cells was assigned a value of 100.*

Treatment	Relative Resistance
Control	100
cAMP	465
Isoproterenol	439
5-HT	586
Forskolin	834

restricting paracellular movement. The authors assayed the flux of free fluorescein (MW 376) and fluorescein-conjugated dextrans of 4 kDa and 71 kDa across brain ECs in culture. In low-resistance ECs there is leakage even of the large 71-kDa dextran. In the high-resistance ECs, flux of any of three dextrans is not detectable. An assay of the flux of sucrose across the monolayer revealed a tenfold reduction in paracellular movement of sucrose in ECs treated with ACM and cAMP/PDE1 compared with untreated cultures. Similar findings were generated for cholecystokinin, gastrin, nerve growth factor, and BSA.

The early work of electron microscopists has revealed that another well-established property of brain ECs is the paucity of intracellular vesicles compared with peripheral ECs. This presumably manifests as a low degree of pinocytosis. The significance of pinocytosis in the normal and pathologically disrupted BBB is still unclear. It is thought that increased plasma protein exudation into the brain parenchyma during disruption of the BBB by ischemia or hypertension, for example, is due to increased pinocytosis. In any case, a functionally "true" in vitro model should have a low rate of pinocytosis. Fluid-phase pinocytosis was measured in brain ECs by incubating the cells in a variety of fluorescent tracers, such as fluorescein isothiocynanate-dextran. The amount of fluorescein isothiocynanate-dextran taken up by brain ECs was markedly lower than that in peripheral ECs. However, this low rate of pinocytosis in brain ECs was observed in the absence of ACM and cAMP/PDE1, and thus far, quantitative studies have indicated that neither of these factors alters pinocytosis. Thus, it appears that brain ECs in culture maintain this phenotypic characteristic, whereas other additions are required to induce the formation of high-resistance tight junctions.

Having replicated in culture some of the key features of the BBB, the authors began developing techniques for discretely modulating the permeability of brain EC tight junctions. Based on the dramatic effect of cAMP on electrical resistance, it appeared that agents that reduce intracellular cAMP or antagonize the effect of cAMP should enhance permeability. We were unable to test the effects of these agents in vitro for the following reason. Modulation of cAMP in these cells is difficult to achieve since cAMP must be present in the cells to maintain the brain EC phenotype. It is impossible to antagonize cAMP while it is present in pharmacologic amounts in the cell; the removal of cAMP rapidly causes a decrease in resistance, hence, the reversion to low-resistance "non-BBB" ECs. Therefore, tests were not conducted on the effects of these agents on electrical resistance of ECs. Instead, this information was used to establish a roster of putative BBB permeators to test in vivo whose receptor-mediated effects are transduced via cAMP. There are contradictory reports in the literature regarding the effect of cyclic nucleotides on EC permeability. Elevations of intracellular cyclic nucleotide levels enhanced barrier properties of ECs cultured from human umbilical vein (Stelzner et al. 1989; Yamada et al. 1990). In vivo studies by Joo and colleagues have suggested that elevated cyclic nucleotide levels cause increased macromolecular transport across the BBB (Joo 1972; Joo et al. 1983). In the authors' studies, agents that increase intracellular cyclic 5'-guanosine monophosphate (cGMP) reduce electrical resistance. For example, 8-bromo-cGMP (500 µM) and nitroprusside (10 µM) decrease resistance by about 40 percent in 1 hour. The discrepancies may relate to differences in the effects of the cyclic nucleotides in different EC types, or they could reflect inconsistency in in vitro and in vivo results. We are pursuing the effects of the cyclic nucleotides on the permeability properties of cultured brain ECs and have started to test the effect of these compounds on BBB permeability in vivo.

IN VIVO EFFICACY OF POSSIBILE BBB PERMEATORS

The most careful and thorough analysis of a compound's capacity to enhance blood-to-brain transfer is to measure changes in either the extraction fraction or a transfer rate constant (Fenstermacher et al. 1981). The authors reasoned that, even after determining these parameters for each compound, it would still be necessary to test the efficacy of the compound of interest in a behavioral assay—that is, in an assay where peripheral administration of a CNS active drug that normally is impermeant or weakly permeant results in some observable behavioral change. Therefore, the screening system includes a somewhat crude brain tracer uptake assay and at least two behavioral assays.

Toxicity studies are routinely conducted to determine a nondebilitating, sublethal dose of the test compound. This dose is coadministered via the mouse tail vein along with a tracer cocktail containing ^{3}H-sucrose and ^{125}I-BSA. The animals are perfused 15 or 60 minutes later, and the brains are removed, weighed, and assayed by liquid scintillation spectrometry. The disintegrations per minute per wet weight is averaged for a minimum of four animals per experimental group. Standard error of the mean (SEM) values are less than 10 percent. The between-experiment error for the control groups is also less than 10 percent. The fold increase in tracer content is calculated by dividing the average treated DPM by that of the control DPM. Compounds that cause an increase of 1.5-fold or more are considered candidates for testing in the behavioral assays. These assays are designed to demonstrate delivery of a drug into the brain parenchyma at levels sufficient to have a therapeutic effect. Morphine and the naturally occurring peptides, endorphin and enkephalin, bind to μ-opioid receptors in the brain and suppress the sensation of pain. This analgesic effect can be demonstrated with mice in the hot-plate assay. Mice are placed on a surface uniformly heated to 55 °C. The time it takes for the mouse to respond to the heat stimulus by licking its paws is measured. Morphine (MW 700) delivered intravenously at doses of 1 to 10 mg/kg has an analgesic effect in that it increases the latency of response to the heat stimulus measured 15 minutes after injection. The latency is expressed as percent-analgesia. The purpose of these experiments is to test the ability of putative BBB openers to shift the morphine dose-analgesic response curve in the leftward direction, indicating enhanced delivery of morphine to the brain parenchyma as reflected by increased paw-lick latency time. Similar experiments are conducted using the less permeant but significantly more costly enkephalin.

Adenosine agonists that bind to the adenosine-1 receptor subtype (A1) are negatively coupled to adenylate cyclase and, thus, should decrease intracellular cAMP and increase permeability. Cyclopentyladenosine (CPA) (100 μg/kg, 1 hour) increased sucrose and BSA uptake into the mouse brain by 2.6- and 1.9-fold, respectively. A second A1 agonist, R-phenylisopropyladenosine (R-PIA), but not its inactive stereoisomer, S-PIA (25 μg/kg, 1 hour), increased sucrose and BSA uptake by 2.4- and 2.2-fold, respectively. In the morphine behavioral assay, CPA and R-PIA increased the percent-analgesia by threefold and eightfold, respectively; the S-PIA isomer had no effect in this assay.

Agents that increase cGMP also showed positive effects in the tracer and behavioral assay. Dipyridamole (50 mg/kg, 15 minutes) and nitroprusside (3 mg/kg, 15 minutes) caused increases in sucrose uptake by 1.7- and 2.3-fold, respectively, and both agents increased the percent morphine-induced analgesia. Dipyridamole also caused a 4.4-fold increase in enkephalin-induced analgesia.

We also looked at the 5-HT class of compounds. Recently, it has become clear that there is a large family of 5-HT receptor subtypes whose occupation affects different intracellular second messengers (Schmidt and Peroutka 1989). Occupation of 5-HT1a, 1b, and 1d receptors causes inhibition of adenylate cyclase, whereas occupation of 5-HT3 receptors stimulates the enzyme. Agonists acting at 5-HT1c and 5-HT2 receptors stimulate phosphatidylinositol turnover (Litosch and Fain 1985; Sanders-Bush and Conn 1987). An effect of 5-HT on BBB permeability has been reported (Westergaard 1977; Sharma et al. 1990). The authors' preliminary studies suggest an effect of 5-HT on tracer uptake. In addition, amitriptyline, which inhibits 5-HT reuptake, has been shown to increase BBB permeability in rodents and primates (Preskorn et al. 1981, 1983; Sarmento et al. 1990). Consistent with these reports is our finding that amitriptyline increased tracer uptake and doubled the percent increase in morphine-induced analgesia.

Thus, the authors are presently in various stages of assaying for efficacy of these classes of compounds. In addition to the morphine-induced analgesia assay, a second behavioral test has been included with different pharmacological and physiological end points. Furthermore, many of these compounds may have profound effects on cardiovascular function, rendering them unsuitable as clinically useful prototypical BBB permeators. Many of these agents have multiple physiologic effects; nevertheless, the authors have established a set of assays that, considered as a whole, will provide meaningful leads for novel BBB permeators.

CONCLUSION

The BBB represents a major obstacle in therapeutic drug delivery to the brain. Presently, there are two practices used for enhancing drug delivery to brain parenchyma. One is chemical modification of the drug of interest to increase its lipophilicity and, hence, increase its passage into the brain. Although this is a clinically effective approach, it is not always chemically possible to achieve. A second approach was pioneered by Rapoport and colleagues (1972) and used clinically by Neuwelt and colleagues (1981). It entails the intracarotid administration of hyperosmotic mannitol and has been used successfully to deliver methotrexate to brain tumors.

The authors are interested in developing a noninvasive technique that would enable the delivery of a variety of drugs (i.e., avoiding the need for individual drug modification) and have developed an in vitro model that allows assessment of a critical component of drug delivery to the brain: changes in resistance as a function of changes in tight junction formation. Key features of this model are the requirements for ACM and cAMP/PDE1. The dependence of the brain EC phenotype on cAMP has focused the investigation on the receptor-mediated modulation of cAMP to reveal putative BBB permeators. Furthermore, the BBB model allows examination of the novel aspects of brain ECs at the molecular level. Such studies will provide the ability to more precisely antagonize the intracellular events that regulate tight junction formation and disruption.

The acid test for a true BBB permeator is efficacy at the physiological level. The authors are examining, by a variety of in vivo assays, the use of A1 and 5-HT receptor agonists and substances that increase cGMP as putative BBB permeators. These studies, in conjunction with information about brain ECs derived from the in vitro model, serve two related purposes. One is to remove a major obstacle in the drive to discover new agents for treatment of brain dysfunction, and the second is to provide a noninvasive, safe, and reversible technology that is clinically useful for drug delivery to the CNS.

REFERENCES

Audus, K.L., and Borchardt, R.T. Characterization of an in vitro model for studying drug transport and metabolism. *Pharm Res* 3:81-87, 1986.

Bauer, H.C.; Tontsch, U.; Amberger, A.; and Bauer, H. Gamma-glutamyl-transpeptidase (GGTP) and Na^+K^+-ATPase activities in different subpopulations of cloned cerebral endothelial cells: Responses to glial stimulation. *Biochem Biophys Res Commun* 168:358-363, 1990.

Beck, D.W.; Roberts, R.L.; and Olson, J.J. Glial cells influence membrane-associated enzyme activity at the blood-brain barrier. *Brain Res* 381:131-137, 1986.

Bowman, P.D.; Ennis, S.R.; Rarey, K.E.; Betz, A.L.; and Goldstein, G.W. Brain microvessel endothelial cells in tissue culture: A model for study of blood-brain barrier permeability. *Ann Neurol* 14:396-402, 1983.

Brightman, M.W., and Reese, T.S. Junctions between intimately apposed cell membranes in the vertebrate brain. *J Cell Biol* 40:648-677, 1969.

Crone, C., and Olesen, S.P. Electrical resistance of brain microvascular endothelium. *Brain Res* 241:49-55, 1982.

DeBault, L.E., and Cancilla, P.A. Gamma-glutamyl transpeptidase in isolated brain endothelial cells: Induction by glial cells in vitro. *Nature* 207:653-655, 1980.

DeBault, L.E.; Kahn, L.E.; Frommes, S.P.; and Cancilla, P.A. Cerebral microvessels and derived cells in tissue culture: Isolation and preliminary characterization. *In Vitro* 15:473-487, 1979.

Ehrlich, P. *Das Sauerstoff Bedurfnis des Organismus. Eine Farbenanalytischer Studie.* Berlin: Hirschwald, 1885.

Fenstermacher, J.D.; Blasberg, R.G.; and Patlak, C.S. Methods for quantifying the transport of drugs across brain capillary systems. *Pharmacol Ther* 14:217-248, 1981.

Janzer, R.C., and Raff, M.C. Astrocytes induce blood-brain barrier properties in endothelial cells. *Nature* 325:253-257, 1987.

Joo, F. Effect of ^{6}N,O^6-dibutyryl cyclic 3',5'-adenosine monophosphate on the pinocytosis of brain capillaries of mice. *Experientia* 28:1470-1471, 1972.

Joo, F.; Temesvari, P.; and Dux, E. Regulation of the macromolecular transport in the brain microvessels: The role of cyclic GMP. *Brain Res* 278:165-174, 1983.

Larson, D.M.; Carson, M.P.; and Haudenschild, C.C. Junctional transfer of small molecules in cultured bovine brain microvascular endothelial cells and pericytes. *Microvasc Res* 34:184-199, 1987.

Lillien, L.E.; Sendtner, M.; Rohrer, H.; Hughes, S.M.; and Raff, M.C. Type-2 astrocyte development in rat brain cultures is initiated by a CNTF-like protein produced by type-1 astrocytes. *Neuron* 1:485-494, 1987.

Litosch, J., and Fain, J.N. 5-Methyltryptamine stimulates phospholipase C-mediated breakdown of exogenous phosphoinositides by blowfly salivary gland membranes. *J Biol Chem* 260:16052-16055, 1985.

Maxwell, K.; Berliner, J.A.; and Cancilla, P.A. Induction of gamma-glutamyl transpeptidase in cultured cerebral endothelial cells by a product released by astrocytes. *Brain Res* 410:309-314, 1987.

Meresse, S.; Dehouck, M.-P.; Delorme, P.; Bensaid, M.; Tauber, J.-P.; Delbart, C.; Fruchart, J.C.; and Cecchelli, R. Bovine brain endothelial cells express tight junctions and monoamine oxidase activity in long-term culture. *J Neurochem* 53:1363-1371, 1989.

Meyer, J.; Mischeck, U.; Veyhl, M.; Henzel, K.; and Gall, H.-J. Blood-brain barrier characteristic enzymatic properties in cultured brain capillary endothelial cells. *Brain Res* 514:305-309, 1990.

Neuwelt, E.A.; Diehl, J.T.; Vu, H.L.; Hill, S.A.; Michael, A.J.; and Frenkel, E.P. Monitoring of methotrexate delivery in patients with malignant brain tumors after osmotic blood brain barrier disruption. *Ann Intern Med* 94:449-454, 1981.

Oldendorf, W.H.; Cornford, M.E.; and Brown, J.W. The large apparent work capability of the blood-brain barrier: A study of the mitochondrial content of capillary endothelial cells in brain and other tissues of the rat. *Ann Neurol* 1:409-417, 1977.

Preskorn, S.H.; Irwin, G.H.; Simpson, S.; Friesen, D.; Rinne, J.; and Jerkovich, G. Medical therapies for mood disorders alter the blood-brain barrier. *Science* 213:469-471, 1981.

Preskorn, S.H.; Raichle, M.E.; and Hartman, B.K. Antidepressants alter cerebrovascular permeability and metabolic rate in primates. *Science* 217:250-252, 1982.

Rapoport, S.I.; Bachman, D.S.; and Thompson, H.K. Chronic effects of osmotic opening of the blood-brain barrier in the monkey. *Science* 176:1243-1245, 1972.

Reese, T.S., and Karnovsky, M.J. Fine structural localisation of a blood-brain barrier to exogenous peroxidase. *J Cell Biol* 34:207-217, 1967.

Sanders-Bush, E., and Conn, P.J. Neurochemistry of serotonin neuronal systems: Consequences of serotonin receptor activation. In: Meltzer, H.Y., ed. *Psychopharmacology. The Third Generation of Progress.* New York: Raven Press, 1987. pp. 95-103.

Sarmento, A.; Albino-Teixeira, A.; and Azevedo, I. Amitriptyline-induced morphological alterations of the rat blood-brain barrier. *Eur J Pharmacol* 176:69-74, 1990.

Schmidt, A.W., and Peroutka, S.J. 5-Hydroxytryptamine receptor "families." *FASEB J* 3:2242-2249, 1989.

Shah, M.V.; Audus, K.A.; and Borchardt, R.T. The application of bovine brain microvessel endothelial cell monolayers grown onto polycarbonate membranes in vitro to estimate the potential permeability of solutes through the blood-brain barrier. *Pharm Res* 6:624-627, 1989.

Sharma, H.S.; Olsson, Y.; and Dey, P.K. Changes in blood-brain barrier and cerebral blood flow following elevation of circulating serotonin level in anesthetized rats. *Brain Res* 517:215-223, 1990.

Stelzner, T.J.; Weil, J.V.; and O'Brien, R.F. Role of cyclic adenosine monophosphate in the induction of endothelial barrier properties. *J Cell Physiol* 139:157-166, 1989.

Stevenson, B.R.; Siliciano, J.D.; Mooseker, M.S.; and Goodenough, D.A. Indentification of ZO-1: A high molecular weight polypeptide associated with the tight junction (zonula occludens) in a variety of epithelia. *J Cell Biol* 103:755-766, 1986.

Stewart, P.A.; and Wiley, M.J. Developing nervous tissue induces formation of blood-brain barrier characteristics in invading endothelial cells: A study using quail-chick transplantation chimera. *Dev Biol* 84:183-192, 1981.

van Bree, J.B.M.M.; de Boer, A.G.; Danhof, M.; Ginsel, L.A.; and Breimer, D.D. Characterization of an "in vitro" blood-brain barrier: Effects of molecular size and lipophilicity on cerebrovascular endothelial transport rates of drugs. *J Pharmacol Exp Ther* 247:1233-1239, 1988.

Westergaard, E. The blood-brain barrier to horseradish peroxidase under normal and experimental conditions. *Acta Neuropathol* 39:181-187, 1977.

Yamada, Y.; Furumichi, T.; Furui, H.; Yokoi, T.; Ito, T.; Yamauchi, K.; Yokota, M.; Hayashi, H.; and Saito, H. Roles of calcium, cyclic nucleotides, and protein kinase C in regulation of endothelial permeability. *Arteriosclerosis* 10:410-420, 1990.

AUTHORS

Heidi C. Horner, Ph.D.
Scientist

Kari Barbu, B.S.
Research Associate

Frederique Bard, Ph.D.
Scientist

Deborah Hall, Ph.D.
Scientist

Mary Janatpour, B.S.
Research Associate

Katy Manning, B.S.
Research Associate

Janine Morales, B.S.
Research Associate

Seth Porter, Ph.D.
Scientist

Paulette E. Setler, Ph.D.
Executive Vice President of Research and Development

Laura Tanner, Ph.D.
Scientist

Lee R. Rubin, Ph.D.
Staff Scientist

Athena Neurosciences
800F Gateway Boulevard
San Francisco, CA 94080

Pathways Into, Through, and Around the Fluid-Brain Barriers

Richard D. Broadwell

INTRODUCTION

As reflected in the biomedical literature, the past 25 years have witnessed a burgeoning interest in delivering blood-borne, non-lipid-soluble micromolecules and macromolecules (e.g., peptides, proteins) and chemotherapeutic substances into the brain to combat infections, tumors, enzyme and neurotransmitter deficiencies, toxins, and the like associated with disease or dysfunction of the central nervous system (CNS). Coupled to this interest are the CNS entry of psychotherapeutic drugs and the overwhelming health and socioeconomic consequences of drug abuse and addiction. The scientific investigations focus on the fluid-brain barriers, cells that inhibit the ready passage of non-lipid-soluble molecules between the environment external to the CNS (i.e., air, blood) and the CNS milieu. These fluid-brain barriers include (1) the blood-brain barrier (BBB) associated with capillary, venule, and arteriole nonfenestrated endothelia of cerebral blood vessels; (2) the blood-cerebrospinal fluid (CSF) barrier associated with epithelia of the choroid plexus and other circumventricular organs (e.g., median eminence, area postrema); (3) the nose-brain barrier associated with epithelia of the nasal mucosa; and (4) the arachnoid mater-CSF barrier. Each of the barriers is believed to be attributed to circumferential belts of intercellular tight junctional complexes that preclude the extracellular movement of non-lipid-soluble micromolecules and macromolecules bidirectionally between the external environment and the CNS.

Despite reports advocating experimental manipulation to open the fluid-brain barriers transiently, most notably the BBB (Brightman et al. 1973; Rapoport 1985, 1988), these barriers under normal conditions are not absolute. Each is circumvented in a noninvasive fashion by large-molecular-weight endogenous and exogenous proteins moving within patent extracellular routes and/or traversing intracellular pathways related to adsorptive and receptor-mediated endocytic processes. These potentially viable intracellular and extracellular avenues are considered in the following discussion. The cellular secretory process (Palade 1975) and membrane behavior from a cell biological perspective are emphasized with regard to fission and fusion of cell membranes among constituents of the endomembrane system of organelles (e.g., Golgi complex, endosomes, lysosomes, and the plasmalemma).

DISTINGUISHING CHARACTERISTICS OF THE FLUID-BRAIN BARRIERS

The BBB and the blood-CSF barrier are the two most well-studied fluid-brain barriers in mammals. Circumferential belts of tight junctional complexes among nonfenestrated cerebral endothelia (Reese and Karnovsky 1967) and among choroid plexus epithelia (Brightman 1968) represent the distinguishing characteristic of these two cellular barriers. Similar junctional complexes exist among cells of the arachnoid mater (Balin et al. 1986; Broadwell and Sofroniew, submitted for publication; Nabeshima et al. 1975); however, junctional complexes among epithelial cells of the nasal mucosa and median eminence are believed not to be circumferentially tight to the extracellular passage of many molecules (see below). In vitro preparations suggest that tight junctions among cerebral endothelia may be initiated developmentally by astrocytes (see Brightman and Kadota, this volume).

Cells comprising the individual fluid-brain barriers all internalize or retrieve their cell surface membrane, a normal cell biological event for exchanging or recycling old, worn-out plasmalemma for newly synthesized plasma membrane. This cell function is associated with fluid- or bulk-phase endocytosis and permits extracellular macromolecules not binding to the plasmalemma to enter the barrier cells nonselectively and indiscriminately within 40 to 70 nm-wide endocytic vesicles of plasmalemmal origin (figure 1). The fate of such endocytosed macromolecules (e.g., horseradish peroxidase [HRP], serum proteins, uncharged molecules) is degradation within acid hydrolase-containing secondary lysosomes (Balin et al. 1986, 1987; Balin and Broadwell 1988; Broadwell 1989; Broadwell and Salcman 1981). The transcellular transport or transcytosis of fluid-phase macromolecules does not occur through the fluid-brain barriers (for a discussion, see Balin and Broadwell 1988; Broadwell 1989). The "enzymatic" barrier provided by intracellular secondary lysosomes is enhanced by extralysosomal enzymes like monoamine oxidase; this particular enzyme in BBB endothelia hydrolyzes dopamine derived by decarboxylation of blood-borne L-dopa within the endothelium, thus denying entry of dopamine to the CNS through the BBB (Bertler et al. 1963, 1966).

Although the recognized fluid-brain barrier cells are not categorized functionally as phagocytes per se, other cell types located behind and intimately associated with the fluid-brain barriers are likely phagocytic in function. These additional cell types serve as an auxiliary line of defense once the initial endothelial cell

231

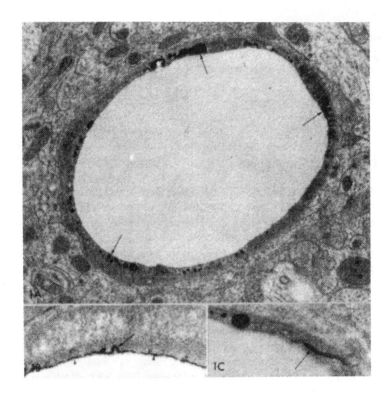

FIGURE 1. *The endocytic activity of the endothelium at the luminal front in rodent and primate brains is demonstrable upon exposure to the fluid-phase tracer HRP administered intravenously. Within 5 minutes postinjection, BBB endothelia exhibit a plethora of peroxidase-labeled dense bodies, tubules, and vesicles (A, arrows); endocytic vesicles harboring peroxidase reaction product very likely are derived from pits or invaginations (B, arrow) in the luminal plasmalemma coated with peroxidase reaction product (B, arrowheads). Tubular profiles (C, arrow) labeled with reaction product are not identified as establishing membrane continuity with the luminal and abluminal plasma membranes simultaneously (Balin et al. 1987); however, some tubules are confluent with peroxidase-labeled dense bodies, and both types of organelles stain positively for acid hydrolase activity (Balin et al. 1987; Broadwell and Salcman 1981), indicating that they are secondary lysosomes. Peroxidase reaction product is not evident on the abluminal surface or within the perivascular clefts of cerebral endothelia deep in the CNS removed from non-BBB sites (e.g., pial surface, circumventricular organs) in animals injected intravenously with the tracer.*

barrier is breached (Balin et al. 1986; Broadwell 1989; Broadwell and Brightman 1976; Broadwell and Salcman 1981; Broadwell and Sofroniew, submitted for publication). Potential phagocytic cells associated with the fluid-brain barriers include perivascular pericytes, microglia, and macrophages; arachnoid and subarachnoid macrophages; and macrophages lying on the surfaces of ependymal and choroid plexus epithelia. The subarachnoid and perivascular phagocytes in the rodent and primate CNS label with the blood-borne, fluid-phase tracer HRP, suggesting that this probe molecule is successful in circumventing the fluid-brain barriers by extracellular routes (see below).

The internalization of cell surface membrane and endocytosis are demonstrable circumferentially in choroid plexus and median eminence epithelia as evidenced by exposure of these epithelia to blood-borne and CSF-borne peroxidase and sequestration of HRP reaction product within epithelial vesicles, endosomes, tubular profiles, multivesicular bodies, and dense body lysosomes (Balin and Broadwell 1988; Broadwell et al. 1987a). BBB endothelia do not exhibit a demonstrable endocytic activity circumferentially. Organelles in BBB endothelia identical to those in choroid epithelia label with *blood-borne* peroxidase, but they fail to do so when the abluminal plasmalemma of BBB endothelia is bathed for 5 minutes through 12 hours in peroxidase delivered into the CNS by ventriculocisternal perfusion (Balin et al. 1986, 1987; Broadwell 1989; Broadwell et al. 1983a). Pits or invaginations in the abluminal plasmalemma of cerebral endothelia readily fill with CSF-borne peroxidase (figure 2) and have been misinterpreted as endothelial vesicles engaged in the transcytosis of protein from blood to brain and from brain to blood under normal and experimental conditions (for references and an indepth discussion, see Broadwell 1989). A comparison of membrane behavior at the luminal vs. abluminal front of the BBB suggests that, unlike epithelia of the blood-CSF barrier, the endothelia of the BBB are polarized with regard to the internalization or recycling of cell surface membrane and endocytosis of macromolecules (Broadwell 1989; Broadwell et al. 1983a; Villegas and Broadwell, in press). This polarity in the BBB suggests further that transcytosis of macromolecules through nonfenestrated cerebral endothelia, if indeed the process occurs significantly, is vectorial, from blood to brain but not from brain to blood. Characteristics of the mammalian fluid-brain barriers considered above are summarized in the list below.

• Cell types

— Blood-brain barrier: Nonfenestrated endothelia

– Circumferential belts of tight junctional complexes (Reese and Karnovsky 1967)

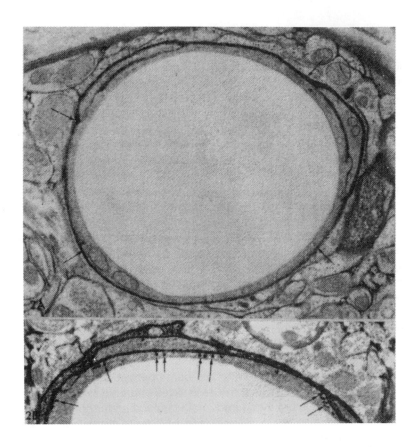

FIGURE 2. *Exposure of the abluminal surface (A, arrows) of cerebral endothelia for 5 minutes to 12 hours to peroxidase-delivered by ventriculocisternal perfusion yields no concentration of peroxidase-labeled organelles comparable to those that label with blood-borne HRP (figures 1A, 1C). This observation suggests that the endocytic activity and internalization of abluminal surface membrane are insignificant or minor at best. Invaginations or pits in the abluminal plasmalemma label with peroxidase reaction product and may be misinterpreted as endocytic vesicles (B, arrows). Abluminal surface pits also can fill with blood-borne peroxidase that has circumvented the BBB extracellularly under normal conditions (figure 6) or that has moved through the experimentally manipulated barrier; abluminal pits labeled in this fashion are misinterpreted as vesicles engaged in transendothelial transport and exocytosis of the tracer from blood to brain (Broadwell 1989; Broadwell et al. 1983a; Broadwell and Sofroniew, submitted for publication).*

- Secondary lysosomes containing acid hydrolases (Broadwell and Salcman 1981; Balin et al. 1987)

- Extralysosomal hydrolytic enzymes (e.g., monoamine oxidase) (Bertler et al. 1963, 1966)

— Blood-CSF barrier

- Choroid plexus epithelium

— Circumferential belts of tight junctional complexes (Brightman 1968)

— Secondary lysosomes containing acid hydrolases (Balin and Broadwell 1988)

- Arachnoid mater

— Circumferential belts of tight junctional complexes (Balin et al. 1986; Broadwell and Sofroniew, submitted for publication; Nabeshima et al. 1975)

— Phagocytes

- Circumventricular organ/subarachnoid macrophages (Balin et al. 1986; Broadwell 1989; Broadwell and Sofroniew, submitted for publication; Villegas and Broadwell, in press)

- Perivascular cells: pericytes, microglia, macrophages (Balin et al. 1986; Broadwell 1989; Broadwell and Brightman 1976; Broadwell and Salcman 1981; Broadwell et al. 1988, 1989; Broadwell and Sofroniew, submitted for publication; Villegas and Broadwell, in press)

- Supraependymal macrophages, Kolmer cells (Villegas and Broadwell, in press)

- Polarity of the BBB. The endothelium is polarized with regard to demonstrable internalization or recycling of its cell surface membrane and endocytosis of non-lipid-soluble macromolecules. These events occur from the blood side but not from the brain side of the endothelium (Broadwell 1989; Broadwell et al. 1983a, 1988; Villegas and Broadwell, in press).

- Blood-brain barrier vs. brain-blood barrier. BBB is not absolute, whereas its counterpart—the *brain-blood barrier*—may be. Potential adsorptive and

235

receptor-mediated transcytoses of macromolecules through the barrier is from blood to brain but not from brain to blood; hence, transcytosis through the endothelium appears to be vectorial (Broadwell 1989; Broadwell et al. 1988; Villegas and Broadwell, in press).

- Blood-CSF barrier is not polarized. Internalization of cell surface membrane associated with fluid-phase and adsorptive endocytoses is circumferential in epithelial cells of the choroid plexus and median eminence (Balin and Broadwell 1988; Brightman 1968; Broadwell et al. 1987a; Villegas and Broadwell, in press). Adsorptive transcytosis through these epithelial cells is bidirectional (Balin and Broadwell 1988; Villegas and Broadwell, in press).

CIRCUMVENTING THE FLUID-BRAIN BARRIERS: INTRACELLULAR PATHWAYS

Non-lipid-soluble micromolecules and macromolecules from the periphery are capable of circumventing the fluid-brain barriers by intracellular routes related to three separate and distinct endocytic processes. The three endocytic processes from the least to the most specific are fluid- or bulk-phase endocytosis, adsorptive endocytosis, and receptor-mediated endocytosis (table 1). All three processes involve the internalization of the external molecule in association with cell surface membrane. Fluid-phase endocytosis has been discussed above. Adsorptive endocytosis concerns molecules such as lectins (e.g., wheat germ agglutinin [WGA]) that bind to carbohydrate moieties on the cell surface and positively charged (cationized) molecules that bind to negatively charged cell surface components. Receptor-mediated endocytosis is identified with the binding of a ligand (e.g., insulin, transferrin) to a cell surface receptor specific for that ligand; the binding then triggers the internalization of the receptor-ligand complex (Dautry-Varsat and Lodish 1984). The suspected intracellular pathways circumventing the fluid-brain barriers are considered below and are listed below.

1. Cerebral endothelium: adsorptive and receptor-mediated transcytoses of specific blood-borne macromolecules (Broadwell 1989; Broadwell et al. 1988; Villegas and Broadwell, in press)

2. Choroid plexus epithelium: bidirectional, adsorptive transcytosis of protein between the blood and CSF (Balin and Broadwell 1988; Villegas and Broadwell, in press)

3. Primary olfactory neurons: anterograde axoplasmic transport and transsynaptic transfer (adsorptive transcytosis) of extracellular protein (Broadwell and Balin 1985)

TABLE 1. *Endocytic process*

Types	Examples	Specificity	Organelles
Fluid phase	HRP, ferritin	Nonspecific	Vesicles, endosomes, lysosomes
Adsorptive phase	WGA, ricin, cationized probes	Specific oligo-saccharides	Vesicles, endosomes, lysosomes, Golgi complex
Receptor-mediated	Insulin, transferrin	Specific receptors	Vesicles, endosomes, lysosomes, Golgi complex (?)

4. Neurosecretory cells, motor and autonomic neurons: retrograde axoplasmic transport and transsynaptic transfer (adsorptive transcytosis) of blood-borne protein (Broadwell and Brightman 1976, 1979; Fishman and Carrigan 1988; Villegas and Broadwell 1989, in press) and virus (Ugolini et al. 1989)

Fluid-Phase Endocytosis

Native HRP, arguably the most well-known and utilized fluid-phase tracer, has no difficulty in gaining entry to cells in general by fluid-phase endocytosis. Peroxidase is a 40,000 molecular-weight glycoprotein that sticks but does not bind to membranes. When administered intravenously, HRP is endocytosed by axon terminals supplying circumventricular organs and peripheral tissues (i.e., ganglia, muscle) possessing permeable blood vessels. Peroxidase taken into the axon terminals first appears in vesicles the size of synaptic vesicles and subsequently undergoes retrograde axoplasmic transport in vesicles, vacuoles, and tubular profiles for sequestration in dendrites and perikarya. Neuronal systems so labeled with *blood-borne* peroxidase include cranial and spinal cord motor and preganglionic autonomic neurons and hypothalamic neurosecretory cells; the latter are afferent to the neurohypophysis and perhaps other circumventricular organs (Broadwell and Brightman 1976, 1979, 1983). Retrogradely transported HRP is not secreted from the parent perikarya and dendrites; peroxidase-labeled organelles undergoing retrograde transport eventually fuse with perikaryal secondary lysosomes or become secondary lysosomes after fusing with primary lysosomes derived from the inner saccule of the Golgi complex (Broadwell 1980; Broadwell and Brightman 1979; Broadwell et al. 1980).

The retrograde labeling of well-defined neuronal perikarya positioned behind the BBB suggests that toxins, neurovirulent viruses, and other substances can enter the same neuronal groups, as does blood-borne peroxidase, from cerebral and extracerebral blood. First-order olfactory neurons in the nasal mucosa exposed extracellularly to HRP likewise will endocytose the tracer protein, which subsequently undergoes anterograde axoplasmic transport in lysosomes to axon terminals innervating the glomeruli of the olfactory bulb (Balin et al. 1986; Broadwell and Balin 1985); organelles transporting peroxidase into the olfactory terminals do not secrete their contents. The transcytosis of fluid-phase markers is not well documented for cells of the fluid-brain barriers or for any cell type;[1] however, a retrograde transneuronal transfer of herpes virus (Ugolini et al. 1989) and the C fragment of tetanus toxin (Fishman and Carrigan 1988) are reported from the periphery through lower motoneurons into the cortex and brain stem. The transcytosis of virus and toxins may be related more to adsorptive or receptor-mediated endocytosis than to fluid-phase endocytosis.

Adsorptive Transcytosis

Potential transcytosis of lectins and cationized molecules is not specific for cells of the fluid-brain barriers; the potential exists for all cells exposed to the molecules, those located within the CNS as well as those situated peripherally. To date, WGA (MW 36,000) conjugated to HRP is the only molecule documented morphologically to be associated with adsorptive transcytosis through the fluid-brain barriers, specifically cerebral endothelia and choroid epithelia (Balin and Broadwell 1988; Broadwell 1989; Broadwell et al. 1988; Villegas and Broadwell, in press). Biochemical data advocate cationized serum proteins as additional molecules for adsorptive transcytosis through BBB endothelia (Pardridge et al. 1990; Triguero et al. 1989; Pardridge, this volume). Lectins and cationized molecules, therefore, may represent excellent vehicles for brain delivery of molecules normally excluded entry by the fluid-brain barriers (see below).

Subsequent to the binding of WGA to n-acetylglucosamine and sialic acid moieties on the plasmalemma of cells (Gonatas and Avrameas 1973), the intracellular pathway that WGA-HRP follows through cells of the fluid-brain barriers and neurons projecting outside the BBB initially is similar to that of fluid-phase molecules. Organelles sequestering WGA-HRP early on include endocytic 40 to 70 nm vesicles, tubular profiles, vacuoles that may represent endosomes or a prelysosomal compartment, and dense bodies comparable morphologically to secondary lysosomes. With the passage of time (e.g., 1 to 3 hours) and unlike with fluid-phase molecules, the innermost saccule of the Golgi complex also labels with reaction product for WGA-HRP. This labeling of the inner Golgi saccule coincides with transcytosis of the lectin conjugate from blood to brain through BBB endothelia (Broadwell et al. 1988; Villegas and Broadwell, in press), with transsynaptic transfer of WGA-HRP from the periphery in the anterograde direction through primary olfactory neurons afferent to the olfactory bulb (Broadwell and Balin 1985) and with transsynaptic transfer in the retrograde direction through hypothalamic neurosecretory neurons (Balin and Broadwell 1987; Villegas and Broadwell 1989, in press).

The signals for transcytosis of WGA-HRP through BBB endothelia are (1) sequestration of reaction product for blood-borne WGA-HRP within the inner Golgi saccule of cerebral endothelia; (2) reaction product filling the perivascular clefts; (3) labeling of perivascular phagocytes throughout the CNS, suggesting that adsorptive transcytosis through the BBB is global; (4) WGA-HRP reaction product in the innermost Golgi saccule of perivascular phagocytes; and (5) WGA-HRP occupying extracellular clefts and processes in the neuropil beyond the basal lamina surrounding the perivascular phagocytes and endothelia (figure 3) (Broadwell et al. 1988; Villegas and Broadwell, in press).

Adsorptive transcytosis of WGA-HRP figures prominently with the Golgi complex and, therefore, with the Palade (1975) scheme of the cellular secretory process. The innermost Golgi saccule, which exhibits acid phosphatase activity enzyme cytochemically, gives rise to primary lysosomes and additional vesicles/vacuoles involved in delivering membrane and macromolecules, such as enzymes, to other organelles; this Golgi saccule also is charged with packaging molecules for export and exocytosis at the cell surface (for references, see Balin and Broadwell 1988; Broadwell and Balin 1985; Broadwell and Oliver 1981, 1983). WGA-HRP labeling of the Golgi complex may be a consequence of overwhelming the cellular endosomal compartment by the internalization of cell surface membrane tagged with the lectin conjugate.

The endosome compartment is the common denominator among fluid-phase, adsorptive, and receptor-mediated endocytic processes; it represents a clearing center and first intracellular stop in the endocytic pathway for internalized cell surface membrane associated with lectin, the ligand-receptor complex, and fluid-phase molecules (Dautry-Varsat and Lodish 1984; Gonatas et al. 1984; Helenius et al. 1983; Steinman et al. 1983). The endosome serves to dissociate internalized membrane from the attached lectin/ligand so that the membrane can recycle to the cell surface, leaving the lectin/ligand within the endosome. In fluid-phase endocytosis, internalized cell surface membrane likewise recycles from endosomes to the plasmalemma after endocytic vesicles have deposited their contents in endosomes. Broadwell and

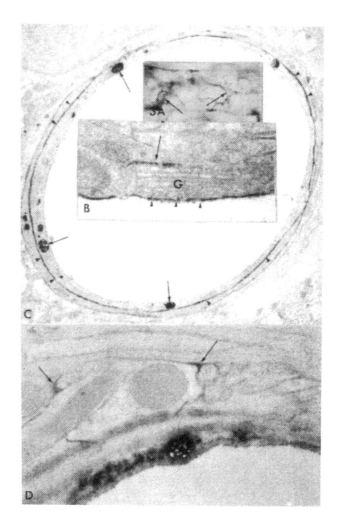

FIGURE 3. *The lectin WGA conjugated to HRP and administered intravenously to rodents labels perivascular phagocytes (A, arrows) throughout the CNS at 3 to 6 hours postinjection. Prior to 3 hours, reaction product is identified ultrastructurally on the luminal surface membrane (B, arrowheads) and within the inner saccule of the Golgi complex (B, arrow), vesicles, tubules, and dense bodies (C, arrows) of BBB endothelia. Reaction product occupies the perivascular clefts (C, arrowheads) and extracellular spaces (D, arrows) in the neuropil beyond the endothelial basal lamina at postinjection times of 3 hours and longer (Broadwell 1989; Broadwell et al. 1983a; Villegas and Broadwell, in press).*

colleagues (Balin and Broadwell 1988; Broadwell and Balin 1985; Villegas and Broadwell, in press) speculated that, when individual endosomes are overloaded with endocytic membrane associated with WGA-HRP, the "normal" intracellular endocytic pathway may be perturbed. As a consequence, internalized membrane with attached lectin may be diverted to the inner Golgi saccule wherein specific enzymes reside that contribute to the processing of membrane macromolecules, such as the addition or replacement of sialic acid (Bennett and O'Shaughnessy 1981; Bennett et al. 1981) to which WGA binds on the cell surface. Membrane and WGA-HRP recycled through the inner Golgi saccule would be packaged for export to other organelles (e.g., endosomes, secondary lysosomes, and plasmalemma) as well as for exocytosis.

Although Broadwell and colleagues have yet to identify the transcytosis of macromolecules from brain to blood through BBB endothelia (see below and Broadwell 1989; Broadwell et al. 1983a; Villegas and Broadwell, in press), transcytosis of WGA-HRP does occur bidirectionally through choroid plexus epithelia and perhaps without necessary involvement of the Golgi complex. WGA-HRP delivered into the lateral cerebral ventricle is endocytosed avidly by choroid epithelia at the microvillus face of the cells and is transcytosed through the epithelia within 10 minutes for binding to fenestrated endothelia located at the opposite pole of the epithelia; this transcytosis occurs in advance of WGA-HRP labeling of the innermost Golgi saccule and is speculated to utilize the endosome compartment as an intermediary in the transcytotic pathway (Balin and Broadwell 1988). If Broadwell and colleagues are correct, the transcytotic pathway through choroid epithelia is similar to that reported for immunoglobulin-G through intestinal epithelia (Rodewald and Kraehenbuhl 1984). The author and his group also find that the transcytosis of blood-borne WGA-HRP through choroid epithelia is not without difficulty. The event requires 17 to 24 hours to be identified ultrastructurally and is minor at best, with the signal for transcytosis of the lectin conjugate represented by WGA-HRP labeling of the microvillus border and of phagocytic (Kolmer) cells residing on the surface of the microvilli (Villegas and Broadwell, in press). The binding of blood-borne WGA-HRP to luminal and abluminal surfaces of fenestrated endothelia supplying the choroid plexus is so prominent that extracellular availability of the lectin for adsorptive endocytosis by choroid epithelia appears compromised (Balin and Broadwell 1988). Suspected membrane trafficking within choroid epithelia is diagrammed in figure 4.

Receptor-Mediated Transcytosis

Data advocating the receptor-mediated transfer across BBB endothelia abound for ligands, specifically a host of peptides (e.g., insulin, transferrin, and vasopressin); however, the data are more biochemical (Banks and Kastin 1985; Banks et al. 1987; Barrera et al. 1989; Duffy and Pardridge 1987;

CSF

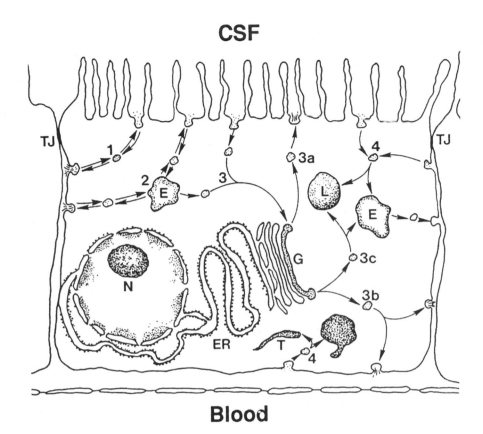

Blood

FIGURE 4.   *Three potential intracellular pathways through epithelia of the choroid plexus are proposed for the transcytosis of CSF-borne and blood-borne proteins and peptides that bind to the plasmalemma. Such macromolecules would enter the choroid epithelium by adsorptive endocytosis (e.g., lectins) or receptor-mediated endocytosis (e.g., ligands). The transcytotic pathways are vesicular transport (1) bidirectionally between the basolateral surface and the apical or microvillus surface, or indirect (2) by way of endosomes (E), or by recruitment of the Golgi complex (G), either directly from the cell surfaces or indirectly from endosomes (3). The transmost or inner Golgi saccule gives rise to a host of transporting vesicles; some of the vesicles are destined to engage in exocytosis at the apical surface (3a) or basolateral surface (3b) of the choroid epithelium,*

242

whereas others represent primary lysosomes (3c) that ferry acid hydrolytic enzymes to endosomes (prelysosomes) and secondary lysosomes (L). Blood-borne/CSF-borne macromolecules entering the choroid epithelium in vesicles derived from the plasmalemma by fluid-phase endocytosis (e.g., native HRP, ferritin), adsorptive endocytosis (WGA, cationized probes), or receptor-mediated endocytosis (e.g., ligands) are most likely directed to endosomes or secondary lysosomes (pathway 4); internalized plasmalemma possessing receptors freed from ligand/lectin deposited in endosomes may recycle to the cell surface. The endoplasmic reticulum (ER) and tubular profiles (T) do not participate in the transepithelial transport and exocytosis of extracellular macromolecules (Balin and Broadwell 1987; Broadwell et al. 1983b; Cataldo and Broadwell 1986). Because the choroid epithelium is not polarized with regard to its endocytic activity and internalization of cell surface membranes, a bidirectional transcytosis of extracellular macromolecules through the epithelium between blood and CSF is conceivable. N, nucleus; TJ, tight junctional complex.

Fishman et al. 1987; Pardridge 1986) than morphological (Broadwell 1989; Broadwell et al. 1983a; Villegas and Broadwell, in press), but are not without controversy (Meisenberg and Simmons 1983; Ermisch et al. 1985). One laboratory is of the belief that selected peptides may be involved in a bidirectional transfer across the BBB (Banks et al. 1988, 1989). These data should be interpreted with caution for reasons to be considered shortly.

The potential pathways for receptor-mediated transcytosis through and membrane trafficking within BBB endothelia are diagrammed in figure 5; the pathways are (1) direct vesicular transport from the luminal to the abluminal side, (2) indirect vesicular transport utilizing the endosome compartment as an intermediary, and (3) vesicular transport by way of the Golgi complex. Similar pathways would apply for receptor-mediated transcytosis through epithelia of the blood-CSF barrier (figure 4).

Data of ferrotransferrin (f-TRF; MW 35,000) conjugated to peroxidase for receptor-mediated transcytosis through the BBB are, at best, suggestive and raise important questions regarding the process in BBB endothelia (Broadwell 1989; R.D. Broadwell, A. Wolf, M. Tangoren, B.J. Baker, and C. Oliver, unpublished data; Tangoren et al. 1988). Immunohistochemistry has demonstrated that endothelia possessing the receptor for f-TRF are

Brain

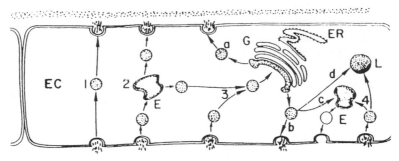

Blood

FIGURE 5. *Potential transcytotic routes through endothelial cells (EC) of the BBB and membrane events associated with fluid-phase, adsorptive, and receptor-mediated endocytic processes are represented in pathways 1-4. A direct transendothelial vesicular transfer (1) or an indirect route (2) through the endosome compartment (E) may apply for the receptor-mediated transcytosis of blood-borne ligands (e.g., transferrin, insulin); available data suggest the indirect route is the more plausible of the two (see text). Macromolecules entering the endothelium by adsorptive endocytosis are channeled to endosomes (2) and either directly or indirectly to the inner saccule (3) of the Golgi complex (G); this Golgi saccule is responsible for packaging macromolecules for exocytosis at the abluminal (a) and luminal (b) faces of the endothelium. Alternatively, some Golgi-derived vesicles represent primary lysosomes charged with delivering acid hydrolases to endosomes (E; pathway c) and secondary lysosomes (L; pathway d). Fluid-phase macromolecules and some macromolecules taken into the endothelium by receptor-mediated and adsorptive endocytic processes are directed to endosomes and secondary lysosomes (4) for degradation. In pathway 4, the internalized cell surface membrane may recycle to the luminal plasmalemma as vesicles from the endosome compartment. Reports that the endoplasmic reticulum (ER) of the cerebral endothelium may be involved with the transcytosis of blood-borne macromolecules (Mollgard and Saunders 1975, 1977) are not confirmed (Broadwell et al. 1983b; Cataldo and Broadwell 1986). Endocytosis and retrieval of cell surface membrane at the abluminal front are not conspicuous in comparison to the same events at the luminal plasmalemma (see text for discussion).*

restricted to cerebral vessels (Jefferies at al. 1984). Receptor recognition of f-TRF may promote the transport and delivery of transferrin and iron from plasma into brain. The f-TRF-HRP used by Broadwell and colleagues is run on gel electrophoresis and chromatographed to ensure that the conjugate administered into the carotid artery of rats (6 mg in 0.5-1.0 cc saline) is not contaminated with free HRP. At 1 hour postinjection, reaction product for f-TRF-HRP is observed within endothelial endocytic vesicles, tubules, spherical endosomes, and dense bodies and within the perivascular clefts and perivascular phagocytes. Subarachnoid macrophages, the circumventricular organs, and Golgi saccules in BBB endothelia are free of reaction product.[2] Infrequently, reaction product fills a presumptive "exocytic vesicle" or pit positioned at the abluminal plasmalemma. The data suggest a priori that the entire f-TRF-HRP conjugate may have undergone receptor-mediated transcytosis through the BBB; however, at this time this interpretation must be viewed with caution. Because of the specificity of the endothelial transferrin (TRF) receptor in brain, blood-borne TRF may be an ideal vehicle for ferrying substances across the barrier.

If receptor-mediated transcytosis of f-TRF-HRP does occur through cerebral endothelia, the treatment of f-TRF by this endothelium differs from that in other cell types. In the hepatocyte, for example, the f-TRF associated with the cell surface f-TRF receptor is internalized and directed to endosomes, wherein iron is dissociated from the transferrin peptide and transferred to the iron-storing protein ferritin; the iron-free apotransferrin remains bound to its membrane receptor and is recycled with it to the cell surface (Dautry-Varsat and Lodish 1983). The iron-free apotransferrin is released to bind additional iron when the receptor-apotransferrin complex encounters the neutral pH of the extracellular medium.

Broadwell and colleagues hypothesize that the fate of f-TRF in the endosome of BBB endothelia is dissociation of the ligand from its receptor, which is recycled to the luminal surface; f-TRF is anticipated to be transferred to a vesicle of endosome origin for export and exocytosis at the abluminal front (R.D. Broadwell, A. Wolf, M. Tangoren, B.J. Baker, and C. Oliver, unpublished data; Broadwell 1989). Iron would dissociate from the TRF once exocytosis into the perivascular space commences. Perivascular phagocytes are in position to endocytose the free TRF. This scheme excludes consideration of a direct transendothelial vesicular transport comparable to that diagramed in figure 5. To date, direct transendothelial vesicular transport is only a suggestion in the BBB literature without confirmation. Immunocytochemistry utilizing a monoclonal antibody against a BBB protein (Sternberger and Sternberger 1987) fails to support movement of luminal surface membrane to abluminal surface; the antibody recognizes a luminal membrane antigen that is internalized but is not directed to the abluminal surface (N. Sternberger and C. Shear, personal communication, November 1990).

THE ENIGMA OF TRANSCYTOSIS THROUGH THE BBB

The event of transcytosis through the BBB implies that the membrane of exporting vesicles engaged in exocytosis at the abluminal front of the endothelium fuses with the plasmalemma. In so doing, exocytic vesicle membrane is added necessarily to abluminal surface membrane. The Palade (1975) scheme of the cellular secretory process states that exocytosis and endocytosis are complementary events—events well recognized in bona fide secretory cells such as the neuron and those of endocrine and exocrine glands. With the addition of secretory vesicle or granule membrane to the plasmalemma for exocytosis to commence, the endocytic process signals the retrieval of cell surface membrane as a compensatory response to exocytosis, thereby ensuring that the overall surface area of cell membrane remains static with each exocytic event. The endocytic activity at the luminal front of the BBB is demonstrable upon even brief exposure to blood-borne tracer (figure 1) but not so at the abluminal front exposed for 5 minutes through 24 hours to native peroxidase or WGA-HRP filling the perivascular clefts following ventriculocisternal perfusion of the proteins (Balin et al. 1986; Broadwell 1989; Broadwell et al. 1983a; Villegas and Broadwell, in press). In the latter preparation, peroxidase-labeled endosomes and dense bodies are exceedingly rare within the endothelia, and labeled tubular profiles and Golgi saccules are nonexistent (figure 2). Presumptive exocytic and endocytic vesicles at the abluminal face are impossible to discern morphologically and unequivocally from static pits studding the abluminal plasmalemma. Abluminal surface pits are appreciated readily in preparations incubated to reveal the alkaline phosphatase activity inherent to the plasma membranes and fill with peroxidase that has gained access to the perivascular clefts from the blood through patent extracellular routes (considered below), from ventriculocisternal perfusion (figure 2), or from experimental manipulation of the BBB (Broadwell 1989).

The enigma of a *significant* transcytosis of blood-borne proteins and peptides through the BBB concerns how this endothelial barrier compensates for the absence of a demonstrable endocytic activity subsequent to exocytosis at its abluminal plasma membrane. Such a discrepancy in the cellular secretory process applied to the BBB requires clarification for defining transcytosis through the BBB. The problem is not encountered with the bidirectional transcytosis through the blood-choroid epithelial barrier, because the choroid epithelium demonstrates endocytic activity circumferentially. The apparent absence of macromolecular transcytosis through the cerebral endothelium from brain to blood suggests that the CNS possesses a brain-blood barrier that indeed may be absolute, whereas its counterpart—the BBB—is not.

EXTRACELLULAR PATHWAYS

Extracellular pathways circumventing the fluid-brain barriers (listed below) are comparable in the CNS of rodents and a subhuman primate (Balin et al. 1986; Broadwell 1989; Broadwell and Sofroniew, submitted for publication). The most highly documented extracellular route is through the circumventricular organs (e.g., median eminence, organum vasculosum of the lamina terminalis, subfornical organ, and area postrema), all of which contain fenestrated capillaries and, therefore, lie outside the BBB. Blood-borne macromolecules, specifically fluid-phase molecules, escaping fenestrated vessels supplying the circumventricular organs move extracellularly into adjacent brain areas located behind the BBB (for references, see Broadwell and Brightman 1976; Broadwell et al. 1987a; Gross 1987).

- Permeable blood vessels

  — Circumventricular organs (e.g., median eminence, area postrema) (Broadwell and Brightman 1976; Broadwell et al. 1983a, 1987a, 1987b, 1989).[3]

  — Pial surface (Balin et al. 1986; Broadwell 1989; Broadwell et al. 1991; Broadwell and Sofroniew, submitted for publication).[3]

- Patent intercellular junctional complexes

  — Nasal epithelium; absence of a nose-brain barrier (Balin et al. 1986).

  — Ependymal lining of median eminence and area postrema (Broadwell et al. 1983a, 1987a; Gotow and Hashimoto 1979, 1981; Richards 1978).

- Intracerebral transplants

  — Blood vessels supplying solid tissue grafts of peripheral origin are leaky and are indigenous to the grafted tissue; the grafts are deficient in a BBB and a *brain-blood barrier* (Broadwell et al. 1991).

  — Blood vessels supplying cell suspension grafts of peripheral origin are leaky and are of host origin; the vessels have forfeited their BBB and *brain-blood barrier* characteristics (Broadwell et al. 1991).

Additional extracellular avenues into the CNS are believed to be associated with sites possessing patent intercellular junctional complexes: the nasal mucosa, the epithelial linings of the median eminence and area postrema, and possibly the endothelia of large vessels on the pial surface and/or occupying the Virchow-Robin spaces. The degeneration-regeneration of cells in the nasal mucosa allows the intercellular clefts of this epithelium to be patent to fluid-phase macromolecules instilled in the nares (i.e., air borne, applied topically) or delivered to the epithelium from the blood through leaky capillaries. The extracellular route continues along the olfactory nerve into the subarachnoid space at the level of the olfactory bulb (Balin et al. 1986). The absence of a nose-brain barrier is of importance when the nose is considered a site for delivery of drugs, viruses, and environmental toxins associated with neurological disease (Barthold 1988; Langston 1985; Talamo et al. 1989).

Junctional complexes among ependymal cells lining the area postrema and median eminence are suspected of being discontinuous and not circumferentially tight, unlike the tight junctional complexes among BBB endothelia and epithelia of the choroid plexus; the apparent absence of a blood-CSF barrier at these two circumventricular organs heralds the bidirectional exchange of micromolecules and macromolecules between the blood and CSF (Broadwell et al. 1983a, 1987a; Gotow and Hashimoto 1979, 1981; Richards 1978). Even if the junctional complexes among ependymal cells in the median eminence and area postrema were circumferentially tight, blood-borne, fluid-phase substances leaking from vessels in the circumventricular organs could move extracellularly around the tight junctions and enter the CSF through gap junctions among ependymal cells adjacent to the median eminence and area postrema.

The absence of a BBB to blood-borne macromolecules at the pial surface of the brain was reported initially in mice injected intravenously with the fluid-phase tracer HRP (Balin et al. 1986) and recently confirmed in rat and monkey (Broadwell 1989; Broadwell and Sofroniew, submitted for publication). The latter studies suspect that the "leak" lies at the level of larger vessels on the pial surface and/or within the Virchow-Robin spaces. Blood-borne peroxidase that has entered the subarachnoid space by this route easily moves extracellularly through the pia mater and glial limitans into the extracellular clefts of the underlying neuropil and through the Virchow-Robin spaces for widespread distribution within the perivascular clefts (figure 6). The circumventricular organs also contribute to the dissemination of blood-borne HRP through the perivascular clefts. Subarachnoid macrophages followed by perivascular phagocytes lying superficially and deep within the brain parenchyma label with blood-borne HRP in that order. Fluid-phase markers may be propelled through the perivascular clefts in vivo by the pulsatile activity of arterioles (Rennels et al.

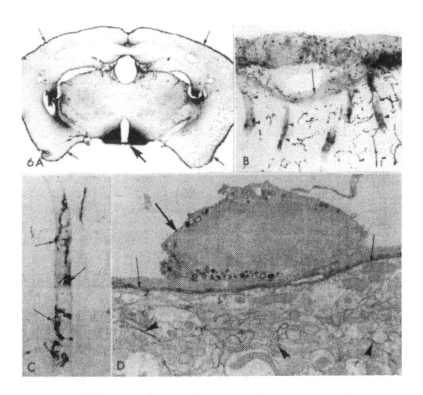

FIGURE 6. *Blood-borne HRP enters the rodent and primate brain extracellularly through permeable vessels supplying the pial surface (A and B, small arrows) and circumventricular organs, such as the median eminence (A, large arrow). Once on the pial surface (B and D, arrows), blood-borne peroxidase can enter the perivascular clefts (B, arrowheads) and move deeper into the CNS; peroxidase is endocytosed by phagocytic cells on the pial surface (D, large arrow) and in the perivascular spaces (C, arrows). Blood-borne peroxidase on the pial surface is able to pass extracellularly among cells of the pia mater and glial limitans to enter the subpial neuropil (D, arrowheads).*

1985). The patent extracellular pathways serve to explain how perivascular phagocytes throughout the rodent and monkey CNS become exposed to and label with blood-borne peroxidase in less than 1 hour postinjection (Balin et al. 1986; Broadwell 1989; Broadwell and Sofroniew, submitted for publication). CNS sites leaky to fluid-phase molecules circumventing the BBB are not insignificant; they allow the ingress of blood-borne, fluid-phase, endogenous molecules the size of IgM (MW 165,000) (Broadwell and Sofroniew, submitted for publication) and represent nonimmunologically privileged sites in the CNS (Broadwell 1989; Broadwell and Sofroniew, submitted for publication; Santos and Valdimarsson 1982). Absence of a BBB in the circumventricular organs and subarachnoid space is compensated for partially by populations of microglia, macrophages, and class II cells of the major histocompatibility complex (MHC) occupying these sites (R.D. Broadwell, B.J. Baker, A. Wolf, and J.S. Villegas, unpublished data).

WGA-HRP as an adsorptive-phase tracer also may follow the extracellular avenues into brain from the blood despite avid binding of the WGA molecule to the plasma membrane of cells (Balin and Broadwell 1988; Broadwell and Balin 1985; Villegas and Broadwell, in press). Whether blood-borne, receptor-mediated phase molecules not binding to specific endothelial receptors gain access to extracellular routes circumventing the BBB remains to be determined.

INTRACEREBRAL TRANSPLANTS AND THE BLOOD-BRAIN BARRIER

Immunohistochemistry with antibodies directed against MHC class I antigen on the luminal surface of endothelia has demonstrated that blood vessels inherent to intracerebrally placed grafts of CNS or peripheral origin are sustained and anastomose with host cerebral vessels (Broadwell et al. 1991). Consequently, solid brain tissue grafted intracerebrally presents a BBB to blood-borne macromolecules (Broadwell 1988; Broadwell et al. 1987b, 1989, 1991). Cell suspensions of astrocytes or neurons injected intracerebrally are supplied with host CNS vessels and a BBB to circulating protein (Broadwell et al. 1991). Solid tissue of the anterior pituitary gland (Broadwell et al. 1987b, 1991), adrenal medullary gland (Rosenstein 1987), muscle, skin, and superior cervical ganglia (Rosenstein and Brightman 1986; Wakai et al. 1986) grafted intracerebrally do not exhibit a BBB nor do intracerebral cell suspensions of peripheral origin (e.g., fibroblasts, PC12 cells). The latter are supplied exclusively with host BBB vessels that lose their BBB properties and become fenestrated and/or have patent interendothelial junctional complexes (Broadwell et al. 1991). Not only will peripheral tissue/ cell suspension grafts create a "window" in the BBB for entry of blood-borne substances, such as chemotherapeutics, to the brain, but also the absence of a BBB in these grafts necessarily means the absence of a *brain-blood barrier* as well. This fact introduces a significant problem to the intracerebral application of peripheral tissue/cell suspension grafts for production and release of a neurotransmitter or peptide in clinical treatment for neurodegenerative disorders (e.g., Parkinson's disease). Any neurotransmitter or peptide anticipated to be secreted from intracerebral, peripheral tissue/cell suspension grafts would likely fail to enter the surrounding host neuropil in large enough concentration to effect a significant clinical improvement; rather, the secreted product most likely would enter the non-BBB vessels supplying the graft and be removed within the general circulation. Broadwell and coworkers have confirmed that the presence or absence of blood-brain and brain-blood barriers within intracerebrally positioned grafts is dictated by the grafted tissue/cells and not by the surrounding host tissue contributing vessels to the graft (Broadwell et al. 1991).

SUMMARY AND CONCLUSIONS

The potential intracellular and extracellular pathways that blood-borne substances may follow for circumventing the fluid-brain barriers and entry to the CNS are numerous. The extracellular avenues, patent to blood-borne protein the size of IgM, and movement of blood-borne macromolecules through perivascular clefts deep into the CNS complicate the interpretation and identification of bona fide transcytosis through the BBB. The often-stated belief in literature reviews of the BBB that nonfenestrated cerebral endothelia fail to engage in endocytosis and possess few vesicles under normal conditions is invalid. Endocytic vesicle formation and vesicular traffic among constituents of the endomembrane system are no different in BBB endothelia than in other cell types. Available biochemical and morphological data advocate the transcytosis of blood-borne protein and peptides through nonfenestrated cerebral endothelia. However, absence of demonstrable endocytic activity at the abluminal front compared with a very prominent endocytic activity at the luminal surface of BBB endothelia argues against bidirectional membrane trafficking through the BBB and supports the concept of a *brain-blood barrier*. The latter is no less significant functionally than the BBB and may be more so in deterring transendothelial transfer of peptides and proteins bidirectionally through the nonfenestrated cerebral endothelium. The difficulty in interpreting transcytosis through BBB endothelia is not encountered for epithelia of the blood-CSF barrier at the level of the choroid plexus. Choroid epithelia engage in endocytosis circumferentially; hence, the potential for transcytosis and circumvention of the blood-CSF barrier through an intraepithelial route exists bidirectionally in the choroid plexus.

NOTES

1. The potential for native HRP to undergo transcellular transport following fluid-phase endocytosis exists in the epithelium of the seminal vesicle (Mata and David-Ferriera 1973) and in somatotrophs of the anterior pituitary gland (Broadwell and Oliver 1983); HRP introduced extracellularly to both cell types in vivo becomes sequestered within the innermost Golgi

251

saccule of the cells for packaging, export, and possible exocytosis. In these cell types, native HRP may behave as a membrane-bound marker (comparable with a lectin or ligand) rather than as a soluble or fluid-phase marker. The binding may involve the carbohydrate moieties of the peroxidase molecule. Available data suggest that HRP (Straus 1981) may bind to mannose-6-phosphate receptors on the cell surface (Sly et al. 1981).

2. In vitro studies suggest that the transferrin receptor in some cell types may recycle through the Golgi complex (Fishman and Fine 1987; Snider and Rogers 1985; Woods et al. 1986).

3. These sites lie outside the barrier and, therefore, are not immunologically privileged sites within the CNS.

REFERENCES

Balin, B.J., and Broadwell, R.D. Lectin-labeled membrane is transferred to the Golgi complex in mouse pituitary cells in vivo. *J Histochem Cytochem* 35:489-498, 1987.

Balin, B.J., and Broadwell, R.D. Transcytosis of protein through the mammalian cerebral epithelium and endothelium. I. Choroid plexus and the blood-cerebrospinal fluid barrier. *J Neurocytol* 17:809-826, 1988.

Balin, B.J.; Broadwell, R.D.; and Salcman, M. Evidence against tubular profiles contributing to the formation of transendothelial channels through the blood-brain barrier. *J Neurocytol* 16:721-728, 1987.

Balin, B.J.; Broadwell, R.D.; Salcman, M.; and El-Kalliny, M. Avenues for entry of peripherally administered protein to the CNS in mouse, rat, and monkey. *J Comp Neurol* 251:260-280, 1986.

Banks, W.A., and Kastin, A.J. Permeability of the blood-brain barrier to neuropeptides: The case for penetration. *Psychoneuroendocrinology* 10:385-399, 1985.

Banks, W.A.; Kastin, A.J.; and Durham, D.A. Bidirectional transport of interleukin-1 alpha across the blood-brain barrier. *Brain Res Bull* 23:433-437, 1989.

Banks, W.A.; Kastin, A.J.; Fasold, M.B.; Barrera, C.M.; and Augereau, G. Studies of the slow bidirectional transport of iron and transferrin across the blood-brain barrier. *Brain Res Bull* 21:881-885, 1988.

Banks, W.A.; Kastin, A.J.; Horvath, A.; and Michals, E.A. Carrier-mediated transport of vasopressin across the blood-brain barrier of the mouse. *J Neurosci Res* 18:326-332, 1987.

Barrera, C.M.; Banks, W.A.; and Kastin, A.J. Passage of Tyr-MIF-1 from blood to brain. *Brain Res Bull* 23:439-442, 1989.

Barthold, S.W. Olfactory neural pathway in mouse hepatitis virus nasoencephalitis. *Acta Neuropathol (Berl)* 76:502-506, 1988.

Bennett, G.; Kan, F.W.K.; and O'Shaughnessy, D. The site of incorporation of sialic acid residues into glycoproteins and the subsequent fate of these molecules in various rat and mouse cells types as shown by radio-autography after injection of (^{3}H)N-acetylmannosamine. II. Observations in tissues other than liver. *J Cell Biol* 88:16-31, 1981.

Bennett, G., and O'Shaughnessy, D. The site of incorporation of sialic acid residues into glycoproteins and the subsequent fates of these molecules in various rat and mouse cell types by radioautography after injection of (^{3}H)N-acetylmannosamine. I. Observations in hepatocytes. *J Cell Biol* 88:1-15, 1981.

Bertler, A.; Falck, B.; Owman, C.H.; and Rosengren, E. Localization of monoaminergic blood-brain barrier mechanism. *Pharmacol Rev* 18:369-385, 1966.

Bertler, A.; Falck, B.; and Rosengren, E. The direct demonstration of a barrier mechanism in brain capillaries. *Acta Pharmacol Toxicol (Copenh)* 20:317-321, 1963.

Brightman, M.W. The intracerebral movement of proteins injected into blood and cerebrospinal fluid of mice. *Prog Brain Res* 29:19-31, 1968.

Brightman, M.W.; Hori, M.; Rapport, S.I.; Reese, T.S.; and Westergaard, E. Osmotic opening of tight junctions in cerebral endothelium. *S Comp Neurol* 152:317-326, 1973.

Broadwell, R.D. Cytochemical localization of acid hydolases in neurons of the mammalian central nervous system. *J Histochem Cytochem* 28:87-89, 1980.

Broadwell, R.D. Addressing the absence of a blood-brain barrier within transplanted brain tissue. *Science* 24:473, 1988.

Broadwell, R.D. Transcytosis of macromolecules through the blood-brain barrier. A critical appraisal and cell biological perspective. *Acta Neuropathol (Berl)* 79:117-128, 1989.

Broadwell, R.D., and Balin, B.J. Endocytic and exocytic pathways of the neuronal secretory process and trans-synaptic transfer of wheatgerm agglutinin-horseradish peroxidase in vivo. *J Comp Neurol* 242:632-650, 1985.

Broadwell, R.D.; Balin, B.J.; and Cataldo, A.M. Fine structure and cytochemistry of the mammalian median eminence. In: Gross, P.M., ed. *Circumventricular Organs and Body Fluids.* Boca Raton, FL: CRC Press, 1987a. pp. 61-85.

Broadwell, R.D.; Balin, B.J.; and Salcman, M. Transcytosis of blood-borne protein through the blood-brain barrier. *Proc Natl Acad Sci U S A* 85:632-636, 1988.

Broadwell, R.D.; Balin, B.J.; Salcman, M.; and Kaplan, R.S. Brain-blood barrier? Yes and no. *Proc Natl Acad Sci U S A* 80:7352-7356, 1983a.

Broadwell, R.D., and Brightman, M.W. Entry of peroxidase to neurons of the central and peripheral nervous system from extra-cerebral and cerebral blood. *J Comp Neurol* 166:257-284, 1976.

Broadwell, R.D., and Brightman, M.W. Cytochemistry of undamaged neurons transporting exogenous protein in vivo. *J Comp Neurol* 185:31-73, 1979.

Broadwell, R.D., and Brightman, M.W. Horseradish peroxidase: A tool for study of the neuroendocrine cell and other peptide secreting cells. *Meth Enzymol* 103:187-218, 1983.

Broadwell, R.D.; Brightman, M.W.; and Oliver, C. Neuronal transport of acid hydrolases and peroxidase within the lysosomal system of organelles: Involvement of agranular reticulum-like cisterns. *J Comp Neurol* 190:519-532, 1980.

Broadwell, R.D.; Cataldo, A.M.; and Salcman, M. Cytochemical localization of glucose-6-phosphatase activity in cerebral endothelial cells. *J Histochem Cytochem* 31:818-822, 1983b.

Broadwell, R.D.; Charlton, H.M.; Balin, B.; and Salcman, M. Angioarchitecture of the CNS, pituitary gland, and intracerebral grafts revealed with peroxidase cytochemistry. *J Comp Neurol* 260:47-62, 1987b.

Broadwell, R.D.; Charlton, H.M.; Ebert, P.; Hickey, W.F.; Shirazi, Y.; Villegas, J.; and Wolf, A.L. Allografts of CNS tissue possess a blood-brain barrier: II. Angiogenesis in solid tissue and cell suspension grafts. *Exp Neurol* 112:1-28, 1991.

Broadwell, R.D.; Charlton, H.M.; Ganong, W.F.; Salcman, M.; and Sofroniew, M. Allografts of CNS tissue possess a blood-brain barrier. I. Grafts of medical preoptic area in hypogonadal mice. *Exp Neurol* 105:135-151, 1989.

Broadwell, R.D., and Oliver, C. The Golgi apparatus, GERL, and secretory granule formation within the hypothalamo-neurohypophysial system of control and hyperosmotically stressed mice. *J Cell Biol* 90:474-484, 1981.

Broadwell, R.D., and Oliver, C. An enzyme cytochemical study of the endocytic pathways in anterior pituitary cells of the mouse in vivo. *J Histochem Cytochem* 31:325-335, 1983.

Broadwell, R.D., and Salcman, M. Expanding the definition of the blood-brain barrier to protein. *Proc Natl Acad Sci U S A* 78:7820-7824, 1981.

Broadwell, R.D., and Sofroniew, M. Immunohistochemical identification of serum proteins circumventing the blood-brain barrier. *J Neurosci*, submitted for publication.

Cataldo, A.M., and Broadwell, R.D. Cytochemical identification of cerebral glycogen and glucose-6-phosphatase activity under normal and experimental conditions. I. Choroid plexus and ependymal epithelia, endothelia, and pericytes. *J Neurocytol* 15:511-524, 1986.

Dautry-Varsat, A., and Lodish, H.F. The Golgi complex and the sorting of membrane and secreted proteins. *Trends Neurosci* 6:484-490, 1983.

Dautry-Varsat, A., and Lodish, H.F. How receptors bring proteins and particles into cells. *Sci Am* 250:52-58, 1984.

Duffy, K.R., and Pardridge, W.M. Blood-brain barrier transcytosis of insulin in developing rabbits. *Brain Res* 420:32-38, 1987.

Ermisch, A.; Rhule, H.J.; Landgraf, R.; and Hess, J. Blood-brain barrier and peptides. *J Cereb Blood Flow Metab* 5:350-357, 1985.

Fishman, J.B., and Fine, R.E. A trans Golgi-derived exocytic coated vesicle can contain both newly synthesized cholinesterase and internalized transferrin. *Cell* 48:157-164, 1987.

Fishman, J.B.; Rubin, J.B.; Handrahan, J.V.; Connor, J.R.; and Fine, R.E. Receptor-mediated transcytosis of transferrin across the blood-brain barrier. *J Neurosci Res* 18:299-304, 1987.

Fishman, P.S., and Carrigan, D.R. Motoneuron uptake from the circulation of the binding fragment of tetanus toxin. *Arch Neurol* 45:558-561, 1988.

Gonatas, N.K., and Avrameas, S. Detection of plasma membrane carbohydrates with lectin peroxidase conjugates. *J Cell Biol* 59:436-445, 1973.

Gonatas, N.K.; Steiber, A.; Hickey, W.F.; Herbert, S.H.; and Gonatas, J.O. Endosomes and Golgi vesicles in adsorptive and fluid phase endocytosis. *J Cell Biol* 99:1379-1390, 1984.

Gotow, T., and Hashimoto, P.H. Fine structure of the ependymal and intercellular junctions in the area postrema of the rat. *Cell Tissue Res* 201:207-225, 1979.

Gotow, T., and Hashimoto, P.H. Graded differences in tightness of ependymal intercellular junctions within and in the vicinity of the rat median eminence. *J Ultrastruct Res* 76:292-311, 1981.

Gross, P.M. *Circumventricular Organs and Body Fluids.* Vols. I-III. Boca Raton, FL: CRC Press, 1987.

Helenius, A.; Mellman, I.; Wall, D.; and Hubbard, A. Endosomes. *Trends Biochem Sci* 8:245-249, 1983.

Jefferies, W.A.; Brandon, M.R.; Hunt, S.V.; Williams, A.F.; Gatter, K.C.; and Mason, D.Y. Transferrin receptor on endothelium of brain capillaries. *Nature* 312:162-163, 1984.

Langston, J.W. MPTP and Parkinson's disease. *Trends Neurosci* 8:79-83, 1985.

Mata, L.R., and David-Ferriera, J.F. Transport of exogenous peroxidose to Golgi cisternae in the hamster seminal vesicle. *J Microscop* 17:103-110, 1973.

Meisenberg, G., and Simmons, W.H. Peptides and the blood-brain barrier. *Life Sci* 32:2611-2623, 1983.

Mollgard, K., and Saunders, N.R. Complex tight junctions of epithelial and endothelial cells in early foetal brain. *J Neurocytol* 4:453-468, 1975.

Mollgard, K., and Saunders, N.R. A possible transepithelial pathway via endoplasmic reticulum in foetal sheep choroid plexus. *Proc R Soc Lond [Biol]* 199:321-326, 1977.

Nabeshima, S.; Reese, T.S.; Landis, D.M.D.; and Brightman, M.W. Junctions in the meninges and marginal glia. *J Comp Neurol* 164:127-169, 1975.

Palade, G. Intracellular aspects of the process of protein synthesis. *Science* 189:347-358, 1975.

Pardridge, W.M. Receptor-mediated peptide transport through the blood-brain barrier. *Endocr Rev* 7:314-330, 1986.

Pardridge, W.M.; Triguero, D.; and Buciak, J.L. B-endorphin chimeric peptides: Transport through the blood-brain barrier in vivo and cleavage of disulfide linkage by brain. *Endocrinology* 126:977-984, 1990.

Rapoport, S.I. Tight junctional modification as compared to increased pinocytosis as the basis CF osmotically-induced opening of the blood-brain barrier. Further evidence of the tight junctional mechanism and against pinocytosis. *Acta Neurol Scand* 72:107, 1985.

Rapoport, S.I. Osmotic opening of the blood-brain barrier. *Ann Neurol* 24:677-680, 1988.

Reese, T.S., and Karnovsky, M.J. Fine structural localization of a blood-brain barrier to exogenous peroxidase. *J Cell Biol* 34:207-217, 1967.

Rennels, M.L.; Gregory, T.F.; Blaumanis, O.R.; Fujimoto, K.; and Grady, P.A. Evidence for a 'paravascular' fluid circulation in the mammalian central nervous system, provided by the rapid distribution of tracer protein throughout the brain from the subarachnoid space. *Brain Res* 326:47-63, 1985.

Richards, J.G. Permeability of intercellular junctions in brain epithelia and endothelia to exogenous amine: Cytochemical localization of extracellular 5-hydroxydopamine. *J Neurocytol* 7:61-70, 1978.

Rodewald, R., and Kraehenbuhl, J.P. Receptor-mediated transport of IgG. *J Cell Biol* 99:159s-164s, 1984.

Rosenstein, J.M. Adrenal medulla grafts produce blood-brain barrier dysfunction. *Brain Res* 414:192-196, 1987.

Rosenstein, J.M., and Brightman, M.W. Alternations of the blood-brain barrier after transplantation of autonomic ganglia into the mammalian central nervous system. *J Comp Neurol* 250:339-351, 1986.

Santos, T.Q., and Valdimarsson, H. T-dependent antigens are more immunogenic in the subarchnoid space than in other sites. *J Neuroimmunol* 2:215-222, 1982.

Sly, W.S.; Fischer, H.D.; Gonzalez-Horiega, A.; Grubb, J.H.; and Alatowieg, M. Role of 6-phosphomannosyl-enzyme receptor in intracellular transport of adsorptive pinocytosis of lysosomal enzymes. In: Hand, A.R., and Oliver, C., eds. *Methods in Cell Biology*. Vol. 23. New York: Academic Press, 1981. pp. 191-197.

Snider, M.D., and Rogers, O.C. Intracellular movement of cell surface receptors after endoyctosis: Resialylation of asialo-transferrin receptor in human erythroleukemia cells. *J Cell Biol* 100:826-834, 1985.

Steinman, R.M.; Mellman, I.S.; Muller, W.A.; and Cohn, Z.A. Endocytosis and the recycling of plasma membrane. *J Cell Biol* 96:1-27, 1983.

Sternberger, N., and Sternberger, L. Blood-brain barrier protein recognized by monoclonal antibody. *Proc Natl Acad Sci U S A* 84:8169-8173, 1987.

Straus, W. Cytochemical detection of mannose-specific receptors for glycoproteins with horseradish peroxidose as a ligand. *Histochem* 73:39-45, 1981.

Talamo, B.R.; Rudel, R.A.; Kosik, K.S.; Lee, V.M.Y.; Neff, S.; Adelman, L.; and Kauer, J.S. Pathological changes in olfactory neurons in patients with Alzheimer's disease. *Nature* 337:736-739, 1989.

Tangoren, M.; Broadwell, R.D.; Moriyama, E.; Oliver, C.; and Wolf, A. How significant is the blood-brain barrier? (Abstract.) *Soc Neurosci* 14:617, 1988.

Triguero, D.; Buciak, J.B.; Yang, J.; and Pardridge, W.M. Blood-brain barrier transport of cationized immunoglobulin G: Enhanced delivery compared to native protein. *Proc Natl Acad Sci U S A* 86:4761-4765, 1989.

Ugolini, G.; Kuypers, H.G.; and Strick, P.L. Transneuronal transfer of herpes virus from peripheral nerves to cortex and brainstem. *Science* 243:89-91, 1989.

Villegas, J.S., and Broadwell, R. Retrograde trans-synaptic transfer of a blood-borne protein. *Soc Neurosci Abstr* 15:821, 1989.

Villegas, J.S., and Broadwell, R.D. Transcytosis of protein through the mammalian cerebral epithelium and endothelium. II. Adsorptive transcytosis and blood-brain and brain-blood barriers. *J Neurocytol*, in press.

Wakai, S.; Meiselman, S.E.; and Brightman, M.W. Focal circumvention of blood-brain barrier with grafts of muscle, skin and autonomic ganglia. *Brain Res* 386:209-222, 1986.

Woods, J.W.; Dorizaux, M.; and Farquhar, M.G. Transferrin receptors recycle to cis and middle as well as trans Golgi cisternae in IgG secreting myeloma cells. *J Cell Biol* 103:277-286, 1986.

ACKNOWLEDGMENT

This research was supported in part by U.S. Public Health Service grant NS-18030 from the Stroke and Trauma Program, National Institute of Neurological Disorders and Stroke, National Institutes of Health.

AUTHOR

Richard D. Broadwell, D.Phil.
Professor of Neurological Surgery and Director of Laboratories of Neurological Surgery
Division of Neurological Surgery
Department of Surgery

University of Maryland School of Medicine
634 MSTF Building
10 South Pine Street
Baltimore, MD 21201

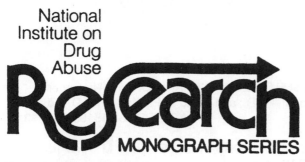

National
Institute on
Drug
Abuse

Research

MONOGRAPH SERIES

While limited supplies last, single copies of the monographs may be obtained free of charge from the National Clearinghouse for Alcohol and Drug Information (NCADI). Please contact NCADI also for information about availability of coming issues and other publications of the National Institute on Drug Abuse relevant to drug abuse research.

Additional copies may be purchased from the U.S. Government Printing Office (GPO) and/or the National Technical Information Service (NTIS) as indicated. NTIS prices are for paper copy; add $3 handling charge for each order. Microfiche copies are also available from NTIS. Prices from either source are subject to change.

Addresses are:

NCADI
National Clearinghouse for Alcohol and Drug Information
P.O. Box 2345
Rockville, MD 20852
(301) 468-2600
(800) 729-6686

GPO
Superintendent of Documents
U.S. Government Printing Office
Washington, DC 20402
(202) 275-2981

NTIS
National Technical Information Service
U.S. Department of Commerce
Springfield, VA 22161
(703) 487-4650

For information on availability of NIDA Research Monographs 1 through 70 (1975-1986) and others not listed, write to NIDA, Community and Professional Education Branch, Room 10A-54, 5600 Fishers Lane, Rockville, MD 20857.

71 OPIATE RECEPTOR SUBTYPES AND BRAIN FUNCTION. Roger M. Brown, Ph.D.; Doris H. Clouet, Ph.D.; and David P. Friedman, Ph.D., eds.
GPO out of stock   NTIS PB #89-151955/AS $31

72 RELAPSE AND RECOVERY IN DRUG ABUSE. Frank M. Tims, Ph.D., and Carl G. Leukefeld, D.S.W., eds.
GPO Stock #017-024-01302-1 $6   NTIS PB #89-151963/AS $31

73 URINE TESTING FOR DRUGS OF ABUSE. Richard L. Hawks, Ph.D., and C. Nora Chiang, Ph.D., eds.
GPO Stock #017-024-01313-7 $3.75   NTIS PB #89-151971/AS $23

74 NEUROBIOLOGY OF BEHAVIORAL CONTROL IN DRUG ABUSE. Stephen I. Szara, M.D., D.Sc., ed.
GPO Stock #017-024-01314-5 $3.75   NTIS PB #89-151989/AS $23

75 PROGRESS IN OPIOID RESEARCH. PROCEEDINGS OF THE 1986 INTERNATIONAL NARCOTICS RESEARCH CONFERENCE. John W. Holaday, Ph.D.; Ping-Yee Law, Ph.D.; and Albert Herz, M.D., eds.
GPO out of stock   NCADI out of stock
                                          Not available from NTIS

76 PROBLEMS OF DRUG DEPENDENCE, 1986: PROCEEDINGS OF THE 48TH ANNUAL SCIENTIFIC MEETING, THE COMMITTEE ON PROBLEMS OF DRUG DEPENDENCE, INC. Louis S. Harris, Ph.D., ed.
GPO out of stock   NCADI out of stock
                                          NTIS PB #88-208111/AS $53

77 ADOLESCENT DRUG ABUSE: ANALYSES OF TREATMENT RESEARCH. Elizabeth R. Rahdert, Ph.D., and John Grabowski, Ph.D., eds.
GPO Stock #017-024-01348-0 $4   NCADI out of stock
                                          NTIS PB #89-125488/AS $23

78 THE ROLE OF NEUROPLASTICITY IN THE RESPONSE TO DRUGS. David P. Friedman, Ph.D., and Doris H. Clouet, Ph.D., eds.
GPO out of stock   NTIS PB #88-245683/AS $31

79 STRUCTURE-ACTIVITY RELATIONSHIPS OF THE CANNABINOIDS. Rao S. Rapaka, Ph.D., and Alexandros Makriyannis, Ph.D., eds.
GPO out of stock   NTIS PB #89-109201/AS $31

80 NEEDLE SHARING AMONG INTRAVENOUS DRUG ABUSERS: NATIONAL AND INTERNATIONAL PERSPECTIVES. Robert J. Battjes, D.S.W., and Roy W. Pickens, Ph.D., eds.
GPO out of stock   NTIS PB #88-236138/AS $31

81 PROBLEMS OF DRUG DEPENDENCE, 1987: PROCEEDINGS OF THE 49TH ANNUAL SCIENTIFIC MEETING, THE COMMITTEE ON PROBLEMS OF DRUG DEPENDENCE, INC. Louis S. Harris, Ph.D., ed.
GPO Stock #017-024-01354-4 $17   NTIS PB #89-109227/AS
                                                 Contact NTIS for price

82 OPIOIDS IN THE HIPPOCAMPUS. Jacqueline F. McGinty, Ph.D., and David P. Friedman, Ph.D., eds.
GPO out of stock   NTIS PB #88-245691/AS $23

83 HEALTH HAZARDS OF NITRITE INHALANTS. Harry W. Haverkos, M.D., and John A. Dougherty, Ph.D., eds.
GPO out of stock   NTIS PB #89-125496/AS $23

84 LEARNING FACTORS IN SUBSTANCE ABUSE. Barbara A. Ray, Ph.D., ed.
GPO Stock #017-024-01353-6 $6   NTIS PB #89-125504/AS $31

85 EPIDEMIOLOGY OF INHALANT ABUSE: AN UPDATE. Raquel A. Crider, Ph.D., and Beatrice A. Rouse, Ph.D., eds.
GPO Stock #017-024-01360-9 $5.50   NTIS PB #89-123178/AS $31

86 COMPULSORY TREATMENT OF DRUG ABUSE: RESEARCH AND CLINICAL PRACTICE. Carl G. Leukefeld, D.S.W., and Frank M. Tims, Ph.D., eds.
GPO Stock #017-024-01352-8 $7.50   NTIS PB #89-151997/AS $31

87 OPIOID PEPTIDES: AN UPDATE. Rao S. Rapaka, Ph.D., and Bhola N. Dhawan, M.D., eds.
GPO Stock #017-024-01366-8 $7   NTIS PB #89-158430/AS $45

88 MECHANISMS OF COCAINE ABUSE AND TOXICITY. Doris H. Clouet, Ph.D.; Khursheed Asghar, Ph.D.; and Roger M. Brown, Ph.D., eds.
GPO Stock #017-024-01359-5 $11   NTIS PB #89-125512/AS $39

89 BIOLOGICAL VULNERABILTY TO DRUG ABUSE. Roy W. Pickens, Ph.D., and Dace S. Svikis, B.A., eds.
GPO Stock #017-022-01054-2 $5   NTIS PB #89-125520/AS $23

90 PROBLEMS OF DRUG DEPENDENCE 1988: PROCEEDINGS OF THE 50TH ANNUAL SCIENTIFIC MEETING, THE COMMITTEE ON PROBLEMS OF DRUG DEPENDENCE, INC. Louis S. Harris, Ph.D., ed.
GPO Stock #017-024-01362-5 $17

91 DRUGS IN THE WORKPLACE: RESEARCH AND EVALUATION DATA. Steven W. Gust, Ph.D., and J. Michael Walsh, Ph.D., eds.
GPO Stock #017-024-01384-6 $10   NTIS PB #90-147257/AS $39

92 TESTING FOR ABUSE LIABILITY OF DRUGS IN HUMANS. Marian W. Fischman, Ph.D., and Nancy K. Mello, Ph.D., eds.
GPO Stock #017-024-01379-0 $12   NTIS PB #90-148933/AS $45

93 AIDS AND INTRAVENOUS DRUG USE: FUTURE DIRECTIONS FOR COMMUNITY-BASED PREVENTION RESEARCH. C.G. Leukefeld, D.S.W.; R.J. Battjes, D.S.W.; and Z. Amsel, D.Sc., eds.
GPO Stock #017-024-01388-9 $10   NTIS PB #90-148941/AS $39

94 PHARMACOLOGY AND TOXICOLOGY OF AMPHETAMINE AND RELATED DESIGNER DRUGS. Khursheed Asghar, Ph.D., and Errol De Souza, Ph.D., eds.
GPO Stock #017-024-01386-2 $11   NTIS PB #90-148958/AS $39

95 PROBLEMS OF DRUG DEPENDENCE 1989: PROCEEDINGS OF THE 51ST ANNUAL SCIENTIFIC MEETING, THE COMMITTEE ON PROBLEMS OF DRUG DEPENDENCE, INC. Louis S. Harris, Ph.D., ed.
GPO Stock #017-024-01399-4 $21   NTIS PB #90-237660/AS $67

96 DRUGS OF ABUSE: CHEMISTRY, PHARMACOLOGY, IMMUNOLOGY, AND AIDS. Phuong Thi Kim Pham, Ph.D., and Kenner Rice, Ph.D., eds.
GPO Stock #017-024-01403-6 $8   NTIS PB #90-237678/AS $31

97 NEUROBIOLOGY OF DRUG ABUSE: LEARNING AND MEMORY. Lynda Erinoff, Ph.D., ed.
GPO Stock #017-024-01404-4 $8   NTIS PB #90-237686/AS $31

98 THE COLLECTION AND INTERPRETATION OF DATA FROM HIDDEN POPULATIONS. Elizabeth Y. Lambert, M.S., ed.
GPO Stock #017-024-01407-9 $4.75   NTIS PB #90-237694/AS $23

99 RESEARCH FINDINGS ON SMOKING OF ABUSED SUBSTANCES. C. Nora Chiang, Ph.D., and Richard L. Hawks, Ph.D., eds.
GPO Stock #017-024-01412-5 $5   NTIS PB #91-141119 $23

100 DRUGS IN THE WORKPLACE: RESEARCH AND EVALUATION DATA.
VOL. II. Steven W. Gust, Ph.D.; J. Michael Walsh, Ph.D.; Linda B. Thomas,
B.S.; and Dennis J. Crouch, M.B.A., eds.
GPO Stock #017-024-01458-3 $8

101 RESIDUAL EFFECTS OF ABUSED DRUGS ON BEHAVIOR. John W.
Spencer, Ph.D., and John J. Boren, Ph.D., eds.
GPO Stock #017-024-01426-7 $6   NTIS PB #91-172858/AS $31

102 ANABOLIC STEROID ABUSE. Geraline C. Lin, Ph.D., and Lynda Erinoff,
Ph.D., eds.
GPO Stock #017-024-01425-7 $8   NTIS PB #91-172866/AS $31

103 DRUGS AND VIOLENCE: CAUSES, CORRELATES, AND
CONSEQUENCES. Mario De La Rosa, Ph.D.; Elizabeth Y. Lambert, M.S.;
and Bernard Gropper, Ph.D., eds.
GPO Stock #017-024-01427-3 $9   NTIS PB #91-172841/AS $31

104 PSYCHOTHERAPY AND COUNSELING IN THE TREATMENT OF
DRUG ABUSE. Lisa Simon Onken, Ph.D., and Jack D. Blaine, M.D., eds.
GPO Stock #017-024-01429-0 $4   NTIS PB #91-172874/AS $23

105 PROBLEMS OF DRUG DEPENDENCE, 1990: PROCEEDINGS OF THE
52ND ANNUAL SCIENTIFIC MEETING, THE COMMITTEE ON PROBLEMS
OF DRUG DEPENDENCE, INC. Louis S. Harris, Ph.D., ed.
GPO Stock #017-024-01435-4 $22

106 IMPROVING DRUG ABUSE TREATMENT. Roy W. Pickens, Ph.D.; Carl
G. Leukefeld, D.S.W.; and Charles R. Schuster, Ph.D., eds.
GPO Stock #017-024-01439-7 $12

107 DRUG ABUSE PREVENTION INTERVENTION RESEARCH:
METHODOLOGICAL ISSUES. Carl G. Leukefeld, D.S.W., and William J.
Bukoski, Ph.D., eds.
GPO Stock #017-024-01446-0 $9   NTIS PB #92-160985
                                        Paperback $35 Microfiche $17

108 CARDIOVASCULAR TOXICITY OF COCAINE: UNDERLYING
MECHANISMS. Pushpa V. Thadani, Ph.D., ed.
GPO Stock #017-024-01446-0 $7   NTIS PB #92-106608
                                        Paperback $35 Microfiche $17

109 LONGITUDINAL STUDIES OF HIV INFECTION IN INTRAVENOUS DRUG USERS: METHODOLOGICAL ISSUES IN NATURAL HISTORY RESEARCH. Peter Hartsock, Dr.P.H., and Sander G. Genser, M.D., M.P.H., eds.
GPO Stock #017-024-01445-1 $4.50

110 THE EPIDEMIOLOGY OF COCAINE USE AND ABUSE. Susan Schober, Ph.D., and Charles Schade, M.D., M.P.H., eds.
GPO Stock #017-024-01456-7 $11

111 MOLECULAR APPROACHES TO DRUG ABUSE RESEARCH: VOLUME I. Theresa N.H. Lee, Ph.D., ed.
Not for sale at GPO   NTIS PB #92-135743
                                         Paperback $35 Microfiche $17

112 EMERGING TECHNOLOGIES AND NEW DIRECTIONS IN DRUG ABUSE RESEARCH. Rao S. Rapaka, Ph.D.; Alexandros Makriyannis, Ph.D.; and Michael J. Kuhar, Ph.D., eds.
GPO Stock #017-024-01455-9 $11

113 ECONOMIC COSTS, COST-EFFECTIVENESS, FINANCING, AND COMMUNITY-BASED DRUG TREATMENT. William S. Cartwright, Ph.D., and James M. Kaple, Ph.D., eds.
Not for sale at GPO

114 METHODOLOGICAL ISSUES IN CONTROLLED STUDIES ON EFFECTS OF PRENATAL EXPOSURE TO DRUG ABUSE. M. Marlyne Kilbey, Ph.D., and Khursheed Asghar, Ph.D., eds.
GPO Stock #017-024-01459-1 $12

115 METHAMPHETAMINE ABUSE: EPIDEMIOLOGIC ISSUES AND IMPLICATIONS. Marissa A. Miller, D.V.M., M.P.H., and Nicholas J. Kozel, M.S., eds.
GPO Stock #017-024-01460-5 $4

116 DRUG DISCRIMINATION: APPLICATIONS TO DRUG ABUSE RESEARCH. Richard A. Glennon, Ph.D.; Torbjörn U.C. Järbe, Ph.D.; and Jerry Frankenheim, Ph.D., eds.

117 METHODOLOGICAL ISSUES IN EPIDEMIOLOGICAL, PREVENTION, AND TREATMENT RESEARCH ON DRUG-EXPOSED WOMEN AND THEIR CHILDREN. M. Marlyne Kilbey, Ph.D., and Khursheed Asghar, Ph.D., eds.

118 DRUG ABUSE TREATMENT IN PRISONS AND JAILS. Carl G. Leukefeld, D.S.W., and Frank M. Tims, Ph.D., eds.

119 PROBLEMS OF DRUG DEPENDENCE 1991: 53RD ANNUAL SCIENTIFIC MEETING, THE COMMITTEE ON PROBLEMS OF DRUG DEPENDENCE, INC. Louis S. Harris, Ph.D., ed.

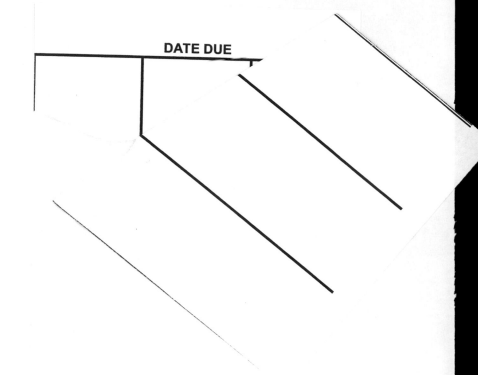

DATE DUE

ISBN 0-16-037914-8